A LOW-COST APPROACH TO PCR

Appropriate Transfer of Biomolecular Techniques

Eva Harris

edited by
Nazreen Kadir

New York   Oxford
OXFORD UNIVERSITY PRESS
1998

Oxford   New York
Athens   Auckland   Bangkok   Bogotá   Buenos Aires   Calcutta
Cape Town   Chennai   Dar es Salaam   Delhi   Florence   Hong Kong   Istanbul
Karachi   Kuala Lumpur   Madrid   Melbourne   Mexico City   Mumbai
Nairobi   Paris   São Paulo   Singapore   Taipei   Tokyo   Toronto   Warsaw

and associated companies in
Berlin   Ibadan

Copyright © 1998 by Oxford University Press, Inc.

Published by Oxford University Press, Inc.
198 Madison Avenue, New York, New York 10016

Oxford is a registered trademark of Oxford University Press

Library of Congress Cataloging-in-Publication Data
Harris, Eva, 1965–
A low-cost approach to PRC : appropriate transfer of biomolecular techniques /
by Eva Harris ; edited by Nazreen Kadir
p.   cm.
Includes bibliographical references and index.
ISBN 0-19-511926-6
1. Polymerase chain reaction—Laboratory manuals.
2. Molecular biology—Technology transfer.
I. Kadir, Nazreen.   II. Title.
QP606.D46H37   1998
572.8—dc21   98-16653

9 8 7 6 5 4 3 2 1
Printed in the United States of America
on acid-free paper

This book is dedicated to
my father,
Zellig S. Harris,
and
all those who persevere in working
toward a better life for all
¡Siempre adelante!

Preface

Since this is an unusual book, its genesis deserves some explanation. Although my training is in basic research, I have always felt the need to take science out of the "ivory tower" and apply it to real-life problems. While certain disciplines of science, such as public health and medicine, are readily applicable to problems in the "real world," it is less obvious how to make basic molecular biology research directly relevant. Yet I was fascinated by the beauty of the biological system and had often thought of the cell as an instructive example for human society, with its components interacting in a harmonious and nondiscriminatory manner, exhibiting remarkable energy efficiency and unity of purpose. I also enjoyed the process of scientific investigation—the rigor, the precision, and the creativity involved in designing and testing hypotheses.

It seemed to me that there must be a way to combine basic research, which leads ultimately to the control of important human diseases, with applied research, which targets more direct questions, all within a socially relevant context. It soon became apparent to me that this would entail creating a new path, since neither the traditional academic sciences nor industry offered this possibility. How exactly to go about doing this was not clear, but it was obvious that there was work to be done—and there still is—and my philosophy has always been to simply go out and do it, following the principles of responsibility, equality, scientific knowledge, and humanity.

After graduating from Harvard University, I decided to take a year off before continuing on with graduate school, even if it meant deferring admission and turning down the National Science Foundation fellowship that I had been awarded. I was determined to find out how my recently earned degree in biochemical sciences could be useful in solving real-world problems. I spent several months in Nicaragua, because at the time, it was possible to work as a volunteer in one of several technical fields. However, none of the organizations that placed volunteers knew exactly what to do with me and my insistence on working in the biological sciences. I ended up on the doorstep of the Ministry of Health, barely speaking Spanish and clutching excerpts from my favorite textbook, "The Molecular Biology of the Cell"[1]—somewhat taken aback by the strutting head rooster, who was clearly more at home in the laboratory compound than I was. Needless to say, my experiences in sophisticated laboratories in Paris, Basel, Woods Hole, and Boston had not prepared me for the urgent needs of a country struggling with serious problems in infectious diseases, vitamin A deficiency, and lead and pesticide poisoning, where laboratories operated with intermittent electricity and running water only twice a week. However, I found a number of ways to contribute, teaching science and technical English and helping out in the parasitology and virology laboratories. By the time I left, after a deeply moving several months, I was determined to find some way to continue supporting the work of my Nicaraguan colleagues.

When I began the doctoral program in Molecular and Cell Biology at the University of California (U.C.), Berkeley, I struck a deal with my advisor, Jeremy Thorner, to allow me to continue to collaborate with Nicaraguan scientists and to work there one month every year as long as I fulfilled my dissertation requirements on schedule. This arrangement worked well, and I received an excellent education in yeast genetics and basic research methodologies while completing the work expected of me. I also continued to collaborate with my Nicaraguan colleagues, researching new techniques, searching the literature for relevant articles, raising funds for reagents, and collecting unused equipment and materials discarded from U.C. Berkeley laboratories to send to the Ministry of Health. On one of my trips, my Nicaraguan colleagues expressed interest in learning about molecular biology, which seemed like a good idea albeit far removed from their reality. I searched for a link that would allow us to design a course on molecular biology yet still address relevant problems. The polymerase chain reaction (PCR) proved to be the answer. At that time, 1989, the PCR technique was just beginning to be widely used. With the advice of my long-term friend and colleague, Cristián Orrego, I organized a hands-on workshop that included a theoretical introduction to the principles of molecular biology and a practical section where course participants learned classical cloning techniques and used PCR both to identify their own DNA, extracted from a hair root or a drop of blood, and to detect the parasite *Leishmania*. Since none of the co-instructors nor course participants had ever seen DNA before, it was a great moment when we all observed the DNA fragments of the expected size in the agarose gels.

With the enthusiasm generated from the first workshop, the help from fellow graduate students at U.C. Berkeley, and continuing financial support from the New England Biolabs Foundation (NEBF), I organized a second, equally successful course in Nicaragua. By this time, our work was becoming known through publications and international conferences and was generating great interest. So much so that, when I finished my doctorate in 1993, I decided to take a year before continuing

---

1. Alberts, B., Bray, D., Lewis, J., Raff, M., Roberts, K., and Watson, J.D. (1983) *The Molecular Biology of the Cell.* New York, Garland Publishing, Inc.

with my planned postdoctoral fellowship at Stanford University to "make good" on some of the promises I had made to colleagues in other Latin American countries. Nina Agabian at the University of California, San Francisco, offered me a place in her laboratory to develop this vision into a more coherent program, and this became the first home of the Applied Molecular Biology/Appropriate Technology Transfer (AMB/ATT) Program. In July 1998, it moved to the School of Public Health at U.C. Berkeley, where I am currently a member of the faculty.

To make a long story short, over the following several years, AMB/ATT courses were given in Ecuador, Cuba, Guatemala, Stanford University, University of Florida, and Bolivia and were solicited in many more countries. When the work was profiled in *Science* (November 25, 1994), it precipitated an avalanche of letters, invited lectures and articles, material donations, and small grants from foundations such as the American Society for Biochemistry and Molecular Biology and NEBF. However, despite the popularity and recognition of this work both in the United States and abroad, it has continued to be very difficult to raise funds. The MacArthur Foundation Fellowship I was recently awarded for this work is a tremendous support, as is an international training grant that we received from the Fogarty International Center at the National Institutes of Health. My colleagues and I have recently established a nonprofit organization (Sustainable Sciences Institute) to expand this project. Nevertheless, this work relies heavily on donated materials and volunteer time from colleagues willing to help develop and adapt the techniques and to prepare and teach the workshops; I am deeply indebted to the many wonderful people who have given of themselves so selflessly to make this program a success.

In terms of the technique, PCR is ideal since in essence it is so simple, so powerful, and so adaptable to a low-cost methodology. However, to perform it properly and avoid artifactual results, a thorough understanding of the principles and practice is essential. That is the reason for this book. For me, transfer of technology must be undertaken responsibly, and it entails far more than sending out a protocol. This is even more critical with PCR, since performing the technique badly can have disastrous consequences in terms of cross-contamination. Over the years we have developed a method for the sustainable transfer of DNA-based technologies and have learned both general principles and essential details that make this approach successful. Thus, to make this experience widely available requires not only the protocols themselves but also a description of the theoretical basis of the technique, the practical details of the method, and the philosophy behind the technology transfer program.

This book is directed to a number of different audiences, including (1) scientists and educators from developing countries who wish to become involved in the transfer of molecular biology (or other technology) to their country; (2) scientists in developed countries who are involved in scientific and educational projects in developing countries; (3) high school, undergraduate, or continuing education programs in the United States; (4) international agencies and foundations as well as policy makers in developing countries who would like to more fully understand the principles and applications of PCR technology; and (5) scientists interested in learning about alternative applications of molecular biology. It is meant to serve as a practical guide and as a prototype, or model, for other technology transfer efforts. The main purpose is to make this exciting technology accessible and, hopefully, to contribute to the generation of more workshops, educational and scientific projects, collaborations, and friendships that are as rewarding and meaningful for others as they have been for me.

E.H.

University of California, San Francisco
July 1998

Acknowledgments

First, I would like to thank my friends and colleagues who have made specific contributions to this book:

Alejandro Belli, for designing the book cover and illustrations and for ten great years of collaboration in creating the AMB/ATT Program;

Richard Cash, for his thoughtful Afterword and for many years of friendship, advice, and collaboration on countless projects;

Lee Riley, for contributing the Foreword, the *Leptospira* extraction protocol, and editorial comments, and for advice and stimulating discussions;

Cristián Orrego, for teaching me PCR years ago, for editorial comments, and for many helpful discussions;

Nazreen Kadir, for her thorough editing of the manuscript and her encouragement;

Nataniel Mamani, for his generous contribution of ingenious equipment designs, building instructions, and photographs—his laboratory is a living example of truly appropriate technology;

T. Guy Roberts, for his tireless efforts in adapting and refining the equipment designs and assembly instructions, as well as for his many contributions to AMB/ATT projects over the years;

John F. Kennedy, for his contribution of an equipment design, for refurbishing equipment for collaborating laboratories overseas, and for informative discussions about sustainability and appropriate technology;

Ian Pacham, for his assistance in adapting certain equipment designs;

Elaine Conolly, for her work on the glossary and for her friendship and support;

Albert Ko, for the *Leptospira* extraction protocol and for advice on field adaptation of laboratory procedures; and

Olga Torres, for preparing the nonradioactive DNA probe protocol for *V. cholerae* colony blots that was included in our 1995 PCR Workshop in Guatemala.

I would like to express my deep gratitude to the following people for their contribution to developing the AMB/ATT Program:

To my special friends who have been there all through the years and who have selflessly donated countless hours in course preparation and as workshop instructors: Alejandro Belli, Christine Rousseau, Elinor Fanning, T. Guy Roberts, Ken Beckman, and Leila Smith;

To the wonderful people who have participated as workshop instructors and worked tirelessly to make every course a tremendous success: Susana Revollo, Deborah Lans, Giovanni Garcia, Gabriela Terrazas, Giovanna Gonzalez, Maria Rosa Cortez, Josefina Coloma, Wilson Paredes, David Moraga, Josefa Moran, Olga Torres, Alvaro Molina, Renata de Cabrera, Teresita Aguilar, Ricardo Luján, Mario Valcarcel, Eugenia Rojas, Javier Pérez, Marcelo Nazábal, Maria del Carmen Dominguez, Adelaide Villareal, Minerva Yaniz, Angel Perez, and Shelley Waters;

To my long-time collaborators Alcides Gonzalez, Angel Balmaseda, Alejandro Belli, Juan José Amador, Erick Sandoval, Betzabé Rodriguez, Sonia Valle, Xiomara Palacios (Nicaragua); Susana Revollo, Roger Carvajal, Nataniel Mamani, Alberto Gianella, Carlos Peredo (Bolivia); Jorge Gavilondo, Manuel Limonta (Cuba); Mauricio Espinel, Marcelo Aguilar, Ronald Guderian, Hernan Avilés, Luis Enrique Plaza, Irina Moleon-Borodowsky (Ecuador); Olga Torres, Ana Maria Xet-Mull, Leticia Castillo (Guatemala); Martin López (Perú); and Laura Kramer (U.C. Davis);

For advice and support, to Nina Agabian, Ed Wakil, George Newport, Debi Dean, Jan Dungan, Jeff Schatz, Jeremy Thorner, and Ichiro Matsumura;

For their interest in this work, to Marcia Barinaga and Barbara Culliton;

For excellent laboratory assistance, to John Selle, Deborah Lans, Jerry Kropp and Gloria Guevara. Thanks again to Gloria and to the InterAmerican Health Foundation for shipping our supplies to Nicaragua.

For financial support to write this book, special thanks to Byron Waksman and the Foundation for Microbiology; Nahum Gusik and the Gusik Foundation; Davida Coady and the San Carlos Foundation, and Ruth Sager and Arthur Pardee.

For donations and grants in support of the AMB/ATT Program, many thanks to the New England Biolabs Foundation, particularly Martine Kellett, Don Comb, and Vickie Cataldo; the MacArthur Foundation, especially Catharine Stimpson; the American Society for Biochemistry and Molecular Biology, particularly Steven Dahms; Roche Molecular Systems, especially Tom White; Perkin-Elmer Corporation, Promega Corporation, Gibco BRL Life Sciences, Boehringer Mannheim, Bio-Rad Laboratories, and Amersham Corporation.

I would like to thank Kirk Jensen, Executive Editor, Nancy Hoagland, Editorial, Design, and Production Manager, and MaryBeth Branigan, Production Editor, at Oxford University Press for their valuable assistance, and Steven Dunham and Doug Mortensen at Harvest Graphics for their excellent work.

For invaluable support and friendship, I am indebted to Ruth Sager, Arthur Pardee, and Esther Altschul.

Finally, my eternal gratitude to my mother, Naomi Sager, for being with me through thick and thin and for excellent editorial assistance; to my father, Zellig Harris, for illuminating discussion and inspiration; to my lifetime compañero, Pablo Rodriguez, for his understanding and optimism; and all three, for their uncompromising values and unconditional love and support.

Contents

Foreword

Emerging infectious diseases are currently a fashionable topic for books, politicians, government funding agencies, international health organizations, and research institutions. In actuality, in developing countries, the so-called emerging infectious diseases have been emerging for hundreds of years. What has emerged is the sudden realization and recognition by those in developed countries that these problems exist and are important. Unfortunately, the recognition that there is a need to do something about these diseases is often couched in the rationale that if something were not done, hordes of infectious diseases would arrive at their shores and cause unimaginable havoc. Eva Harris recognized many years ago that technology and science do not have to be limited by such a rationale. The only rationale that is needed is that these infectious diseases kill thousands of children and adults every day in thousands of places outside of North America and Western Europe, and one has to take science to where the disease is.

Over the last ten years, Harris has developed and led a training program called the Applied Molecular Biology/Appropriate Technology Transfer (AMB/ATT) Program in several Latin American countries. After receiving her Bachelor of Arts degree (*magna cum laude*) from Harvard University (1987), she entered the University of California at Berkeley in 1988 and received her doctoral degree in Molecular and Cell Biology (1993) in the field of yeast genetics. She initiated a new molecular pathogenesis research project related to dengue virus while at the University of California in San Francisco, and has recently joined the faculty of the School of Public Health at U.C. Berkeley. Harris is a 1997 recipient of the coveted MacArthur "genius" award in recognition of her work in Latin America. Her applied research serves as a paradigm of what science can do to address infectious disease public health problems in developing countries. While the term "appropriate technology" connotes many meanings, depending on one's previous experiences with programs of a similar designation; as applied here, it is a completely novel, grassroots designation, born out of the imagination and insight of Harris and her friends and colleagues. Their motivation is a common interest and goal to make science accessible to those who can use it to make a difference in their communities.

Transfer of the polymerase chain reaction (PCR) technique plays a prominent role in the AMB/ATT workshops, and this book will serve as a hands-on reference for similar programs. The introduction of the various techniques in Nicaragua, Ecuador, Bolivia, Guatemala, and Mexico has already spawned several independent studies by investigators in those countries, which should facilitate improved understanding and control of infectious disease problems that were previously not possible and would not have been possible without Harris's involvement and insight. For instance, she has adapted a PCR-based method that can rapidly differentiate dengue viruses according to serotypes and has field-tested it in a number of Latin American countries. It was this technique, which she introduced into Nicaragua in 1995, that led to the discovery that a large-scale epidemic (2,480 persons became ill, 750 were hospitalized, and 16 died) of a febrile illness, initially thought to be dengue, was actually leptospirosis. After Nicaraguan scientists demonstrated that dengue virus was not the cause, investigation by the U.S. Centers for Disease Control and Prevention and by the Cuban Pedro Kouri Institute of Tropical Medicine identified *Leptospira* from patients with fatal cases. Leptospirosis is an illness treatable with easily obtained, inexpensive antibiotics. During the epidemic, the ability to rapidly rule out dengue was critical in the final determination of the etiology and the institution of control measures for this illness, which is now emerging as a major infectious disease problem in the developing world.

Since its introduction in the late 1980s, the PCR technique has revolutionized not only molecular biology research but also fields in which the use of molecular biology techniques was never previously considered. Its application in fields as diverse as linguistics, anthropology, archaeology, phylogeny, and medicine has helped to propel each of these fields into new directions and introduced concepts and ideas previously not imagined. Dozens of books on the technique and its myriad variations have appeared during the last decade. However, many of these applications remain within the confines of research and academic environments. Now, Harris's book takes the technology to address real, daily, and ordinary problems of millions of people around the world.

This book makes accessible an elegantly simple technique to address infectious disease problems that face children and adults of developing countries. Harris makes a compelling argument for its use in areas of the world that cannot practically or financially apply even conventional laboratory methods, and she guides the reader through the steps of its application in clear, precise language, avoiding jargon that frequently obfuscates techniques books. She not only writes the book as a guide for potential users in developing countries, but also as a guide for scientists in developed countries who may wish to work abroad. While the specific examples of the PCR applications outlined in the book become immediately useful, they are written in a sufficiently informed and technically solid manner that readers can generalize the information to apply the technique in new areas and situations. Such a style is consistent with the general theme of this book, which emphasizes sustainability and transfer of a usable, practical, and important technology.

Of course, the PCR technique by itself will not contribute to solving the public health problems related to infectious diseases. It is the will, understanding, and skills of health care and public health professionals and workers that will ultimately aid them in the exploitation of the data generated from the technique to implement appropriate disease control strategies. In this regard, this book is unique, because it is not designed solely as a techniques book. For every application of the PCR technique, it details how the data generated from the application can be used to deal with the problem at hand and points out caveats and limitations of each application. Therefore, the book will facilitate laboratories in many areas of the world to generate databases related to infectious diseases that can then be used by epidemiologists, public health workers, health policy professionals, and other health professionals to develop new strategies for disease control.

PCR technology is a constantly evolving technology, but the book itself is not likely to be made obsolete due to the author's emphasis on immutable features of the technique and its underlying principles. Thus, with its focus on the accessibility and sustainability of PCR applications in areas of the world where they are most needed, this book is bound to remain timely far into the future.

Lee W. Riley, M.D.

School of Public Health, University of California, Berkeley
Berkeley, California
January 1998

I

PCR and Technology Transfer

1

Introduction

This book is based on experience gained over the past ten years during the development of the Applied Molecular Biology/Appropriate Technology Transfer (AMB/ATT) Program. The objectives of the AMB/ATT Program are to simplify and demystify molecular biology techniques to make them accessible in developing countries for application to relevant issues in public health and biomedical sciences (Harris, 1996; Harris et al., 1996). This process includes adapting the techniques themselves to existing conditions, training scientists and health professionals in the theory and practice of molecular biology techniques, and assisting local scientists to apply these techniques to their own areas of interest. The low-cost methodology and the participatory didactic approach that was developed as part of the program can be applied and transferred to any environment with limited resources. Chapter 4 describes this program in detail.

1.1 Molecular Biology and the Polymerase Chain Reaction

Molecular biology has expanded tremendously since its beginning in the early 1950s (Cairns et al., 1966; Watson and Crick, 1953a, 1953b), from a branch of the biological basic sciences to the point where DNA is now a household term. The Polymerase Chain Reaction (PCR), a procedure that exponentially amplifies a piece of DNA of specific size and sequence, has revolutionized molecular biology worldwide since its invention in 1985. It is currently imperative to be "fluent" in the language of molecular biology and, more specifically, to become familiar with PCR technology in a number of settings, including universities and other teaching institutions (including high schools), hospitals, health clinics, public health departments, and disease surveillance centers. PCR has allowed genetic analysis to become widely accessible, and its diverse applications continue to expand fields of scientific inquiry, both on conceptual and practical levels (White, 1996). For instance, the phenomenal progress within the last few years in sequencing the human genome as well as that of other organisms and infectious agents is due largely to PCR technology.

Despite the sophistication of automated PCR-based genome sequencing and other complex applications, PCR is really a very simple technique. Interestingly, molecular biology has advanced to such an extent that the most sophisticated technology is, in a sense, the most simplified. One of the most powerful aspects of PCR is the relative ease with which genetic information can be obtained. For example, the same procedure that allows detection of a pathogenic organism in a diagnostic sample can also furnish information about the pathogen's genome that permits classification at the level of genus, species, or strain. Simple PCR-based fingerprinting techniques can identify individual strains of microorganisms, which facilitates the investigation of disease outbreaks, the understanding of transmission patterns, and the examination of the biological significance of genetic differences, all of which aid in the control and prevention of infectious diseases.

Molecular biology techniques such as PCR can be more specific, sensitive, versatile, rapid, accessible, and safer than alternative methods in many situations, as discussed in chapter 2. Most important, PCR can be less costly than other techniques, but only when adapted to local human and material resources; this approach is described in chapter 3. While this book focuses on the application of molecular biology techniques to the diagnosis and epidemiology of human diseases (chapters 4 and 5), the same approach can be applied to the detection and characterization of nucleic acid sequences in the fields of genetic diseases, agriculture, conservation genetics, biodiversity, molecular evolution, and many other areas.

1.2   Infectious Diseases and International Health

Due to environmental, demographic, economic, political, and biological factors, emerging and re-emerging infectious diseases (such as AIDS, tuberculosis, cholera, and dengue fever) are no longer confined to a particular geographic region or country and are rapidly becoming global health concerns. Of course, many of the so-called "emerging diseases" have existed in the vast majority of the world's population for a long time. In addition, endemic diseases, while perhaps less glamorous to the mainstream media, represent a far greater burden in terms of morbidity and mortality. It is therefore essential that every country have the ability to monitor and control infectious diseases, both for its own well-being and to deliver critical information to global surveillance networks. Laboratory capability as well as clinical and epidemiological expertise is necessary to achieve these objectives. Thus, less-developed countries must obtain access to the most relevant and appropriate modern technologies and maintain effective state-of-the-art diagnostic and epidemiological capabilities on-site (Harris, 1996). Building scientific capacity includes training in a number of areas: research methodology, proficiency in laboratory techniques, and skills in project development, study design, and preparation of funding applications and scientific publications. Training in all these subjects is necessary for the true transfer of technology.

PCR and other molecular biology techniques can serve multiple purposes in infectious disease research and control when used responsibly. In terms of applied research, these tools can be utilized for the detection and/or characterization of infectious agents, as outlined in chapters 4 and 5. Infectious disease diagnosis based on detection of a particular pathogen is useful for individual case management and for national and international surveillance services that compile morbidity and mortality statistics. As previously mentioned, genetic information obtained using molecular biological techniques is critical for understanding the geographical distribution of infectious agents, investigating specific outbreaks, and conducting epidemiological studies aimed at identifying risk factors and designing subsequent control measures for disease prevention. However, it is essential that users know what information they need, what a given technique can provide, and how to interpret and use resulting data.

1.3   Appropriate Application of Technology

In implementing any new technology, it is important to fully understand the limitations as well as the advantages of the techniques of interest. Users must know how to decide when to use and when *not* to use the new techniques in favor of alternative methods. Unfortunately, there is often a pressure to use the most modern techniques available due to a combination of sales tactics by product manufacturers and the desire of investigators to use the latest techniques. However, without comprehensive knowledge, informed decisions about the application of such tools cannot be made. Inappropriate application of new techniques is often uninformative, wasteful, and even counterproductive. For instance, the irresponsible substitution of rigorous clinical laboratory procedures and classical microbiological methods of infectious disease diagnosis with the PCR technique can result in the loss of critical clinical information and vital stocks of isolated pathogens. It cannot be overemphasized that new techniques such as PCR should not simply replace other methods but rather should serve a specific purpose to fill a void and answer questions that cannot be addressed using existing techniques.

For the detection and characterization of infectious pathogens, many types of techniques are available, including microbiological, biochemical, serological, and more recently, molecular biological methods. It is important that as many of these methods as possible be accessible to investigators and health professionals in developing as well as developed countries. Each technique has its advantages and limitations and must be evaluated in the context of each disease application, as discussed in chapter 3. For example, the most useful approaches to massive screening or development of simple dipstick assays are based on serological methods. Microscopic techniques are low-cost, simple, and appropriate for use in primary health clinics. Microbiological or virological methods are essential for isolating pathogens for subsequent analysis. Molecular biology techniques such as PCR can provide specific advantages in terms of rapidity, sensitivity, and genetic information, and are complementary to the already-existing methods.

1.4   General Principles

While this book is based on specific experience in applying PCR to the analysis of infectious diseases in developing countries, several principles have emerged that have wider implications. The same approach to developing a low-cost methodology in the case of PCR can be applied to other techniques; namely, understanding the principles underlying the technique of interest, breaking it down into its constituent parts, and simplifying each component to adapt it to existing conditions, as outlined in section 3.1. Similarly, the framework for evaluation and the criteria for assessment to determine the appropriate application of PCR are generalizable to any new technology, as described in section 3.3. The overall concept presented is that technologies can be made accessible through a knowledge-based approach to simplification, adaptation to existing conditions, and application to relevant problems.

Another widely applicable concept is the approach taken in chapter 4 to maximize the sustainability of the transfer process itself. The use of a phased series of workshops of increasing complexity that incorporates training in both laboratory techniques and grant application preparation skills can serve as a prototype for other fields. The clarity and detail of each protocol and the background information provided for each disease in chapter 5 emphasize a knowledge-based approach that can be transferred to any discipline. The support of local initiative, emphasis on a participatory and responsible transfer process, and incorporation of adequate follow-through, as illustrated in the AMB/ATT Program, should be instructive for other technology transfer efforts.

1.5   Book Structure

The book consists of three interrelated parts. The first section includes a straightforward, comprehensive overview of the PCR technique, a discussion of appropriate application of new technologies and the development of a low-cost methodology, and a description of the AMB/ATT Program as a case study. The second section contains detailed PCR protocols for detection and characterization of twelve infectious disease agents, along with a review of each disease (clinical manifestations and epidemiology, classical methods of diagnosis, and PCR-based procedures). A protocol for the use of nonradioactive DNA probes and one detailing standard molecular biological methods for rapid cloning of PCR products are also included in this section. These protocols were either developed de novo or were adapted from published procedures through first-hand application on-site in collaborating laboratories overseas. The protocols can serve directly as a laboratory manual and as teaching tools or as a model for preparing course material for similar workshops. The third part of the book consists of an extensive Appendix that includes the following: designs for homemade equipment and materials; protocols for in-house preparation of certain molecular biology reagents and solutions; an inventory of equipment and materials required for a PCR laboratory; a guide for preventing contamination and for troubleshooting technical problems; workshop teaching tips and worksheets; useful World Wide Web sites for easy access to pertinent information; and a comprehensive glossary.

In summary, this book is both a prototype for the simplification and sustainable transfer of advanced technologies and a practical guide for the application of PCR to the diagnosis and epidemiology of infectious diseases.

References

Cairns, J., Stent, G.S., and Watson, J.D., eds. (1966) *Phage and the Origins of Molecular Biology*. New York, Cold Spring Harbor Laboratory of Quantitative Biology.

Harris, E. (1996) Developing essential scientific capability in countries with limited resources. *Nat. Med.*, 2:737–739.

Harris, E., Belli, A., and Agabian, N. (1996) Appropriate transfer of molecular technology to Latin America for public health and biomedical sciences. *Biochem. Educ.*, 24:3–12.

Watson, J.D., and Crick, F.H.C. (1953a) Genetical implications of the structure of deoxyribonucleic acid. *Nature*, 171:964–967.

Watson, J.D., and Crick, F.H.C. (1953b) Molecular structure of nucleic acids: A structure for deoxyribose nucleic acid. *Nature*, 171:737–738.

White, T.J. (1996) The future of PCR technology: Diversification of technology and applications. *Trends Biotechnol.*, 14:478–483.

2

PCR Technology

2.1 Description of the Technique

2.1.1 Historical Overview

Just as the discovery of restriction enzymes and the ability to clone fragments of DNA had profound impacts on the biological sciences in the 1970s (Cohen et al., 1973), so too the invention of the polymerase chain reaction (PCR) revolutionized molecular biology in the late 1980s. Kary Mullis first conceptualized the process of PCR in 1985 (Saiki et al., 1985a). In that year, the first clinical application of PCR, in a case of sickle cell anemia, was published (Saiki et al., 1985b). In 1986, the description of the use of PCR for analysis of allelic sequence variation in the HLA locus set the stage for PCR-based forensic analysis (Saiki et al., 1986). During this time, "first-generation" PCR technology began to disseminate in laboratories in the developed world. The next advance was the advent of the thermostable polymerase *Taq*, isolated from the thermophilic bacteria *Thermus aquaticus*, which greatly facilitated the procedure. Prior to the introduction of *Taq* polymerase, fresh polymerase had to be added to the reaction after each cycle, because the incubation temperature (94°C) necessary for denaturation of the DNA template also destroyed the thermolabile polymerases available at the time. In 1988–89, recombinant *Taq* polymerase became available (Lawyer et al., 1989). Recently, there has been an explosion in the number of different thermostable enzymes on the market, the so-called "designer enzymes," each of which is optimized for a slightly different PCR application. Going back to the time line, by 1989, over 1000 PCR-related papers had been published, according to the Medline database. By 1992, the number of PCR-related papers had risen to over 15,000 and has continued to skyrocket ever since. By 1990, "second-generation" thermocyclers and enzymes had become available, and the use of PCR began in developing countries (Harris et al., 1993). PCR has become an essential tool in research laboratories worldwide and the basis for many clinical and forensic tests.

2.1.2   The Molecular Basis of PCR

The fundamental principle of PCR is the amplification of a specific fragment of DNA through successive cycles of exponential multiplication (Figure 2.1) until sufficient product has accumulated to be visualized. In this manner, a single molecule can generate over a billion copies of itself after 30 cycles of exponential replication ($2^{30} = 1,073,741,824$). Each cycle of amplification typically consists of three temperatures, at which the ingredients of the PCR reaction mixture undergo different physical and biochemical processes (denaturation, annealing, and extension) for the template DNA to be replicated (Figure 2.2). The first step is an incubation at 94°C to allow denaturation of the two strands of the template DNA double helix. This is followed by an annealing step[1] to allow hybridization of the primers with their complementary sequences in the target DNA. Finally, the cycle is completed during an extension step at 72°C when the polymerase extends from the primer in the direction 5′ to 3′, replicating the template strand. A standard amplification consists of between 25 and 35 cycles.

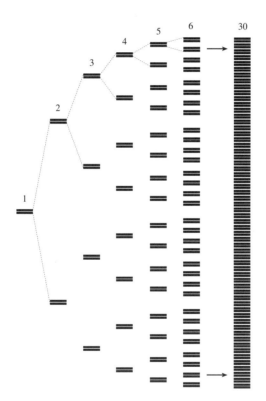

Fig. 2.1. Product accumulation during the exponential amplification of DNA by PCR.

---

1. The annealing temperature is discussed in sections 2.2.1 and 2.2.2.

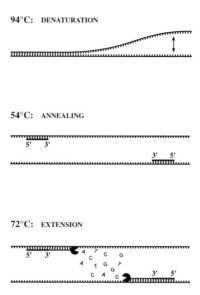

Fig. 2.2. Schematic diagram of the denaturation, annealing, and extension steps in each amplification cycle. Representative temperatures are shown; for additional information, *see* section 2.2.

The amplification process is illustrated in detail in Figure 2.3, which should be carefully reviewed until the concept is clearly understood. In cycle 1, the primers anneal to their complementary sequences on opposite strands of the denatured double helix, and the polymerase replicates the template. In cycle 2, each of the newly synthesized strands, as well as the original strands, serves as a template for the next round of synthesis. An important concept to understand is that when the newly synthesized products (from cycle 1) are used as template, primer A anneals to its complementary site, and the polymerase extends 5′ to 3′, but it runs out of template when it comes to the site of primer G, which is the 5′ terminus of the template. Similarly, primer G anneals to its complementary site, and the polymerase extends 5′ to 3′ but runs out of template when it comes to the site of primer A. Thus, this process generates two single strands limited in length by the location of the two primers. When these strands are used as templates in cycle 3, two short double-stranded products of defined length are generated, specified by the location of primers A and G, in addition to the single-stranded products of defined length and the long strands of undefined length replicated in a linear manner in every cycle. In cycle 4, the two double-stranded products of defined length are replicated, and the exponential amplification of the double-stranded fragments of defined length (referred to as "PCR product") begins. This process is repeated until literally millions of copies are generated. Note that the products of defined length are multiplied exponentially, while the long products generated from the original DNA strands acculmulate in a linear manner.

   The key concept is that a *specific* sequence of DNA of a *defined length* is *replicated exponentially* so that it can be easily detected.

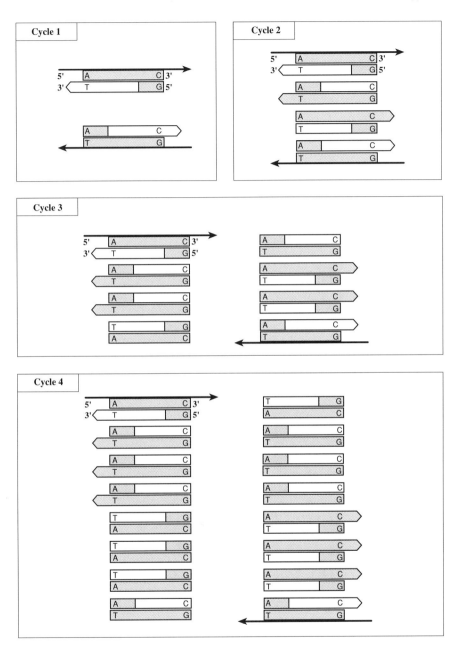

Fig. 2.3. Mechanism of DNA amplification during the first four cycles of PCR. The target sequence is delineated by primer A ($5'$ adenosine) and primer G ($5'$ guanosine); primer A hybridizes to the region at T and primer G hybridizes to a complementary region at C. Shaded areas represent DNA present at the start of the cycle, clear portions indicate product synthesized during the current cycle, and the black line represents genomic DNA.

2.1.3   Advantages and Disadvantages

Table 2.1 lists some of the advantages and limitations of PCR in relation to diagnosis and epidemiology of infectious diseases. This is followed by an explanation of each item on the list.

Advantages

- *Rapidity.* One advantage of PCR is that it can be executed from start to finish in one day. This compares favorably with, for example, the diagnosis of tuberculosis by culture, which takes from 6–8 weeks, or dengue viral isolation from cell culture, which takes 6–14 days.

- *Sensitivity.* Since a single molecule of DNA can often be amplified by PCR to detectable levels, PCR is an extremely sensitive diagnostic tool, detecting fractions of organisms. Even with crude extracts as templates and simple product visualization methods, the level of sensitivity is often just a few organisms.

- *Specificity.* Since DNA constitutes the genetic material unique to each organism, a technique like PCR that identifies the organism by its DNA is the most accurate ("specific") possible.

- *Versatility.* PCR is a remarkably versatile technique; that is, the same experimental procedure is conducted with essentially the same equipment, materials, and chemical and biological reagents in order to amplify any DNA of interest. Thus, once a laboratory is equipped to conduct one PCR protocol or detect one pathogen, the same instruments and reagents can be used for other applications. The protocols can be easily adapted for detection of other pathogens simply by obtaining new primers and reaction conditions at little extra cost.

Table 2.1. Advantages and Disadvantages of the Use of PCR in the Diagnosis and Epidemiology of Infectious Diseases

Advantages	Disadvantages
Rapidity	Risk of cross-contamination
Sensitivity	Equipment accessibility
Specificity	Reagent accessibility
Versatility	Reagent instability
Low cost	Medium throughput
Genetic information	Not suitable for primary clinics
Sample accessibility	Training users
Standardized results	Troubleshooting technical problems
No need for microbiological sterility	Reproducibility
Safety (the pathogen is killed immediately to liberate the DNA)	Detection of nonviable as well as viable organisms
Rapid technology transfer	

- *Low cost.* Although PCR is often marketed as an expensive, sophisticated technique, it is actually quite simple and can be approached using a low-cost methodology (*see* section 3.1). By implementing appropriate technology, alternative techniques, simplification of experimental procedures, "in-house" preparation of reagents, and recycling of materials, the cost per reaction of PCR can be greatly reduced, until it compares favorably with most existing diagnostic techniques.

- *Genetic information.* One of the most useful aspects of PCR is that it can provide important information about the organism under study. Because of the genetic specificity of the primers, an organism can be simultaneously detected and characterized at the genus, complex, or species level. Simple fingerprinting methods allow identification of individual strains for molecular epidemiological studies (Friedman et al., 1995; Riley and Harris, in press; Tibayrenc et al., 1993). Information about toxicity or drug resistance can be determined as well; for example, by targeting bacterial toxin genes or genes known to be involved in antibiotic resistance. Of course, PCR products can be sequenced to extract the maximum genetic information.

- *Sample accessibility.* In addition to clinical samples, specimens from a variety of sources can be analyzed using the same molecular techniques. For instance, pathogenic organisms can be detected in insect vectors, animal reservoirs, plants, and environmental sources such as water supplies and food samples. The organism does not have to be culturable for successful PCR analysis; this permits identification and analysis of otherwise intractable organisms.

- *Standardized results.* Since the results of PCR are recorded as the presence or absence of a DNA fragment of a particular size, there is minimal variability in interpreting results between individual practitioners. This feature contrasts with many of the microscopic techniques, which require highly trained, experienced technicians to identify the morphological characteristics of particular organisms. Thus, it is easier to standardize PCR results.

- *No requirement for microbiological sterility.* A major problem with diagnostic and strain characterization techniques that rely on culturing an organism is the need to maintain microbiological sterility. This can be very difficult in laboratories without access to appropriate sterile culture facilities in dusty, tropical climates. Since PCR requires only minute quantities of DNA and not living organisms, it completely obviates the need for microbiological sterility.

- *Safety.* The first step in the preparation of a sample for PCR is lysing the cells to liberate the DNA; of course, killing the cells in the process. This contrasts with many classical diagnostic procedures, which involve growing large quantities of the pathogen in order to later establish its identity. Clearly, it is safer for the health worker to begin the identification process by killing the pathogenic organism rather than culturing it.

- *Rapid technology transfer.* Since the procedure is essentially the same no matter what DNA is amplified, the initial training in using PCR is fairly rapid.

A week-long intensive training workshop has been developed for this purpose and successfully conducted in a number of countries (*see* chapter 4). It is critical for beginners to maintain contact with experienced PCR practitioners for assistance with troubleshooting technical difficulties that may arise.

Disadvantages

- *Risk of cross-contamination.* The extreme sensitivity of PCR, which is one of its main advantages, also contributes to its major disadvantage; namely, the risk of false-positive artifactual results. In theory, a single product molecule from a previous amplification can contaminate negative samples in a subsequent amplification. To minimize this risk, there are a number of approaches to "carryover" prevention that consist of both simple and sophisticated methods (section 2.2.4).

- *Equipment accessibility.* Although the equipment required to set up a PCR laboratory is minimal in comparison to that required for many other laboratory techniques, there are still certain instruments that are necessary. Many of these can be improvised (section 3.1.1 and Appendix A) or alternative processes implemented (section 3.1.2). Nonetheless, certain critical pieces of equipment may be difficult to acquire due to transportation problems, price inflation, customs delays, and prohibitive taxation, among other factors.

- *Reagent accessibility.* Availability of molecular biology reagents is also subject to the same pitfalls as imported equipment, mentioned above. Ideally, as many reagents as possible should be prepared on-site to minimize dependence on outside sources (section 3.1.4). However, certain items will need to be purchased abroad, and ways must be found to make this process as streamlined and cost-effective as possible.

- *Reagent instability.* One key problem with obtaining and storing certain PCR reagents is their lability. This problem is worsened in tropical climates, where ambient temperature is high. Oligonucleotides (primers) and DNA are actually quite stable at ambient temperature when dried, and can be shipped easily without damage. Since the critical enzyme is a thermostable polymerase, it is hardier than most other enzymes that are much more heat-sensitive; nonetheless, the half-life of the *Taq* is prolonged if it is kept cold. The main problem is with the reverse transcriptase enzymes, which are necessary to convert RNA to DNA for subsequent amplification; these enzymes are notoriously fragile and are difficult to transport safely and conveniently. However, a thermostable reverse transcriptase/polymerase isolated from *Thermus thermophilus* (rTth) is now available, which is by nature much more robust.

- *Medium throughput.* PCR is very useful for many applications, but it is not an ideal technique for routine analysis of large numbers of samples. Using the conventional procedure in individual tubes, 50–60 samples is approximately the comfortable upper limit per amplification run by a single person. Newer adaptations of PCR to the microtiter plate format allow larger number of samples to be analyzed more easily (96 amplifications per plate).

- *Not suitable for primary clinics.* While PCR can be tremendously simplified for use under difficult circumstances, it is not a quick or simple diagnostic method. The technique requires an adequately equipped laboratory with properly trained personnel. It is better suited for a central laboratory in a hospital or university or a reference center than for widespead use in rural clinics.

- *Training users/troubleshooting technical problems.* As with any technique, users must be well-trained, not only in the practical aspects but also in the principles behind the technique. A certain amount of knowledge can be learned fairly quickly, but more time and experience are required to learn to troubleshoot technical problems independently.

- *Reproducibility.* There are a number of ways in which a PCR amplification can go wrong, and many factors can affect reproducibility. These include: poor quality of the sample, the presence of inhibitors or nucleases, lot-to-lot variability of reagents, poor water quality, unanticipated power outages, loss of enzyme activity, and technical problems with the thermocycler. These potential problems must be kept in mind to reliably maintain optimal performance.

- *Detection of nonviable as well as viable organisms.* This attribute of PCR is also an advantage, since live organisms are not necessary for successful detection. However, in situations where one wants to detect only live organisms (e.g., in the evaluation of drug efficacy), culture techniques that detect viability are preferable to PCR.

2.2   Technical Details

This section provides information about the components of the PCR mixture, the thermal cycling parameters, optimization of performance, potential problems, and detection of the products. Further information can be obtained from a number of reference texts, which provide comprehensive introductions to PCR (Dieffenbach and Dveksler, 1995; Erlich, 1989, 1992; Innis et al., 1990; McPherson et al., 1991, 1995; Mullis et al., 1994; Persing et al., 1993; White, 1993).

2.2.1   Components of the PCR Mixture

The basic reagents in the PCR mixture are the buffer, magnesium chloride, primers, deoxynucleotide triphosphates, the thermostable polymerase, and the DNA template. Stabilizers and enhancers are also sometimes included.

Buffer

The typical PCR buffer is fairly standard, although some of the "designer enzymes" have special requirements. Most buffers contain Tris at 10 mM and KCl at 50 mM concentrations; the pH varies from 8.2 to 9.0 (at 25°C). Remember that the pH of Tris drops as the temperature increases, decreasing 0.03 pH units for every additional degree centigrade. So pH 9.0 at 25°C translates to approximately pH 7.6 at 72°C, which is the optimal temperature for polymerase activity. pH 7.0–7.5 is considered optimal for *Taq* polymerase. Some buffers also contain detergent, since the presence of nonionic detergent (Nonidet P-40 or Triton® X-100) increases the processivity[2] of *Taq* polymerase. Sometimes the detergent is included in the storage buffer with the *Taq* itself (e.g., Perkin-Elmer AmpliTaq®) or else in the reaction buffer (e.g., the buffer from Promega Corp.). It is important to use the reaction buffer supplied with the polymerase by the manufacturer, since this combination has been optimized.

Magnesium Chloride

Magnesium is a cation that binds to the polymerase and is an essential cofactor for polymerase activity. The concentration of magnesium can have a profound effect on the amplification results. It is important to titrate the concentration of magnesium in each new amplification in order to determine the optimal amount (usually between 1.0 and 3.0 mM); a change of 0.25 mM can mean the difference between excellent yield of product of the expected length or no product at all. The lower the magnesium concentration, the more stringent the conditions for primer annealing. Magnesium chloride is occasionally included in the buffer at a fixed concentration; be careful to check whether the buffer in use is supplied with or without magnesium. Some enzymes require other divalent cations as well, such as the thermostable r*Tth*, which needs manganese acetate [$Mn(OAc)_2$] for the reverse transcriptase activity.

Primers

Primers are synthetic oligonucleotides, generally 15–30 nucleotides in length, which are complementary to a particular sequence in the genome of the organism of interest. Since the other reagents are common to all PCR reactions, the sequence of the primers is what confers specificity to the amplification. Primers directed to a conserved region of the chromosome will amplify all members of the genus or the gene family, whereas primers specific to a variable region will target only a particular species or gene. Primers used for the detection and epidemiology of infectious pathogens or genetic alterations are usually specific primers of defined sequence complementary to known sequences. PCR can also be used to amplify unknown sequences when the target sequence is only partially available, by using degenerate primers where certain positions in the oligonucleotide contain a mixture of 2, 3, or 4 bases. This book refers exclusively to primers with defined sequences. The optimal primer concentration for PCR is usually between 0.1 and 1.0 μM.

The main rules to follow in designing PCR primers include:

1. The theoretical annealing temperature (T_{ann}) of one primer should equal the T_{ann} of the other(s). The T_{ann} is calculated using the following formula, which

---

2. Enzyme processivity refers to the number of nucleotides that the polymerase incorporates into the replicated strand before the enzyme falls off the template.

assigns 4°C for every GC pair held together by three hydrogen bonds and 2°C for each AT pair bridged by two hydrogen bonds: $4(G + C) + 2(A + T) - 5$.[3]

2. Avoid secondary structure within the oligonucleotide (self-complementary sequences that lead to hairpin formation).

3. Avoid complementarity with other primer(s) in the reaction.

4. Check the genomic sequence of the organism of interest for secondary primer hybridization sites.

A number of primer design programs exist (e.g., OLIGO,® National Biosciences Inc., Plymouth, MN; PRIMER, Whitehead Institute for Biomedical Research, Cambridge, MA); however, primers can certainly be designed manually following the guidelines above.

Deoxynucleotide Triphosphates (dNTPs)

Deoxynucleotide triphosphates are the building blocks of the DNA replicated during PCR. Equal amounts of each of the four dNTPs (dATP, dCTP, dGTP, dTTP) are included in the reaction, usually at a concentration of 0.2 mM (200 µM) each. In order to increase the stringency of certain delicate reactions that require heightened specificity, the nucleotide concentration can be lowered (e.g., to 1.5 mM each; Meredith et al., 1993). To generate labeled probes, radioactive dNTPs or nucleotides conjugated to compounds for nonradioactive detection (such as biotin or digoxigenin) can be incorporated into the product during the PCR amplification.

Thermostable Polymerase

The most common thermostable polymerase and the first to be widely used for PCR is *Taq* DNA polymerase. Initially purified from *Thermus aquaticus* and used in its native form (Saiki et al., 1988), it was soon replaced by a recombinant version made from the cloned *T. aquaticus* gene expressed in *E. coli.* (Lawyer et al., 1989). A number of currently available thermostable polymerases are listed in Table 2.2, with a description of their properties.

These polymerases can replicate approximately 1–4 kilobases per minute, depending upon the particular enzyme. The rate of misincorporation varies between polymerases and is controlled by the presence of a 3'—>5' exonuclease, also called "proofreading activity," which enables the enzyme to check for mismatches during polymerization, remove an erroneous base if it finds one, and replace it with the correct match. Enzyme processivity also varies, ranging from 5–10 nucleotides for low-processivity enzymes, such as the *Taq* Stoffel fragment, to 50–60 nucleotides for high-processivity polymerases like the intact *Taq*. The half-life at elevated temperatures

---

3. For an oligonucleotide of approximately 20 nucleotides, the annealing temperature is calculated by subtracting 5 degrees from the melting temperature [$T_m = 4(G + C) + 2(A + T)$], the temperature at which the two strands separate, or denature.

Table 2.2. Properties of thermostable polymerases

Polymerase	T$_{1/2}$ 95°C	Bacteria	Proof-reading activity	Properties
Taq	40–96 min	Thermus aquaticus	No 3'—>5' exo*	High processivity
Taq Stoffel fragment	80 min	Thermus aquaticus	No 3'—>5' exo	No 5'—>3' exo Low processivity
Ultma®	40 min at 97.5°C	Thermatoga maritima	3'—>5' exo	No 5'—>3' exo High fidelity Low processivity
Vent®	6.7 h	Thermococcus litoralis	3'—>5' exo	High fidelity Low processivity
Deep Vent™	23.0 h	Pyrococcus	3'—>5' exo	High fidelity Low processivity
Pfu	95% active after 1 h	Pyrococcus furiosus	3'—>5' exo	High fidelity Low processivity
rTth	20 min	Thermus thermophilus	No 3'—>5' exo	RT** plus DNA polymerase

*exonuclease
**reverse transcriptase

of 94–95°C differs among the polymerases. Originally, thermophilic bacteria like *T. aquaticus* were isolated from hot springs; more recently, enzymes have been purified from bacteria that grow naturally at even higher temperatures in vents in the ocean floor (e.g., *Thermococcus litoralis*, *Pyrococcus*). rTth is an interesting enzyme that acts as both a reverse transcriptase (in the presence of manganese) and a DNA polymerase (in the presence of magnesium) (Myers and Gelfand, 1991). Thus, by chelating one cation and replacing it with another, one can change the predominant activity of the enzyme. The technique has been further refined by the use of the buffer bicine, which regulates both activities so that reverse transcriptase (RT)-PCR can be conducted in a single tube without the need to open the tube in order to adjust the reagent concentrations. In addition, different thermostable polymerases can be used in combination and optimized for specific purposes. For instance, for long PCR products (up to 42 kilobase fragments have been reported), high-fidelity polymerases are used to minimize misincorporation; however, since these enzymes have low processivity, polymerases with higher processivity are also included in the same reaction to increase the yield.

Stabilizers

In order to stabilize the polymerase, bovine serum albumin (BSA; 0.01%),[4] gelatin (0.01%), or glycerol (1–2%) are sometimes included in the reaction mix.

---

4. 0.1 mg/mL.

Enhancers

A number of chemicals can be used to optimize the performance and sensitivity of PCR, including dimethyl sulfoxide (DMSO), tetramethylammonium chloride (TMAC), and betaine. Most of these compounds function by destabilizing the hydrogen bonds between the bases in opposite strands of the double helix, thereby making it easier for the two strands to be denatured and become accessible for primer binding and subsequent strand replication. In effect, this lowers the T_{ann} of the annealing step.

DNA Template

Different approaches to sample preparation are described in more detail in section 3.1.3. PCR is such a sensitive technique that product amplification can be achieved even with very crude sample preparations. However, the cleaner the template, the higher the sensitivity; therefore, the trade-off is between a longer, more complicated nucleic acid extraction, which will yield maximal sensitivity, and more simple "quick and dirty" protocols, which will result in less sensitive detection. Thus, the choice of sample preparation method depends on the desired sensitivity. Procedures range from protocols that yield purified DNA/RNA, such as standard organic extraction/ethanol precipitation or nucleic acid separation using silica particles, to crude lysates generated with detergents and proteases, chloroform, chelating resins, boiling or autoclaving, or direct extraction. These procedures are discussed in more detail in section 3.1.

2.2.2   Thermal Cycling Parameters

As described above, the principle of PCR is the exponential amplification of a given sequence of DNA by repeated cycles at different temperatures. This cycling can be achieved either manually or automatically.

Thermal Cycling Profile

Each cycle typically consists of an incubation for a certain amount of time at each of three temperatures. As described previously, the first step is an incubation for 30–60 seconds at 94–95°C to allow denaturation of the DNA template, followed by an annealing step of 1–2 minutes for hybridization of the primers with their complementary sequences in the target DNA. The annealing temperature is initially calculated using a formula such as the one described in section 2.2.1, and then empirically tested until the appropriate temperature has been determined. The hybridization step is followed by extension at 72°C for 1–5 minutes, depending on the length of the product, where the polymerase replicates the template strand, extending from the primers. As expected, the number of cycles greatly influences the amount of product generated. A standard amplification consists of between 25 and 35 cycles, with high-sensitivity diagnostic applications occasionally reaching 40 cycles. It is not advisable to increase the number above this level because of the risk of artifacts (i.e., false-positives) and the decreasing activity of *Taq* after this many cycles.

The incubation time at each temperature varies depending on the size of the tube (i.e., 0.5 mL or 0.2 mL). Conversion of a cycling protocol developed for 0.5-mL tubes to one suitable for 0.2-mL thin-walled tubes involves reducing the incubation times by approximately one-half. When a very short product is generated (e.g., approximately 100 base pairs), the cycle is sometimes reduced to only two steps: denaturation and annealing. While the reaction proceeds from the annealing temperature to the denaturation temperature, the polymerase can complete the replication/extension of the short products.

Automatic vs. Manual Cycling

The standard method of conducting the amplification, for those laboratories that can afford it, is by means of an automated thermocycler (Figure 2.4). This instrument can be programmed to execute the amplification profiles for many different PCR assays. The thermocycler contains a metal block into which the tubes with the PCR reaction mixture are placed, and the block varies in temperature in accordance with the amplification protocol. Alternatively, manual amplification can be carried out using water baths set at the different temperatures (Figure 2.5). Under these conditions, the PCR reaction tubes are placed in a floating rack in the water bath at the appropriate temperature for an indicated amount of time and manually transferred between baths until the cycling process is complete. Thus, with automatic cycling, the tubes remain in place while the temperature in the block changes around them, whereas with manual cycling, the tubes are moved from one bath to another to vary the temperature.

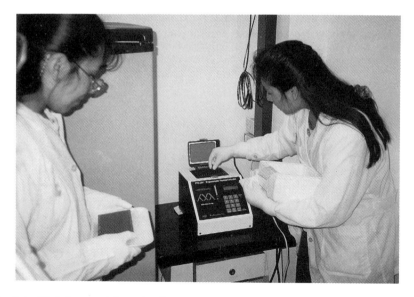

Fig. 2.4. Workshop participant loading an automated thermocycler.

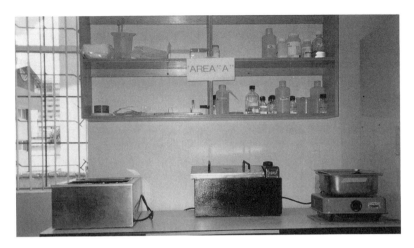

Fig. 2.5. Water baths set up for manual amplification.

Thermocycler Variability

Several thermocyclers are currently on the market, each with a different heating and cooling system, programming procedure, weight, size, ramp time,[5] and fit of the tubes in the heating block. These features will be discussed in more detail in section 3.1.1. The results of a PCR amplification can differ dramatically depending on the thermocycler used (Riley and Harris, in press). The parameters that have the most effect on amplification are the ramp time and thermal transfer.[6] Remember that the thermal profile as programmed in a thermocycler (the theoretical profile) may not necessarily reflect the real temperatures and incubation times that the PCR reaction mixture is subjected to inside the reaction tubes in the block (Hoelzel, 1990). The theoretical profile and the actual conditions are only concurrent if the thermocycler program is controlled by a thermocouple which records the existing temperature in a sample tube in the block.

Reverse Transcriptase PCR (RT-PCR)

One very important variation of PCR is the ability to analyze RNA templates. However, since the thermostable polymerases can only replicate DNA, the RNA must first be converted into DNA by the action of a reverse transcriptase. This RT-PCR can be accomplished in two steps: conversion of RNA to DNA in one

---

5. Length of time spent going from one temperature to the next.
6. Transfer of the thermal energy (temperature) in the metal block to the PCR mixture inside the tubes in the block.

reaction tube followed by PCR amplification of the resulting cDNA in another. A more convenient alternative is the combination of the two procedures in a single tube, which contains all of the reagents necessary for the two reactions, including both of the required enzymes. In this case, the cycling protocol of the PCR amplification is preceded by an incubation step (e.g., 60 minutes at 42°C) to allow reverse transcription to occur. A number of RTs are available, including RAV-2 (Rous associated virus 2; Amersham Corp.), AMV (avian myeloblastosis virus), M-MLV (Moloney murine leukemia virus), and the thermostable r*Tth* (Perkin-Elmer). For unknown reasons, some RTs function more efficiently than others for particular applications; for example, RAV-2 is more efficient at reverse transcribing dengue virus than MMLV (Lanciotti et al., 1992).

2.2.3   Optimization

There are a number of ways to optimize a particular PCR reaction. As mentioned above, the concentration of magnesium significantly affects the amplification; in addition, the concentration of primers, dNTPs, polymerase, and template can be adjusted to optimize yield. The temperature profile, especially the hybridization temperature and the length of the extension, is one of the main factors in a successful reaction. The ramp time and the number of cycles are also important variables in the cycling protocol. The thermocycler itself influences the outcome of the reaction; some function better for diagnostic applications, others for generating characteristic patterns of bands, or fingerprints. The effects of these different parameters are discussed in more detail in Appendix F.

One technique commonly used to improve the specificity of a reaction is the "hot start" method, whereby all of the reaction ingredients are prevented from interacting productively until after the first denaturation step at 94°C (D'Aquila, 1991). This prevents the formation of nonspecific products at lower temperatures, particularly primer-dimers. There are a number of ways to achieve a "hot start." The simplest method is to withold one ingredient, such as the *Taq* polymerase, from the reaction mix and add it back only when the reaction tubes are heated to 85°C; then the cycling begins with the first denaturation at 94°C. Another practice is to separate some of the ingredients (e.g., the primers) from the rest of the reaction mixture using a wax pellet, which is melted and resolidified to form an impermeable barrier between the two solutions. Then, when the amplification begins, the wax layer melts as the temperature approaches 94°C for the first denaturation, and the two solutions are mixed with each other. Several more sophisticated alternatives have been described, including the addition of anti-*Taq* antibodies, which neutralize the polymerase until the antibodies denature at 94°C, releasing an active enzyme. Similarly, AmpliTaq Gold™ is a modified enzyme, which is provided in an inactive form; a pre-PCR heat incubation (9–12 minutes at 95°C) serves to activate the polymerase for the remainder of the amplification. Yet another approach is the use of single-strand binding (SSB) proteins, which bind to the single-stranded template and prevent primers from annealing at lower temperatures and forming nonspecific products; the SSB proteins denature at 94°C and leave the template accessible.

The specificity and sensitivity of PCR can also be increased by the method of nested amplification. In this procedure, after primary amplification is performed, the product is reamplified in a second PCR using primers that hybridize within the first product. There is less chance of nonspecific amplification with this technique, since two sets of primers must recognize different regions of the template to generate the final product. Logically, the sensitivity is augmented by conducting two successive amplifications. These conditions can be modified so as to carry out both amplifications in the same tube (Wilson et al., 1993). Many other "specialty" amplifications have been described, including touchdown PCR and rapid amplification of cDNA ends (RACE) (Frohman et al., 1988). For information about these techniques, the reader is referred to more comprehensive PCR textbooks, such as Dieffenbach and Dveksler (1995), Erlich (1989, 1992), Innis et al. (1990), McPherson et al. (1991, 1995), Mullis et al. (1994), Persing et al. (1993), and White (1993).

2.2.4   Potential Problems

As with any technique, there are a variety of potential technical difficulties. A practical approach to troubleshooting PCR is provided in Appendix F. The following is a brief overview of the types of problems that may occur.

Inhibitors

Numerous compounds are known to inhibit the activity of polymerases, thereby blocking amplification. These include substances that are found in certain types of clinical samples; for example, heme in whole blood and bilirubin and bile salts in feces (Kreader, 1996). Other types of inhibitors include substances added to clinical specimens, such as the anticoagulants heparin and EDTA. Still others may be introduced during the extraction of the PCR sample. Chemicals commonly used in DNA/RNA purification are known inhibitors of PCR (e.g., guanidinium isothiocyanate, phenol, EDTA, and ionic detergents such as SDS). Of course, if the extraction is carried out properly and the purified nucleic acids are adequately washed, there should be no interference with the amplification. It is important to keep these points in mind when deciding what specimens to use, how to conserve them, and which method of sample preparation to follow.

Incomplete Extension

The amplification product may be incompletely formed due to (1) excessive distance between the two primers or insufficient extension time at 72°C; (2) degradation of the DNA or RNA template by nuclease contaminants; (3) secondary structures in the template DNA that physically block the polymerase (hairpins, cloverleafs); (4) high GC content of the template, which hinders complete denaturation of the double helix; (5) suboptimum concentration of polymerase or primers; or (6) low processivity of the polymerase.

Primer-Dimers

Primer-dimers are short products of 40–50 base pairs that are formed by hybridization of the primers to themselves and subsequent extension by the polymerase. These interfere with the reaction by consuming primers, nucleotides and *Taq* activity, and produce an unsightly band during visualization by gel electrophoresis and UV transillumination. Primer-dimers can be minimized by reducing the primer concentration and utilizing "hot start" techniques (previously mentioned), and may be reduced by conducting all operations strictly on ice when preparing the reaction.

Cross-Contamination

There are several approaches to "carryover" prevention (*see* section 3.1.2 and Appendix E). Simple methods for prevention of contamination include the following:

1. Physical separation and use of dedicated color-coded pipettors for preparation of the reaction mix ("white area"), sample (DNA/RNA) preparation ("grey area") and product analysis ("black area")

2. The use of bleach to clean work surfaces and pipettors

3. The use of small aliquots of all reagents

4. Multiple negative controls, to check for contamination at each step in every amplification.

Ideally, the color-coded areas should be physically separate rooms; if space is not available, separate areas (or laminar flow hoods) in different parts of one room should be designated for the different activities. Sophisticated and more expensive methods involve the use of aerosol-resistant pipet tips (ART tips), positive displacement pipets, and selective destruction of PCR products from previous amplifications. The selective destruction of previous PCR products can be achieved in several different ways, including (1) using the nucleotide dUTP instead of dTTP, then treating the next PCR reaction mix with uracil-N-glycosylase to destroy any contaminating uracil-containing product; (2) photochemical modification of the PCR product to make it inaccessible as a PCR template; or (3) irradiation of the new PCR reaction mix with shortwave UV light prior to sample addition.

It is critical to include a number of internal PCR controls in order to assure quality control of the reaction. These are detailed in Appendix E and include several different negative controls, inhibition controls, and positive controls.

Fidelity

One major problem with PCR amplification is the introduction of errors during the replication of the template DNA by *Taq* polymerase. The misincorporation rate of *Taq* is 1/1000 to 1/10,000 nucleotides, which is higher than human and bacterial polymerases but lower than some viral polymerases (e.g., HIV, polio). Several high-fidelity thermostable polymerases exist with lower error rates due to the presence of a 3'—>5' exonuclease proofreading activity (previously discussed). In vitro recombination (shuffling) can also occur when an incomplete product is generated, which then serves as a primer in a subsequent cycle. In general, incorporation of errors during amplification is only problematic when individual products are analyzed by cloning and sequencing. When the population of products is analyzed as a whole by gel electrophoresis, hybridization, restriction enzyme digestion, or sequencing, these errors are not detectable, since they usually only occur in a very small percentage of the product.

2.2.5   Detection of PCR Products

The most straightforward detection of PCR products involves separating the negatively charged DNA molecules in an electric field by migrating them from the negative to the positive poles through a matrix made of agarose or polyacrylamide. The smaller DNA fragments migrate faster than the larger ones, and by analyzing the products simultaneously with DNA markers of known molecular weight, the size of the PCR product(s) of interest can be easily determined. Another method involves crosslinking the product to a nylon or nitrocellulose membrane and hybridizing the captured product with labeled probes that are complementary to the amplified sequence. This procedure can be done in reverse (called reverse capture) by first attaching the complementary probe to the membrane, then hybridizing with the labeled PCR product, washing, and detecting the signal. Similar results can be obtained via solution hybridization in microtiter plates (PCR-ELISA), where the complementary probes are attached to microtiter wells, and the procedure is conducted like an ELISA. The PCR product, labeled with the plant compound digoxigenin, for example, hybridizes to its complementary probe attached to the microwell. After washing the wells, an anti-digoxigenin antibody conjugated to an enzyme (alkaline phosphatase or peroxidase) is added, followed by a colorimetric or chemiluminescent substrate for the enzyme. More complex detection methods include fluorescence quantitation (Vlieger et al., 1992) and Taq-man (Holland et al., 1991; Livak et al., 1995).

2.3   Frequently Used PCR-Based Techniques

Several PCR-based techniques have been extensively used to detect genetic polymorphism, such as small differences in sequence, variations in the distribution of repetitive elements or restriction sites, and differences in genomic organization. Small sequence variations can be detected using allele-specific oligonucleotide (ASO) hybridization, heteroduplex analysis (Delwart et al., 1993; White et al., 1992), and single-strand conformation polymorphism (SSCP) (Orita et al., 1989). Fingerprinting methods include random amplified polymorphic DNA (RAPD) (Williams et al., 1990), arbitrarily primed-polymerase chain reaction (AP-PCR) (Welsh and McClelland, 1990), amplified fragment length polymorphism (AFLP) (Vos et al., 1995), and RNA arbitrarily primed PCR (RAP-PCR) (Welsh et al., 1992). Differences in the expression pattern of messenger RNA can be detected using the powerful differential display (DD) method (Liang and Pardee, 1992). A few of the most frequently used methods are described below.

- In RAPD analysis, a single primer (usually a 10-mer) with an arbitrary sequence is used under low-stringency reaction conditions in order to amplify products from the DNA template. Upon electrophoresis, these products generate a pattern of bands that is specific for a particular strain of the organism of interest. The advantage of using a random primer is that no prior information is needed about the sequence of the targeted organism. The disadvantage is that RAPD is a finicky technique that requires that each amplification be performed under absolutely identical conditions for the results to be reproducible (*see* section 5.1.11).

- ASO hybridization is commonly used to detect specific sequences of DNA; for example, a particular mutation in a gene of interest or natural differences in haplotype loci. A small region of the gene (200–1000 base pairs) is amplified and applied to a nylon membrane, fixed to the membrane, and then hybridized with a labeled probe whose sequence is complementary to the mutated gene or particular haplotype. The probe can be labeled using radioactivity or a nonradioactive label and visualized using colorimetric or chemiluminescent detection procedures. Alternatively, DNA probes representing particular mutations or haplotypes can be fixed to the nylon membrane and then hybridized with labeled PCR product amplified from the sample to be tested. This is also known as "reverse capture" hybridization.

- Heteroduplex analysis (also known as the heteroduplex mobility assay [HMA]) is a technique that allows the detection of novel as well as previously described mutations or sequence differences. Heteroduplex analysis involves the amplification of DNA fragments (300–1000 base pairs) from a potentially polymorphic region. These fragments are denatured and immediately renatured to promote the reannealing of the strands with other amplified fragments in the mixture from the same locus, which may contain sequence differences, thus forming a heteroduplex. When the renatured fragments are electrophoresed on a polyacrylamide gel, the noncomplementary regions of the DNA fragment form gaps that cause the heteroduplex to migrate with a slower mobility in polyacrylamide gels. Mutations and variations in DNA sequence are detected by the presence of bands with altered mobility in the gel matrix.

- SSCP, or single-strand conformational analysis (SSCA), is a commonly used technique to screen for novel mutations or genetic differences. SSCP involves the amplification of small fragments from genomic DNA (200–300 base pairs), denaturation of these fragments, and renaturation prior to electrophoresis. The single-stranded DNAs form secondary structures unique to their nucleotide composition (e.g., hairpins, cloverleafs) and migrate according to their unique secondary structure. Thus, changes in the DNA sequences produce differences in secondary structure, which result in variations in mobility when electrophoresed on a polyacrylamide gel.

2.4   Applications

PCR has become a fundamental tool in many areas of the biological sciences, from clinical applications to molecular epidemiology to basic research. Each of these areas is broad in scope and can justifiably be the subject of separate books. A brief overview of some of these application follows. More detailed information can be obtained from the many PCR texts (Ehrlich and Greenberg, 1994; Erlich, 1992; Innis et al., 1990; McPherson et al., 1991, 1995; Persing et al., 1993).

PCR has been used extensively in the diagnosis and epidemiology of infectious diseases. PCR lends itself to diagnostic applications, in that the specific amplification of the DNA of a particular organism or gene is indicative of its presence in the sample material. Though the technique is very sensitive and rapid, it is not ideal for the large-scale analysis of massive numbers of samples, unless the microplate format is used. The protocols provided in this book are related to the field of infectious diseases, where PCR is used for detection of pathogens in clinical specimens, insect vectors, animal reservoirs, and enviromental samples. Essentially the same amplification technique is applied no matter what the source of the material and regardless of whether the organism is a bacterium, parasite, or virus. Since genetic information can be obtained through amplification of specific sequences, PCR can be used for strain characterization and fingerprinting as well as for finer analysis of point mutations in molecular epidemiological studies. The genetic characterization protocols presented in Part II include typing of dengue virus by RT-PCR, identification of complexes of *Leishmania* parasites, speciation of the malarial parasite *Plasmodium*, and fingerprinting individual strains of *Mycobacterium tuberculosis* and *Trypanosoma cruzi.*

PCR has also been widely applied to the diagnosis and epidemiology of genetic diseases. Genetic polymorphisms or mutations in particular sequences are often detected by sequencing PCR products, hybridizing with ASO probes, or using lower resolution methods such as SSCP, heteroduplex analysis, or denaturing gradient gel electrophoresis (DGGE) (Myers et al., 1989). With respect to cancer, PCR-based techniques have been used extensively to detect mutations in tumor suppressor-like genes such as p53, retinoblastoma (RB), and the breast cancer-associated BRCA1 and BRCA2. PCR protocols have been developed to detect chromosomal abnormalities, including the translocation of chromosomes 9 and 22 (known as the Philadelphia chromosome), which is associated with chronic myelogenous leukemia (Cross et al., 1993). PCR has also been useful for the detection of somatic mutations in oncogenes (Loda, 1994) and tumorigenic viruses, such as human T-cell leukemia viruses I and II (HTLV-I and HTLV-II). Noncancerous genetic diseases are also diagnosed using PCR-based techiques; these methods have been adapted to prenatal diagnosis as well. PCR can be used for allele characterization and identification of carriers and homozygotes of genetic diseases through detection of point mutations, insertions, and deletions in the gene of interest (e.g., cystic fibrosis, sickle cell anemia, β-thalassemia) or dinucleotide and trinucleotide repeat expansion (Huntington's disease, Fragile X, muscular dystrophy).

Another area of application of PCR has been in human genotyping and forensics. Typing of human leukocyte antigen (HLA) loci by PCR followed by oligonucleotide hybridization is used to determine appropriate matches for transplantation, analysis of disease association and risk factors, paternity testing, and genetic identification of suspects in criminal cases. PCR amplification and sequencing of the mitochondrial D loop is often used in forensic applications in human rights work involving identification of disappeared persons in individual cases or mass graves.

PCR is a cornerstone of many genome sequencing projects currently under way; these endeavors simply would not be possible without PCR-based techniques. Fundamental techniques used in genomic sequencing that are based on PCR include the generation of sequence-tagged-sites (STS) for construction of physical maps (Olson et al., 1989), the analysis of cDNA clones for the formation of expressed sequence tags (EST) (Adams et al., 1991), and genetic mapping by amplification of short tandem repeat (STR) sequences (White, 1996). These genome projects are creating enormous sequence databases that are of great use in mapping human disease genes, identifying pathogen virulence factors, and understanding the biology of a variety of organisms (Blackwell, 1997; Olson, 1995; Strauss and Falkow, 1997). Numerous genome projects that have been completed or are underway include vertebrates (human, mouse), invertebrates (*Drosophila melanogaster*), plants (rice, maize, *Arabidopsis thaliana*), yeast (*Saccharomyces cerevisiae, Candida albicans*), parasites (*Plasmodium falciparum, Leishmania major, Trypanosoma cruzi, Trypanosoma brucei, Toxoplasma gondii, Schistosoma mansoni*) and bacteria (*Escherichia coli, Mycobacterium tuberculosis, Bacillus subtilis, Haemophilus influenza, Heliobacter pylori, Chlamydia trachomatis, Neisseria gonorrhea, Vibrio cholerae*), to name a few.

There has also been extensive use of PCR methodologies in agricultural applications; for example, in the detection of agricultural pathogens (e.g., plant viruses, parasites in vegetables, and animal pathogens), screening of transgenic plants, and construction of the appropriate DNA vectors for transgenic and vaccine research.

PCR technology has been of great value in molecular studies of evolution, conservation genetics, and biodiversity. Because of its enormous sensitivity, PCR allows the amplification of minute quantities of very old or degraded DNA (Lawlor et al., 1991). This permits genetic identification of ancient remains of humans and animals for evolutionary studies as well as characterization of a large variety of living organisms from miniscule specimens (for example, DNA recovered from a bird feather or shark tooth). Construction of phylogenetic trees[7] has been greatly facilitated through amplification of genomic sequences, including mitochondrial DNA, followed by sequencing. Because of the minimal equipment requirements for conducting PCR and the portability of essential equipment, PCR has important utilization in the field. There are a number of reports of PCR conducted in unconventional locations.[8]

---

7. Evolutionary trees that display the genetic distance and ancestral relationships between organisms.

8. In one instance, to prove that a particular country was violating a ban on whaling, investigators traveled to the country and analyzed the suspected meat, bought at a local market. They conducted PCR in their hotel room and demonstrated that the meat in question was in fact from illegally hunted whales (Baker et al., 1996; Baker and Palumbi, 1994).

There are countless basic research applications of PCR, including sequence modification (introduction of restriction sites, antigenic epitopes, or promoters; site-specific or random mutagenesis; construction of chimeric genes), cloning of amplified sequences, cycle-sequencing, gene expression studies, construction of phage antibodies (Huse et al., 1989), long fragment PCR (Barnes, 1994), and in situ PCR of cells (Haase et al., 1990) and tissues (Nuovo et al., 1991) in solution or directly on slides (slide-PCR) (Yap and McGee, 1991).

It is also possible to use these amplification techniques for analysis of unknown sequences by chromosome walking, inverse PCR (using template circularization), PCR with primers complementary to repetitive DNA, or expressed sequence tags. Fingerprinting methods using repetitive sequences (IRS) or short arbitrary primers (RAPD) can generate characteristic patterns useful for distinguishing different species or individual strains. Differential display is a powerful PCR-based technique for analyzing populations of mRNA expressed in cells under different conditions (Liang and Pardee, 1992), making it possible to screen for candidate genes of interest that are involved in specific biological processes.

A number of alternative amplification techniques have been described, such as the Ligation Chain Reaction (LCR) (Wu and Wallace, 1989), Self-Sustained Sequence Replication (3SR) (Fahy et al., 1991; Guatelli et al., 1990), and Strand Displacement Amplification (SDA) (Walker et al., 1992a, 1992b), but none has been as widely used as PCR.

References

Adams, M.D., Kelley, J.M., Gocayne, J.D., Dubnick, M., Polymeropoulos, M.H., Xiao, H., Merril, C.R., Wu, A., Olde, B., Moreno, R.F., Kerlavage, A.R., McCombie, W.R., and Venter, J.C. (1991) Complementary DNA sequencing: Expressed sequence tags and human genome project. *Science*, 252:1651–1656.

Baker, C.S., Cipriano, F., and Palumbi, S.R. (1996) Molecular genetic identification of whale and dolphin products from commercial markets in Korea and Japan. *Mol. Ecol.*, 5:671–685.

Baker, C.S., and Palumbi, S.R. (1994) Which whales are hunted—A molecular genetic approach to monitoring whaling. *Science*, 265:1538–1539.

Barnes, W.M. (1994) PCR amplification of up to 35–kb with high fidelity and high yield from λ bacteriophage templates. *Proc. Natl. Acad. Sci. USA*, 91:2216–2220.

Blackwell, J.M. (1997) Parasite genome analysis. Progress in the *Leishmania* genome project. *Trans. R. Soc. Trop. Med. Hyg.*, 91:107–110.

Cohen, S.N., Chang, A.C.Y., Boyer, H.W., and Helling, R.B. (1973) Construction of biologically functional bacterial plasmids *in vitro*. *Proc. Natl. Acad. Sci. USA*, 70:3240–3244.

Cross, N.C., Feng, L., Chase, A., Bungey, J., Hughes, T.P., and Goldman, J.M. (1993) Competitive polymerase chain reaction to estimate the number of BCR-ABL transcripts in chronic myeloid leukemia patients after bone marrow transplantation. *Blood*, 82:1929–1936.

D'Aquila, R.T., Bechtel, L.J., Videler, J.A., Eron, J.J., Gorczyca, P., and Kaplan, J.C. (1991) Maximizing sensitivity and specificity of PCR by pre-amplification heating. *Nucleic Acids Res.*, 19:3479.

Delwart, E.L., Shpaer, E.G., Louwagie, J., McCutchan, F.E., Grez, M., Rubsamen-Waigmann, H., and Mullins, J.I. (1993) Genetic relationships determined by a DNA heteroduplex mobility assay: Analysis of HIV-1 env genes. *Science*, 262:1257–1261.

Dieffenbach, C.W., and Dveksler, G.S., eds. (1995) *PCR Primer: A Laboratory Manual*. New York, Cold Spring Harbor Laboratory Press.

Ehrlich, G.D., and Greenberg, S.J., eds. (1994) *PCR-Based Diagnostics in Infectious Disease.* Boston, Blackwell Scientific Publications.

Erlich, H.A., ed. (1989, 1992) *PCR Technology: Principles and Applications for DNA Amplification.* New York, Stockton Press.

Fahy, E., Kwoh, D.Y., and Gingeras, T.R. (1991) Self-sustained sequence replication (3SR): An isothermal transcription-based amplification system alternative to PCR. *PCR Meth. Appl.,* 1:25–33.

Friedman, C.R., Stoeckle, M.Y., Johnson, W.D., Jr., and Riley, L.W. (1995) Double-repetitive-element PCR method for subtyping *Mycobacterium tuberculosis* clinical isolates. *J. Clin. Microbiol.,* 33:1383–1384.

Frohman, M.A., Dush, M.K., and Martin, G.R. (1988) Rapid production of full-length cDNAs from rare transcripts: Amplification using a single gene-specific oligonucleotide primer. *Proc. Natl. Acad. Sci. USA,* 85:8998–9002.

Guatelli, J.C., Whitfield, K.M., Kwoh, D.Y., Barringer, K.J., Richman, D.D., and Gingeras, T.R. (1990) Isothermal, *in vitro* amplification of nucleic acids by a multienzyme reaction modeled after retroviral replication. *Proc. Natl. Acad. Sci. USA,* 87:1874–1878.

Haase, A.T., Retzel, E.F., and Staskus, K.A. (1990) Amplification and detection of lentiviral DNA inside cells. *Proc. Natl. Acad. Sci. USA,* 87:4971–4975.

Harris, E., López, M., Arévalo, J., Bellatin, J., Belli, A., Moran, J., and Orrego, O. (1993) Short courses on DNA detection and amplification in Central and South America: The democratization of molecular biology. *Biochem. Educ.,* 21:16–22.

Hoelzel, R. (1990) The trouble with "PCR" machines. *Trends Genet.,* 6:237–238.

Holland, P.M., Abramson, R.D., Watson, R., and Gelfand, D.H. (1991) Detection of specific polymerase chain reaction product by utilizing the $5'$—$>3'$ exonuclease activity of *Thermus aquaticus* DNA polymerase. *Proc. Natl. Acad. Sci. USA,* 88:7276–7280.

Huse, W.D., Sastry, L., Iverson, S.A., Kang, A.S., Alting-Mees, M., Burton, D.R., Benkovic, S.J., and Lerner, R.A. (1989) Generation of a large combinatorial library of the immunoglobulin repertoire in phage lambda. *Science,* 246:1275–1281.

Innis, M.A., Gelfand, D.H., Sninsky, J.J., and White, T.J., eds. (1990) *PCR Protocols: A Guide to Methods and Applications.* San Diego, California, Academic Press.

Kreader, C.A. (1996) Relief of amplification inhibition in PCR with bovine serum albumin or T4 gene 32 protein. *Appl. Environ. Microbiol.,* 62:1102–1106.

Lanciotti, R., Calisher, C., Gubler, D., Chang, G., and Vorndam, A. (1992) Rapid detection and typing of dengue viruses from clinical samples by using reverse transcriptase-polymerase chain reaction. *J. Clin. Microbiol.,* 30:545–551.

Lawlor, D.A., Dickel, C.D., Hauswirth, W.W., and Parham, P. (1991) Ancient HLA genes from 7,000–year-old archeological remains. *Nature,* 349:785–788.

Lawyer, F.C., Stoffel, S., Saiki, R.K., Myambo, K., Drummond, R., and Gelfand, D.H. (1989) Isolation, characterization, and expression in *Escherichia coli* of the DNA polymerase gene from *Thermus aquaticus*. *J. Biol. Chem.,* 264:6427–6437.

Liang, P., and Pardee, A.B. (1992) Differential display of eukaryotic messenger RNA by means of the polymerase chain reaction. *Science,* 257:967–971.

Livak, K.J., Flood, S.J., Marmaro, J., Giusti, W., and Deetz, K. (1995) Oligonucleotides with fluorescent dyes at opposite ends provide a quenched probe system useful for detecting PCR product and nucleic acidhybridization. *PCR Meth. Appl.,* 4:357–362.

Loda, M. (1994) Polymerase chain reaction-based methods for the detection of mutations in oncogenes and tumor suppressor genes. *Human Pathol.,* 25:564–571.

McPherson, M.J., Hames, B.D., and Taylor, G.R., eds. (1995) *PCR 2: A Practical Approach.* Oxford, Oxford University Press.

McPherson, M.J., Quirke, P., and Taylor, G.R., eds. (1991) *PCR: A Practical Approach.* Oxford, Oxford University Press.

Meredith, S.E., Zijlstra, E.E., Schoone, G.J., Kroon, C.C., van Eys, G.J., Schaeffer, K.U., el-Hassan, A.M., and Lawyer, P.G. (1993) Development and application of the polymerase chain reaction for the detection and identification of *Leishmania* parasites in clinical material. *Arch. Inst. Pasteur Tunis*, 70:419–431.

Mullis, K.B., Ferre, F., and Gibbs, R.A., eds. (1994) *The Polymerase Chain Reaction*. Boston, Birkhauser.

Myers, R.M., Sheffield, V.C., and Cox, D.R. (1989) Mutation detection by PCR, GC-clamps, and denaturing gradient gel electrophoresis. In *PCR Technology: Principles and Applications for DNA Amplification*, H. A. Erlich, ed., New York, Stockton Press.

Myers, T.W., and Gelfand, D.H. (1991) Reverse transcription and DNA amplification by a *Thermus thermophilus* DNA polymerase. *Biochemistry*, 30:7661–7666.

Nuovo, G.J., MacConnell, P., Forde, A., and Delvenne, P. (1991) Detection of human papillomavirus DNA in formalin-fixed tissues by *in situ* hybridization after amplification by polymerase chain reaction. *Am. J. Pathol.*, 139:847–854.

Olson, M.V. (1995) A time to sequence. *Science*, 270:394–396.

Olson, M., Hood, L., Cantor, C., and Botstein, D. (1989) A common language for physical mapping of the human genome. *Science*, 245:1434–1435.

Orita, M., Iwahana, H., Kanazawa, H., Hayashi, K., and Sekiya, T. (1989) Detection of polymorphisms of human DNA by gel electrophoresis as single-strand conformation polymorphisms. *Proc. Natl. Acad. Sci. USA*, 86:2766–2770.

Persing, D.H., Smith, T.F., Tenover, F.C., and White, T.J., eds. (1993) *Diagnostic Molecular Microbiology: Principles and Applications*. Washington DC, ASM Press.

Riley, L.W., and Harris, E. Double Repetitive Element-Polymerase Chain Reaction method for subtyping *Mycobacterium tuberculosis* strains. In *Basic Techniques in Mycobacterial and Nocardial Molecular Biology*, R. Ollar and N. Connell, eds., Philadelphia, Raven Publishers, in press.

Saiki, R.K., Bugawan, T.L., Horn, G.T., Mullis, K.B., and Erlich, H.A. (1986) Analysis of enzymatically amplified beta-globin and HLA-DQ alpha DNA with allele-specific oligonucleotide probes. *Nature*, 324:163–166.

Saiki, R.K., Gelfand, D.H., Stoffel, S., Scharf, S.J., Higuchi, R., Horn, G.T., Mullis, K.B., and Erlich, H.A. (1988) Primer-directed enzymatic amplification of DNA with a thermostable DNA polymerase. *Science*, 239:487–491.

Saiki, R., Scharf, S., Faloona, F., Mullis, K., Horn, G., Erlich, H., and Arnheim, N. (1985a) A novel method for the prenatal diagnosis of sickle cell anemia. *Am. J. Hum. Genet.*, 37:A172.

Saiki, R.K., Scharf, S., Faloona, F., B., Mullis, K., Horn, G.T., Erlich, H.A., and Arnheim, N. (1985b) Enzymatic amplification of beta-globin genomic sequences and restriction site analysis for diagnosis of sickle cell anemia. *Science*, 230:1350–1354.

Strauss, E.J., and Falkow, S. (1997) Microbial pathogenesis: Genomics and beyond. *Science*, 276:707–712.

Tibayrenc, M., Neubauer, K., Barnabe, C., Guerrini, F., Skarecky, D., and Ayala, F.J. (1993) Genetic characterization of six parasitic protozoa: Parity between random-primer DNA typing and multilocus enzyme electrophoresis. *Proc. Natl. Acad. Sci. USA*, 90:1335–1339.

Vlieger, A.M., Medenblik, A.M., van Gijlswijk, R.P., Tanke, H.J., van der Ploeg, M., Gratama, J.W., and Raap, A.K. (1992) Quantitation of polymerase chain reaction products by hybridization-based assays with fluorescent, colorimetric, or chemiluminescent detection. *Anal. Biochem.*, 205:1–7.

Vos, P., Hogers, R., Bleeker, M., Reijans, M., van de Lee, T., Hornes, M., Frijters, A., Pot, J., Peleman, J., Kuiper, M., and Zabeau, M. (1995) AFLP: A new technique for DNA fingerprinting. *Nucleic Acids Res.*, 23:4407–4414.

Walker, G.T., Fraiser, M.S., Schram, J.L., Little, M.C., Nadeau, J.G., and Malinowski, D.P. (1992a) Strand displacement amplification—An isothermal, in vitro DNA amplification technique. *Nucleic Acids Res.*, 20:1691–1696.

Walker, G.T., Little, M.C., Nadeau, J.G., and Shank, D.D. (1992b) Isothermal in vitro amplification of DNA by a restriction enzyme/DNA polymerase system. *Proc. Natl. Acad. Sci. USA*, 89:392–396.

Welsh, J., Chada, K., Dalal, S.S., Cheng, R., Ralph, D., and McClelland, M. (1992) Arbitrarily primed PCR fingerprinting of RNA. *Nucleic Acids Res.*, 20:4965–4970.

Welsh, J., and McClelland, M. (1990) Fingerprinting genomes using PCR with arbitrary primers. *Nucleic Acids. Res.*, 18:7213–7218.

White, B.A., ed. (1993) *PCR Protocols: Current Methods and Applications.* Totowa, New Jersey, Humana Press.

White, M.B., Carvalho, M., Derse, D., O'Brien, S.J., and Dean, M. (1992) Detecting single base substitutions as heteroduplex polymorphisms. *Genomics*, 12:301–306.

White, T.J. (1996) The future of PCR technology: Diversification of technology and applications. *Trends Biotechnol.*, 14:478–483.

Williams, J.G., Kubelik, A.R., Livak, K.J., Rafalski, J.A., and Tingey, S.V. (1990) DNA polymorphisms amplified by arbitrary primers are useful as genetic markers. *Nucleic Acids Res.*, 18:6531–6535.

Wilson, S., McNerney, R., Nye, P., Godfrey-Faussett, P., Stoker, N., and Voller, A. (1993) Progress toward a simplified polymerase chain reaction and its application to diagnosis of tuberculosis. *J. Clin. Microbiol.*, 31:776–782.

Wu, D.Y., and Wallace, R.B. (1989) The ligation amplification reaction (LAR)—Amplification of specific DNA sequences using sequential rounds of template-dependent ligation. *Genomics*, 4:560–569.

Yap, E.P.H., and McGee, J.O. (1991) Slide PCR: DNA amplification from cell samples on microscopic glass slides. *Nucleic Acids Res.*, 19:4294.

3

Principles of Sustainable Technology Transfer

3.1 A Low-Cost Methodology

New technologies are often perceived as too sophisticated and expensive for implementation in situations of limited resources. However, there are many ways to adapt technology to make it low-cost and more accessible. Designing or modifying equipment to suit conditions is one approach; the use of alternative, simpler techniques in place of more sophisticated, expensive ones is another. Other methods include simplification of protocols, in-house preparation of reagents, recycling, and appropriate use of donated materials. Each of these will be discussed in detail below. Adapting equipment, streamlining protocols, and recycling materials not only make new technologies economically feasible and environmentally friendlier but also create a more sustainable base for their long-term implementation.

3.1.1 Appropriate Technology

Technology can be made appropriate by constructing equipment whenever possible or redesigning equipment to suit existing conditions. One creative example is the policy used by a laboratory at the Universidad Mayor de San Andrés in La Paz, Bolivia,[1] that every investigator and thesis student should construct a piece of laboratory equipment using available resources. The innovations that have resulted from this practice incude a horizontal shaker constructed from a stereo turntable, a centrifuge made from a blender, a wooden incubator with heat provided by light bulbs, a photography station for agarose gels assembled from old Polaroid camera equipment, a transilluminator of ultraviolet light constructed out of a wooden crate, and an apparatus for washing pipet tips made from a plastic jar and a rubber disk (Figure 3.1). Descriptive details and photographs of these devices are presented in Appendix A. To cite another example, because running water is only available intermittently

---

1. N. Mamani and R. Sanchez, personal communication.

in the laboratories in Nicaragua, a donated distilling apparatus was redesigned to use recirculating water for the cooling system so as not to depend on running water for this purpose.[2] A portable rapid thermal cycler can be constructed to achieve the repeated cycling of temperatures that is required for the polymerase chain reaction; the instrument is heated by a light bulb and the system is cooled by a fan.[3] An economical homemade version of a power supply, which provides sufficient fixed voltage to carry out DNA electrophoresis, was described by Kadokami et al. (1984) and can be easily constructed. Likewise, the gel boxes and trays in which the gel electrophoresis is conducted can also be assembled in-house (*see* Appendix A). Naturally, when designing appropriate equipment, the building materials that are available on-site must be taken into consideration.

Since many countries experience rationing of electrical power and frequent power outages, simple methods to store energy are extremely useful. In Pilcopata, Perú, where there is electrical power only 3–4 hours a day, local scientists have installed giant batteries to collect energy when it is available; this stored energy is

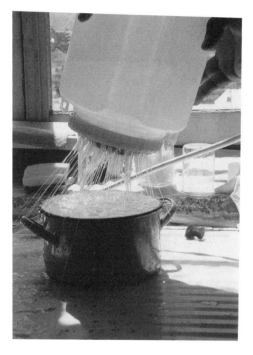

Fig. 3.1. Recycling pipet tips using an apparatus designed for rinsing tips treated with bleach and detergent.

---

2. J. F. Kennedy and E. Harris, unpublished results.
3. M. López, personal communication.

then used to sustain laboratory and computer facilities throughout the day as needed.[4] In Nicaragua, where there are frequent power outages, an emergency generator is kept nearby when procedures requiring electricity are executed (e.g., PCR amplification using a thermocycler).

When it is not possible to design or construct equipment, and when one is able to purchase a piece of equipment, it is important to evaluate what features are most relevant to the prevailing conditions. For instance, in choosing a thermocycler, one critical feature to keep in mind is power failure protection, which ensures that program execution restarts automatically after power interruptions. The newest machines on the market are not necessarily the most appropriate; for example, 0.2-mL tubes are currently popular because many samples can be processed simultaneously due to the small size of the tubes. However, this introduces a dependence on potentially inaccessible materials; namely, the custom-sized 0.2-mL tubes, which are approximately five times more expensive than standard 0.5-mL tubes and much more difficult to obtain. Another important aspect is the number of samples that will be routinely processed; some thermocyclers may be conveniently small and lightweight, but may accommodate too few reaction tubes. Alternatively, other machines may seem attractive because of their large capacity; however, upon analysis, it may turn out that users will rarely, if ever, need to process the maximum number of reactions possible.

Naturally, cost is a primary consideration, especially given the substantial import taxes often levied on imported equipment. The price of thermocyclers varies widely; some smaller, lightweight thermocyclers are about half the price of the sturdier models. The durability of the instrument and ease of maintenance are clearly important aspects as well. Many machines will be used in locations where a service visit by the company's maintenance representative is impossible. Thus, it is essential to conduct a thorough inquiry as to the machine's durability by interviewing other users. Equally critical is the choice of an instrument with simple maintenance features (e.g., intelligible error reports, accessible fuses). Ease of programming is another factor to consider.

Variations among thermocyclers with respect to certain parameters, especially ramp time, tube size, and thermal transfer, produce substantially different results, even when identical protocols are used. Some thermocyclers with faster ramp times have been optimized for diagnostic applications, where high sensitivity is the primary objective. However, these instruments are not optimal for PCR fingerprinting, where a number of amplicons need to be generated to produce a characteristic pattern (fingerprint) for each strain. Thermocyclers with slower ramp times produce a greater number of fragments and thus are better suited for fingerprinting applications. Many thermocyclers allow ramp time to be set by the user; thus, this parameter can be adjusted to optimize performance.

In summarizing the criteria for evaluating a thermocycler, the following features should be considered: power failure protection, tube size (0.5 mL vs. 0.2 mL), number of samples, weight (portability), instrument size (footprint), cost, durability,

---

4. M. López, personal communication.

ease of maintanance, access to technical support, ease of progamming, rapidity (ramp time), and sensitivity.

3.1.2 Alternative Techniques

Alternative means for executing experimental procedures can be implemented so as to obviate the need for inaccessible equipment. For instance, as described in chapter 2, PCR amplification is based on a series of 25–40 cycles, each of which consists of three different temperatures. Currently, most laboratories use thermocyclers to carry out the cycling process. Plastic tubes containing the reaction ingredients are placed in a metal block and the cycling parameters are programmed into the thermocycler's computer. The metal block is then brought to the specified temperatures for the indicated periods the required number of times. However, without access to thermocyclers, PCR can still be carried out successfully in a low-tech, low-cost environment using manual cycling. Water baths, or simply hot plates with beakers of water, are set to the appropriate temperatures, and then the PCR reaction tubes are moved from one bath (temperature) to another the specified number of times in accordance with the cycling protocol (Figure 3.2).

Estimating the concentration of nucleic acids in a solution is a fundamental procedure in molecular biology and is often achieved using a costly ultraviolet (UV) light spectrophotometer (usually several thousand dollars). A "quick and dirty" alternative technique can be accomplished by comparing a series of dilutions of the solution of

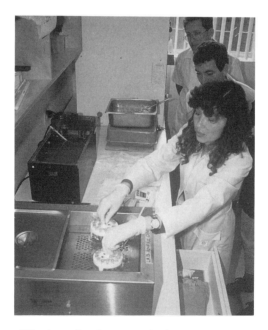

Fig. 3.2. Manual amplification using three water baths set at the appropriate temperatures.

interest with that of a control solution containing a known amount of DNA or RNA. Ethidium bromide is added to the solutions to label the nucleic acids, and 10-microliter drops of each dilution of the control and the unknown solutions are spotted on a UV-transparent plastic dish and examined using a UV transilluminator. The fluorescent intensity of the unknown solution is matched to that of the control, and the concentration of the nucleic acid in the unknown solution is thereby estimated.

DNA probe hybridization techniques often call for a step in which the DNA to be analyzed is physically crosslinked to the solid support (usually a nylon or nitrocellulose membrane). This procedure can be accomplished by either baking the membrane at 80°C in a vacuum oven or by exposing the DNA on the membrane to ultraviolet (UV) light of the appropriate wavelength. A special oven for UV-crosslinking is commercially available; however, without access to this costly equipment, the procedure can be conducted by exposing the membrane (DNA facedown) to ultraviolet light from the same UV transilluminator used to visualize ethidium bromide-stained DNA fragments in agarose gels after electrophoresis. The required time of exposure can be calculated using standard formulas.

Another example of a low-budget alternative technique involves preparation of DNA samples for electrophoretic analysis. In the usual procedure, an aliquot of each sample is mixed with sample loading dye in a separate tube in preparation for application to the gel. Instead of using separate tubes, a simple stage can be constructed for each set of samples to be analyzed (Figure 3.3). A plastic microcentrifuge tube rack is covered with a piece of Parafilm®.[5] Shallow wells are then made

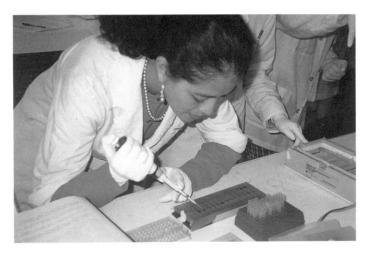

Fig. 3.3. Using a stage constructed from a microcentrifuge tube rack covered with Parafilm® for preparing PCR products for gel loading.

---

5. A wax-like film commonly used for sealing laboratory materials.

and these wells are then labeled with a permanent marker. The samples to be analyzed (e.g., PCR products, restriction digests) are then transferred to the wells in the appropriate order and mixed with sample loading buffer before application to the gel. Thus, a single sheet of Parafilm replaces many disposable plastic tubes. This practice can result in significant savings given the large number of samples routinely analyzed by gel electrophoresis in molecular biology laboratories.

Crushed ice is an important resource for molecular biology laboratories, since many reagents must be kept cold to ensure their integrity. However, large-scale, expensive ice machines are often not available. Instead, plastic bags of water can be frozen and the contents converted into chipped ice using hammers, hand-held ice crushers (Figure 3.4), or small electrical household ice machines.

The use of simple alternatives to more sophisticated techniques is particularly useful for keeping costs down in the prevention of PCR cross-contamination. Since PCR is so sensitive that theoretically as little as one molecule of DNA can be amplified to detectable levels, one danger of the technique is the potential for false-positive results due to the cross-contamination of one sample with another DNA sample or with product from a previous amplification. Modern laboratories and biotechnology companies have devised sophisticated and expensive methods to

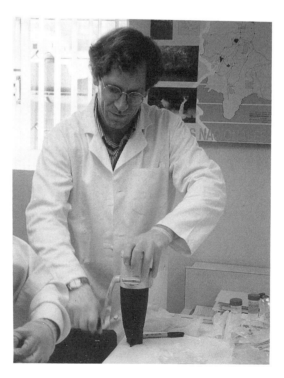

Fig. 3.4. Using a hand-held ice crusher to prepare ice for the day's experiments.

prevent this "carryover" problem. Some of these methods rely on physical prevention of cross-contamination. A common procedure is to use aerosol-resistant pipet tips; each plastic tip contains a cotton plug that prevents molecules of DNA from entering the shaft of the pipettor and then contaminating another reaction. While effective, these tips are tenfold more expensive than regular pipet tips and are not recyclable. Another similar technique involves positive-displacement pipets, where the lower part of the pipet shaft is replaced with each tip. Naturally, these tips are also much more costly than standard pipet tips.

Sophisticated biochemical procedures comprise another approach to carryover prevention. In one method, the PCR amplification is conducted with the deoxynucleotide dUTP instead of dTTP, along with the other three deoxynucleotides dATP, dCTP, and dGTP. The DNA products from this PCR can be used for gel electrophoresis, hybridization analysis, or cloning, even though they contain uracil instead of thymidine. However, this difference can be exploited to specifically destroy the products of a previous amplification before beginning the next PCR. The enzyme uracil N-glycosylase (UNG) is added to the PCR reaction mixture; if there is any contaminating, uracil-containing product from a previous reaction, the UNG will remove the uracil base from the sugar-phosphate backbone, but will not touch the thymidine-containing DNA template of the current reaction. Heating the reaction to 50°C causes the damaged DNA to be cleaved at the abasic sites (in this case, the uracil site); thus destroying the contaminating product. The heat-labile UNG is then destroyed during the first 94°C step of the amplification. While this is a clever manipulation, it involves the use of more molecular biology reagents, which are both expensive and difficult to obtain.

However, there are other, simpler approaches to minimize the risk of cross-contamination, as detailed below. These methods have been implemented effectively in a number of settings, during training courses and in molecular diagnostic laboratories.

- Physical separation of different activities: one isolated area for preparation of the PCR reaction (designated "white"), one for preparation of the sample DNA and addition of the samples to the PCR reaction tubes (designated "grey"), and one for amplifying and analyzing the PCR product (designated "black"). As mentioned in chapter 2, it is preferable to use separate rooms for each color-coded area designated for a different activity. If space is unavailable for this, then separate areas—ideally, different laminar flow hoods—must be dedicated for each activity. This minimizes the chance that the amplified product from one sample can contaminate another reaction before it undergoes the amplification procedure, since the product is analyzed in a different place from where the reactions are set up.

- The use of dedicated sets of pipettors for preparation of the PCR reaction ("white"), manipulation of the sample DNA ("grey"), and analysis of the amplified product ("black"). Designated gloves, racks, pipet tips, tubes, ice buckets, and so forth must also be dedicated to each work area.

- The use of diluted household bleach (1.5% sodium hypochlorite final concentration) to clean instruments and work areas. Bleach destroys the strands of DNA so that they are no longer amplifiable. This common reagent can be used to treat work area surfaces daily and to periodically soak pipettor shafts, followed by thorough rinsing in distilled water (Figure 3.5). Pipettors can also be cleaned between sample manipulation during DNA preparation or between sample addition to PCR reactions. This is done by tamping the tip of the shaft of the pipettor on a paper towel soaked in bleach and then drying it carefully on a second clean paper towel.

- Exposure of pipettors to ultraviolet light for 15 minutes prior to use. UV light destroys DNA; thus, this procedure further reduces the risk of DNA cross-contamination.

- Strict adherence to the rigorous laboratory practices previously described.

- Inclusion of multiple negative controls in each experiment in order to immediately detect any cross-contamination should it occur.

- Use of reagents in small aliquots. If any contamination is detected, all affected solutions can immediately be disposed of without causing excessive loss of expensive reagents.

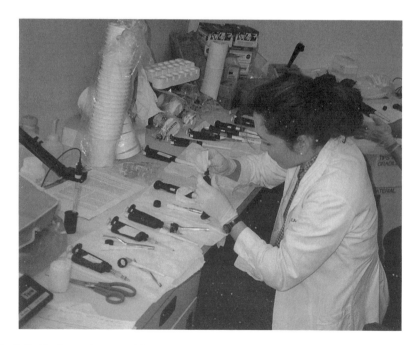

Fig. 3.5. Drying and reassembling pipettor shafts after cleaning with bleach and rinsing.

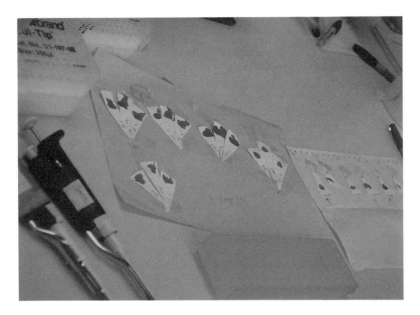

Fig. 3.6. Collection of dried blood spots on filter paper for PCR diagnosis of malaria.

3.1.3 Simplification of Protocols

Often, the experimental protocols themselves can be simplified in order to avoid expensive and complicated steps. Each procedure can be analyzed to determine whether there are simpler ways to achieve a given objective. For example, the PCR analysis of clinical samples involves several operations: specimen collection, DNA/RNA extraction, amplification, and product detection. Each step should be scrutinized and streamlined for improvements to better suit the conditions, as detailed below.

Specimen Collection/Preparation

Specimens can be collected in ways that enhance their stability. For instance, whole blood can be stably transported at ambient temperature when stored dry on filter paper (Figure 3.6). Or, one volume of whole blood can be mixed with an equal volume of guanidine hydrochloride lysis buffer and maintained at ambient temperature for over 1 month. Other types of clinical specimens can be placed in transport medium containing 5% Chelex® 100, which binds magnesium. This increases the stability of DNA and protects it from degradation.[6]

6. Chelex® 100 is an anionic (negatively charged) resin that chelates (binds) positively charged magnesium ions (Walsh et al., 1991). Magnesium ions are required for activity of enzymes that degrade DNA (nucleases); thus, in its absence, nucleases are inactive and DNA is protected. In addition, Chelex 100 chelates positively charged heavy metals (e.g., nickel, cobalt, lead) that can cleave DNA at high temperatures, e.g., while boiling the specimen during the extraction procedure.

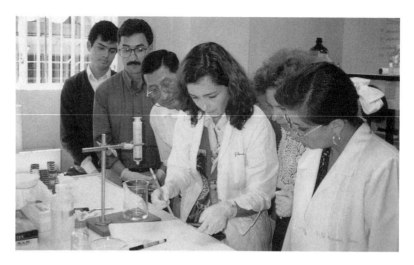

Fig. 3.7. Concentration of bacteria in water samples by syringe filtration prior to preparation of cell lysates for PCR.

In certain situations, there is an additional step during sample preparation prior to nucleic acid extraction. For example, bacteria in environmental water samples must be concentrated before amplification can be conducted. Centrifugation of large volumes of water is one method, but not all laboratories are equipped with a sufficiently large centrifuge. In this case, the bacteria can be concentrated by using the barrel of a large plastic syringe to hold the sample (60 mL) and the plunger to force the water through a small filter attached to the syringe (Figure 3.7). The filter traps the organisms, which are too large to pass through the microscopic pores. Manual pressure can be used to force the water through the filter; if a vaccum pump is available, it can also be used for this purpose. The filter is then subjected to freeze/thaw lysis or a more elaborate DNA extraction procedure and used directly for PCR amplification of genes specific to different pathogenic bacteria, such as *Vibrio cholerae.*[7]

Nucleic Acid Preparation

The underlying principles for the extraction of nucleic acids are (1) the release of DNA and RNA from the organism; (2) separation of the nucleic acids from proteins, lipids, carbohydrates, and cellular debris; (3) the prevention of DNA or RNA degradation (preservation); (4) the removal of inhibitors of the amplification reaction; and (5) the concentration of nucleic acids. As shown in Table 3.1, extraction protocols employ different methods to accomplish these objectives and result in variable levels of nucleic acid purity. Usually, the more elaborate the purification, the cleaner the resulting DNA or RNA, and the higher the sensitivity of the subsequent amplification.

7. E. Harris, unpublished results.

Table 3.1. Nucleic Acid Extraction Methods

	Extraction Method		
Principle	Crude Extraction	Silica Particles	Standard DNA Extraction
Release of nucleic acids	Boiling; freeze/thaw lysis	Lysis buffer (GITC)	Lysis buffer (GITC); NaOH/detergent
Separation of nucleic acids	Not applicable	Silica particles	Protein ppt., organic extraction
Preservation of DNA/RNA	Chelex® 100; freezing; addition of nuclease inhibitors	Freezing	Organic extraction (removal of nucleases)
Removal of inhibitors	Sample dilution	Silica particles	Ethanol precipitation
Level of purity	Crude lysate	High purity	High purity

Crude lysates can be obtained by the use of the following: detergents to rupture cellular membranes, proteases to destroy nucleases, chloroform to destroy cell membranes and proteins, chelating resins to bind magnesium and thereby inactivate nucleases, boiling or autoclaving to lyse the cell and thereby liberate the DNA, or direct extraction, in which the first 94°C incubation of the PCR reaction is sufficient to break open the cells and make the DNA available for amplification. Highly purified nucleic acids can be obtained by using standard organic extraction/ethanol precipitation protocols or silica particles to isolate the DNA/RNA.

While many published protocols call for extensive purification of DNA from samples prior to PCR amplification, it is often possible to substitute a simple procedure that ruptures the cells and releases the DNA. One example is simply boiling the samples or subjecting them to freeze/thaw lysis, which involves repeated cycles of freezing in dry ice or liquid nitrogen and then thawing in a warm water bath. Crude extracts can then be stored in 5% Chelex® 100 until further use (Belli et al., 1998; Walsh et al., 1991).

When high-purity nucleic acids are required, more complex protocols that call for organic extractions and ethanol precipitation can be replaced by a simple procedure using silica particles. These tiny glass particles selectively bind to nucleic acids because of their charged property and can be used to rapidly purify DNA or RNA directly from crude lysis mixtures. For more basic molecular biology applications, this is a method of choice for preparing DNA fragments for cloning. The glass beads can be prepared in the laboratory at low cost (*see* Appendix B).

Amplification

The PCR amplification procedure itself can also be simplified. When the target nucleic acid is RNA, it must first be converted into complementary DNA (cDNA) by the enzyme reverse transcriptase (RT) before subsequent amplification. These two steps can be combined in a single tube to reduce the number of manipulations and the risk of cross-contamination, as in the RT-PCR typing of dengue virus (Harris et al., 1998b; Lanciotti et al., 1992) The same approach can also be used with nested PCR, where one product is amplified and then used as the template for a second amplification. It is possible to design the primers and amplification protocol so as to conduct both amplifications in the same reaction tube, as in the detection of *Mycobacterium tuberculosis* (Wilson et al., 1993) A number of primers can be combined in one tube in what is called a multiplex PCR so as to obtain the maximum amount of genetic information possible in one step (Belli et al., 1998; Harris et al., 1998a, 1998b; Mahoney et al., 1995; Tirasophon et al., 1994, 1995). Many of the protocols presented in chapter 5 are multiplex PCR procedures.

Detection

Once amplification is complete, the products must be detected and visualized. There are many ways to achieve this objective, from simple gel electrophoresis to more complicated product-capture techniques using hybridization strategies or labeled primers coupled with colorimetric or chemiluminescent detection systems. For use in situations of limited resources, the most straightforward and reliable method is simply agarose gel electrophoresis and visualization of ethidium bromide-stained DNA with UV transillumination. The advantage of this method is that it provides information not only about the presence or absence of the expected fragment but also about the size of the product.

One interesting detection technique involves the use of fluorescently-labeled primers in a multiplex PCR reaction, which results in products of different colors when illuminated with ultraviolet light[8] (Embury et al., 1990). The PCR products can be electrophoresed to yield differently colored bands; alternatively, the products can be separated from the rest of the PCR reaction mixture using a homemade centrifugation filter (spin column). The resin used to make the spin column captures the excess primers, allowing only amplified product to pass through. The resulting solution containing purified product can then be observed directly by simply exposing the tube to UV light. The fluorescent color of the solution indicates the product type without the need for electrophoretic analysis.

3.1.4   In-House Preparation of Reagents

Many reagent mixtures and solutions can be prepared in-house instead of purchasing them pre-mixed in commercial kits at higher cost. PCR buffers, magnesium chloride, nucleotide mixtures, and other PCR reagents can be easily prepared. One note of caution, however, is that it is critical to use water of acceptable quality to avoid inhibition of amplification reactions. Likewise, all buffers required for gel electrophoresis can be made in-house to lower operating costs. Recipes for these stock solutions and electrophoresis buffers are provided in Appendix B.

---

8. E. Harris and G. Kropp, unpublished results.

Certain chemicals can be purchased in their crude form and purified in the laboratory instead of buying their more expensive pre-purified versions. One example is glycogen, used as a carrier for nucleic acids during ethanol precipitation. The DNA standards used as size markers on agarose gels can be prepared at lower cost by carrying out restriction digests of stock DNA in the laboratory instead of purchasing pre-made markers. When reagents are purchased, it is more economical to purchase in bulk by combining orders with other laboratories, if possible, or to buy a large stock at once, provided that reliable storage facilities are available.

Some commonly-used materials can also be homemade. For instance, the silica particles used for purifying DNA and RNA can be prepared from powdered flint glass obtained in bulk from ceramic stores (Appendix B). Wax "gems," used to increase specificity in so-called "hot start" PCR (section 2.2.3), can be made by melting wax or Parafilm® and measuring out equal volumes to generate identical wax pellets.

3.1.5   Recycling

Recycling is an extremely important element, not only for economic reasons but also for the integrity of the environment. Much of the plastic- and glassware that are disposed of in more affluent laboratories can be carefully washed and re-used. Plastic tubes, bottles, and pipet tips can be recycled, as long as the decontamination and cleaning procedure is adequate. To recycle plasticware, wash thoroughly with detergent, soak in 1.5% hypochlorite (bleach) for at least 30 minutes, rinse extensively with tap water, and perform a final rinse with distilled water. One essential rule that must be observed is that when pipet tips or tubes are recycled, material from the "white" area (PCR reaction preparation) must be recycled for use in the "white" or "grey" (DNA sample preparation) areas only, while "grey" and "black" (PCR product analysis) area material must be recyled for use in the "black" area only. During certain procedures, gloves can also be reused multiple times; simply labeling them with one's name and the work area is sufficient. Gloves that originate in the "white" area can be used subsequently in the "grey" and then "black" areas but *never* in the opposite direction (Figure 3.8).

When a number of the preceding practices are put into effect, the net result is a more sustainable operation in which resources last much longer. For example, weigh boats used routinely for the same purpose (e.g., weighing agarose) can be labeled and dedicated to that one application instead of using a new weigh boat each time. Agarose gels can be melted down and re-used to pour new gels (3–5 times); since agarose is an expensive reagent, this practice can cut costs considerably. When spatulas are not available, small pieces of aluminum foil can be used instead. There are many more examples of cost-cutting measures.

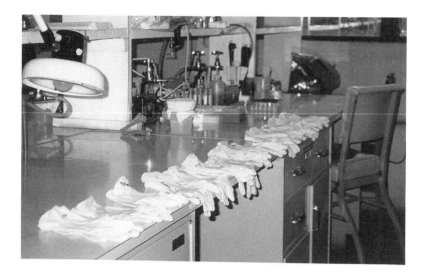

Fig. 3.8. Recycling gloves that have been labeled with workshop participants' name and designated work area color.

3.1.6　Donated Materials

In the developed countries, large amounts of perfectly functional equipment and materials are discarded in high-tech fields such as molecular biology due to rapid obsolescence. One economically attractive and environmentally sound approach to equipping a laboratory involves the collection and shipment of donated materials from more-developed countries to be distributed among colleagues in less-developed countries. This "redistribution" can also be instituted within developed countries, from research laboratories to educational facilities, such as high schools or colleges. It is important to view material aid collection and donation as the re-utilization of high-quality material to fulfill a specific need of the end-user, not simply as a way for laboratories to get rid of old or unused equipment. An essential feature of such programs is that the materials donated must be previously requested by the users, or at least the list of available materials must be reviewed by the end-users, who then choose the particular items of interest to their institution. All equipment must be pretested to ensure optimal working order. Instruction manuals must accompany donated equipment, and workshops in equipment maintenance are strongly suggested.

3.2　Knowledge-Based Participatory Transfer Process

In order to achieve sustainable transfer of knowledge, attention must be given to the transfer process itself. A responsible, equitable, participatory, and knowledge-based approach is essential for a successful outcome. Respect for diverse cultures is a key component as well. It is important that all participants (instructors and course attendees alike) view the undertaking as a serious commitment rather than as a transient event. The objective is to create an ambience of reciprocal exchange, where all participants are considered equal and learn from each other. For the transfer to be fully participatory, it should be a dynamic and creative process in which everyone plays a central role, from the conception of a project to its design, from the planning stages to its execution. While these concepts have been derived from experience in international workshops as part of the AMB/ATT Program (*see* chapter 4), they apply to any situation where there is transfer of knowledge, including high school and college classrooms, community education forums, and international development projects. A number of these principles have also been described in the discussion of community-based action research (Stringer, 1996).

Another fundamental aspect of a successful transfer is that a thorough understanding of the principles underlying the technology be transmitted along with the technology itself in order for a reasonable degree of independence to be achieved. For example, it is important to explain not only the identity and molarity of the ingredients of every solution but also the chemical environment they create and the biochemical reactions they affect. Likewise, it is necessary to describe the mechanical processes performed by the different instruments, so that if a piece of equipment breaks, it can be fixed or another device can be substituted to carry out a similar procedure. Ideally, local scientists should obtain the requisite knowledge to be able to troubleshoot technical problems on-site without depending on outside experts.

While the initial knowledge transfer is often rapid and can be accomplished to a certain extent in an intensive training workshop, the implementation process is gradual and requires sustained long-term follow-up. Appropriate follow-through requires a commitment on the part of the technology "donor" to serve as a resource for scientific consultations, technical guidance, relevant bibliographical information, and often, materials and reagents. Specifically, it is critical that instructors imparting a new technology be willing to serve as long-term advisors, answering technical questions and assisting in the troubleshooting process when necessary by means of electronic mail, fax, or telephone, if not in person. The importance of adequate follow-up cannot be overstated—it is too often ignored, resulting in the failure of many technology transfer efforts.

Clearly, for any concept or technology to take hold, it must be appropriated by individuals who will implement it as their own and be integrated into their work from their perspective. Examples abound where the implementation of new technology died with the departure of its purveyors. The initiative must come from the recipients for the technology to catch on. Thus, it is important to create the opportunity for the recipients of the technology to determine how the technique should be used and to what end. Naturally, this process includes advice from experts in a given field to help shape ideas into a viable project, but the technology should not be presented as a preconceived package transplanted in a top-down hierarchical manner. Finally, it is important to include a positive human element; a professional approach is necessary, but the process can be fun as well (Figure 3.9).

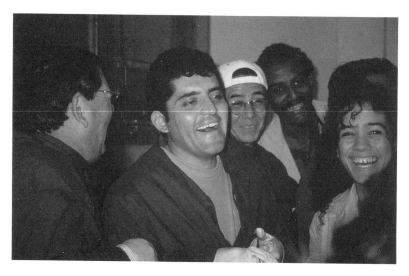

Fig. 3.9. Workshop partipants in the laboratory during an international course.

The AMB/ATT Program described in chapter 4 serves as an example of a successful ongoing knowledge-based technology transfer program that is sustainable and transferable to other locations.

3.3   Appropriate Application

A critical element in the transfer and implementation of any new technology is its appropriate application. The term as used here denotes the judicious assessment of the utility of a given technique with respect to the local conditions and the specific function that the technique is expected to fulfill. This process requires a careful evaluation of the advantages and limitations of the technique in relation to its proposed application. The following section discusses general considerations that influence the successful implementation of a new technology. Next, a general framework for evaluating a new technique is provided and then applied to the analysis of PCR to generate specific assessment criteria. Finally, the application of PCR to several diseases is explored in order to provide examples of the evaluation process.

3.3.1   General Considerations

The most obvious assessment of a new technology is at the technical level; however, many other types of analysis are needed as well. The ability to successfully implement a new technology depends on the convergence of a number of key factors, including economic, political, infrastructural, communication, sociocultural, biological, and environmental concerns, in addition to the immediate technical issues.

These key factors are outlined in Table 3.2, along with examples of specific considerations that fall within each category. Although these factors are likely to be beyond the direct control of the investigator, their existence should be recognized and taken into account.

One of the main obstacles often encountered in implementing a new technology is the lack of adequate infrastructure to support communications, utilities, transportation, information, and public health. Clearly, long-term comprehensive solutions must be sought to increase development capabilities. However, a number of these constraints are easier to overcome on a smaller scale in the immediate term. Some examples of solutions include sharing computers for access to electronic mail, using hand-held radios for domestic communication, storing enough water to last through periods when running water is unavailable, planning experiments carefully around scheduled power outages, maintaining an emergency generator at hand, and setting up simple power storage systems.

Table 3.2. Key Factors in the Appropriate Application of New Techniques

Key Factors	Considerations/Examples
Technical	Does the new technique confer advantage(s) over existing techniques?
	Can the new technique be modified for optimum utility?
	Can technical problems be adequately resolved?
Economic	Is the new technique cost-effective?
	Is there funding for the project?
	Does this funding provide adequate salaries for the investigators?
Political	Is there governmental support of public health and scientific research?
	Is the particular research in question a priority of the government?
	Will the government act on the recommendations made as a result of research/epidemiological studies?
	Will a change in government result in the termination of research activities?
Infrastructural	Is there adequate access to clean water, running water, electricity, computers, transportation, libraries, etc.?
	Can reagents/equipment be imported without prohibitive tariffs and with timely customs clearance?
	Will imported equipment malfunction at prevailing ambient temperatures?
	Can sterile conditions be maintained?
Communication	Is there access to email, the Internet, telephone, and fax?
	Is there communication/contact with other scientists inside and outside the country or are scientists intellectually isolated?
Sociocultural	Do the prevailing work ethics and practices support the introduction of new technology?
	Are there career opportunities and incentives for scientists?
Biological	Does the life cycle of the pathogen of interest permit effective intervention in a timely manner?
Environmental concerns	Can potentially hazardous waste be adequately disposed of?
	Can appropriate biological containment practices be observed/enforced?

3.3.2   An Evaluation Framework

To illustrate the concept of appropriate application, a framework for evaluation is presented below. Again, this a general framework that should be applied to every new technique under consideration.

General Evaluation Framework for a New Technique

1. Identify the local and/or national public health concerns that must be addressed.

2. Prioritize available resources.

3. Determine what clinical or scientific information is desired and what function the new technique should fulfill.

4. Identify the advantages and limitations of existing technologies.

5. Compare these advantages and disadvantages with those of the new technique.

6. Conduct a cost-benefit analysis of the new technique.

7. Investigate the feasibility of obtaining equipment and reagents for the new technique.

8. Determine whether these same equipment and reagents can be used for other purposes.

9. Evaluate how the wasteful/hazardous aspects of the new technique can be minimized.

10. Conduct a thorough literature search to determine which published protocol is best suited for the purpose at hand and how published procedures can be simplified, modified, and adapted to the present circumstances.

11. Explore access to experts in the field who can be contacted for advice on applicability of the technique.

12. Determine how technical problems are to be adequately resolved.

13. Conduct an impartial assessment of the performance of the new technique once it has been implemented.

The first step for the investigator is to define the goal in using a given technique: what information is desired; what specific function should the technique fulfill; how should it be used? For example, PCR is a technique that can be used to obtain routine diagnostic results, epidemiologic information, data for research studies, or as a molecular biological tool to answer basic research questions. At times it may be possible to "kill two birds with one stone", in other words, to obtain diagnostic results that contain useful epidemiological information. But it is critical for the investigator to understand the advantages and disadvantages of the technique with respect to the desired function and information required. Likewise, a comparison of the limitations of existing techniques with those of the new technique is necessary. This step may appear obvious, but there is often a tendency to want to implement a new technique, such as PCR, simply because it is new, modern, "sophisticated," and trendy, without having a clear picture of why the new technique is necessary, if at all, and without a complete understanding of its limitations.

Setting priorities for disease management is important in the case of infectious diseases. The overall public health needs have to be kept in mind in order to avoid getting overly caught up in the technical details of detecting or typing a particular organism. For example, although PCR detection of *M. tuberculosis* may be more rapid, sensitive, and specific than other assays, is increased diagnostic capability really the most critical factor? Where there is competition for resources, it may be that a more effective use of resources is ensuring that those positively diagnosed by conventional methods are successfully treated. However, if resources for clinical treatment and public health control measures are allocated separately from those targeted for diagnostic procedures, and there is no competition for these resources, then achieving optimal diagnostic capability is desirable. Or, it may be that state-of-the-art diagnostic methods are reserved for certain situations. For example, rapid diagnosis of tuberculosis is critical in HIV-infected individuals, and PCR diagnosis is, therefore, particularly useful in such cases. PCR also provides an important capability to distinguish *M. tuberculosis* from other mycobacteria on a genetic basis.

Throughout the process, the investigator has to maintain the ability to objectively judge the utility of a particular technique and not become so vested in its implementation as to bias the assessment of its usefulness or performance. Deciding that a technique is not working for a particular application does not mean that it must be abandoned; instead, it can be used to examine a different problem (*see* tuberculosis example in section 3.3.4).

As experience with a given technique accumulates internationally, problems may appear that were not evident at first, and useful modifications may be reported. It is therefore essential to stay current with the literature through Medline and other electronic databases that provide access to listings of recent publications and abstracts. In addition, many journals are appearing "on-line," and this will increase in the near future (*see* Appendix I). If local libraries do not carry all the relevant journals, copies of articles can be requested by post or electronic mail from contacts in other countries with access to well-stocked libraries.

3.3.3   Assessment Criteria for PCR

The following section illustrates how the foregoing general evaluation framework is applied to the specific analysis of PCR and provides assessment criteria for deciding when to use this technique and for what purposes and when not to use it.

Specific Evaluation Framework for the Use of PCR in Infectious Diseases

1. Determine whether the proposed application of PCR adequately and appropriately addresses the public health and clinical needs of the community in which it will be applied.

2. Set priorities for resource distribution in disease management and control.

3. Determine what information is needed (identification of organisms at the genus, species, or strain level) and what function PCR should fulfill (diagnostic, epidemiologic, or research tool).

4. Identify the advantages and limitations of existing technologies. How rapid, sensitive, and specific are existing methods for pathogen identification and characterization? Which of these qualities are critical? For example, microscopy for detection of *Leishmania* is simple but insensitive and cannot be used for speciation. Culture of *M. tuberculosis* is sensitive and specific but requires 3–6 weeks to process and is compromised by microbial contamination. Serological screening for dengue virus infection using ELISA is fairly inexpensive and allows high throughput, but it is not serotype-specific and cannot detect the pathogen during the first week of illness (the acute phase).

5. Does PCR offer advantage(s) over existing methods? Returning to the examples above, PCR of *Leishmania* is very sensitive and permits simultaneous detection and genetic characterization of the parasite. Under controlled conditions, PCR detection of *M. tuberculosis* can achieve similar levels of sensitivity and specificity as culture, requires only a single day for sample processing, and avoids the problem of microbial contamination. RT-PCR detection of dengue virus can be conducted at low cost and can be used to identify dengue serotypes immediately in viremic samples from acute cases. With respect to genetic information, can data obtained during diagnosis be epidemiologically useful? Are strain identification and molecular fingerprinting useful for studies of transmission patterns and/or risk factors?

6. Is PCR cost-effective? Can in-house preparation of reagents, recycling, etc., reduce the cost of PCR to below that of conventional techniques?

7. Can equipment and reagents for PCR be obtained? What contacts are available with companies and/or with individuals in developed countries who could facilitate the acquisition of necessary equipment and reagents (e.g., *Taq* polymerase) at reasonable cost and time? How can the shipments be efficiently cleared by customs?

8. Since equipment and reagents associated with PCR can be used for multiple purposes, with what other departments in the investigator's institution (university/ministry/hospital) can this technology be shared?

9. How can potentially wasteful or hazardous aspects of the PCR methodology be minimized?

10. Review all of the published PCR protocols for identification and/or typing of the organism of interest by conducting a thorough literature search. Compare the sensitivity, specificity, and simplicity of the various reports. Which assays have been validated in similar circumstances and/or with samples that will be used in the intended application? Which protocols appear to be most easily

reproducible in the given environment? Are certain reagents/equipment already available? Is there local experience with a similar protocol or enzyme?

11. Contact experts in the field for opinions on applicability of PCR to the particular situation. Can they offer advice regarding technical details or experimental design? Is PCR the recommended technique to answer the questions being posed? Is the use of one particular protocol more valuable than others?

12. Can technical problems be adequately resolved?

13. Using objective criteria for evaluation, is PCR sufficiently robust in actual performance to meet the requirements?

3.3.4   Examples of PCR Applied to the Study of Infectious Diseases

Four illustrations are given below of the advantages and disadvantages of PCR applied to the diagnosis and epidemiology of infectious diseases: tuberculosis, malaria, dengue fever, and leishmaniasis. A comprehensive background of each disease is provided in chapter 5.

Tuberculosis

The routine diagnostic assay for verification of tuberculosis (TB) as recommended by WHO is acid-fast bacilli (AFB) smears, which typically range in sensitivity from 30–70% when compared with mycobacterial culture. Using this microscopic method, it is difficult to distinguish *M. tuberculosis* from other Ziehl-Neelsen-positive bacilli. Culture of the bacteria is still preferred as the reference method or "gold standard," but results usually take between 3 and 6 weeks because of the slow growth of the organism. PCR presents an alternative technique that is more rapid than culture (PCR is a one-day procedure), more sensitive than AFB smears, and more specific, in that it allows identification of the species of *Mycobacterium* present in the sample. However, considerable variability has been reported in lab-to-lab reproducibility (Noordhoek et al., 1994; Noordhoek et al., 1996). Overall, the data suggest that PCR is highly sensitive in correctly diagnosing smear-positive cases, but is less sensitive (50–70%) in detecting smear-negative, culture-positive cases. While it is possible to conduct low-cost PCR diagnosis of TB, most commercial kits are extremely expensive, and as currently used, do not replace the conventional tests.

From a public health perspective, the most important issue in reducing transmission of the disease is identifying and treating AFB smear-positive cases, who are coughing up the greatest number of organisms. In rural clinics or poorly equipped public hospitals, the critical objective is to immediately identify active TB cases and begin treatment. In this situation, AFB smears conducted rapidly on-site are recommended over PCR, which would have to be processed at a reference laboratory. However, PCR may be an appropriate diagnostic technique in certain situations in which it is important to diagnose TB cases quickly when it is critical for patient management, such as in HIV$^+$ patients, or where the use of PCR is affordable, such as in private clinics in large cities.

DNA-based techniques can also be used for fingerprinting strains for epidemiological purposes. The standard approach to molecular fingerprinting of *M. tuberculosis* is by repetitive element (IS*6110*)-based restriction fragment length polymorphism (RFLP) (Van Embden et al., 1993). However, a number of simple PCR-based methods have been described recently that can type *M. tuberculosis* isolates by generating patterns of amplified fragments unique to each strain, as reviewed in Suffys et al. (1997). One such technique, double repetitive element (DRE)-PCR (Friedman et al., 1995a) can rapidly and correctly characterize approximately 70% of the RFLP-typed strains; the remaining 30%, which generate too few bands for a definitive identification, can then be analyzed by RFLP (Riley and Harris, in press). A number of important epidemiological questions can be addressed using DRE-PCR. One example is the analysis of strain clustering, which can lead to identification of strains of *M. tuberculosis* with unique biological characteristics (drug resistance, increased virulence) and consequently focus public health efforts on heightened surveillance and control of these strains. Another application is the analysis of transmission patterns in various communities, including hospitals, prisons, and urban centers (Ferreira et al., 1996; Friedman et al., 1995b; Lin et al., 1996; Sepkowitz et al., 1995), which enables the identification of risk factors that can then be the target of intervention and control measures.

Malaria

The diagnosis of malaria is traditionally accomplished by thick smear microscopy. This method is still useful, cheap, low-tech, and relatively sensitive. However, it is only effective when performed by well-trained microscopists spending 15–30 minutes per slide; accuracy can therefore vary considerably from site to site. Nonetheless, for diagnosis of individual cases, the thick smear is still adequate. Since PCR does not achieve much greater sensitivity than thick smear microscopy, there is no reason to replace the thick smear for individual diagnosis.

There are certain applications, however, in which PCR is particularly useful. PCR is advantageous in that it does not require an expert microscopist, and it provides more standardized results. While it is technically possible to morphologically distinguish *Plasmodium* species, this requires substantial expertise; as a result, species misidentification can occur and large proportions of mixed infections can be overlooked. PCR can genetically distinguish the different *Plasmodium* species and has been shown to be very effective in identifying mixed infections (Brown et al., 1992; Harris et al., 1996; Oliveira et al., 1996; Snounou et al., 1993). Thus, one useful application of PCR is in the quality control of routine diagnosis of malaria by microscopy. PCR tests can be used to monitor the effect of treatment on parasite numbers as well (Kain et al., 1993; Kain et al., 1994; Sethabutr et al., 1992).[9] PCR

---

9. For example, PCR was used to amplify parasites from thick smears that had been stored for several years at the Ifaka Centre in Tanzania (Edoh et al., 1997) in order to investigate the clearance of parasites after treatment with sulphadoxine-pyrimethamine (D. Edoh, N. Hurt, M. Burger, personal communication).

assays can also be used for screening known drug resistance genotypes when specific mutations are found to be associated with resistance to a particular drug (Eldin de Pecoulas et al., 1995a, 1995b; Plowe et al., 1995; Wang et al., 1995). Important information about genetic polymorphisms within *Plasmodium* species can be obtained using PCR; this is useful for assessing the extent of genetic variability and for mapping the global distribution of variants (Kain et al., 1991), understanding the population dynamics of the parasite within a single host (Contamin et al., 1996; Kain and Lanar, 1991), and distinguishing treatment failure from reinfection (Kain et al., 1996). Lastly, PCR can be used for detection of *Plasmodium* in the *Anopheles* mosquito vector (Bouare et al., 1996; Schriefer et al., 1991; Stoffels et al., 1995; Tassanakajon et al., 1993).

Dengue Fever

In the case of dengue fever, the situation is different, and nucleic acid-based techniques offer a clear advantage. Classic dengue fever and dengue hemorrhagic fever are caused by four serotypes of dengue virus. The current reference method for typing dengue involves isolation of the virus in cultured cells followed by typing using indirect immunofluorescence. It is a time-consuming and expensive technique for routine use and requires cell culture facilities, which are often unavailable in laboratories in developing countries. The most rapid serological techniques, such as IgM-ELISA, do not furnish information about the serotype of the virus. Other serological methods that allow typing are lengthy and can be hampered by antibody cross-reactivity between the serotypes. Single-step RT-PCR detection and typing of dengue virus offers a sensitive, specific, rapid, and low-cost alternative that requires only one acute-phase serum sample. In addition to providing useful serotype information for epidemiological purposes, this early diagnosis allows for the possibility of mounting a rapid-response effort aimed at mosquito control measures in the affected areas. In addition, it is possible to screen for the presence of dengue virus in its mosquito vector, which increases the possibility of enhancing preparedness and pre-empting epidemics.

Leishmaniasis

Similarly, simultaneous detection and strain characterization of the *Leishmania* parasite by PCR in clinical samples, cultured isolates, and the sandfly vector is extremely useful for both clinical and epidemiological purposes. In the Americas, symptoms of leishmaniasis range from self-curing cutaneous lesions (*L. mexicana* complex), to disfiguring and persistent mucocutaneous manifestations (*L. braziliensis* complex), to the potentially fatal visceral disease (*L. chagasi*). Current diagnostic methods are far from adequate: microscopic examination of dermal scrapings yield low sensitivity (45–50%); culture is time-consuming, with a fairly low sensitivity (65–70%) and high risk of contamination; the Montenegro test is adequately sensitive but does not discriminate between a past or current infection; and animal inoculation is costly and time-consuming. Techniques for species identification, such as isoenzyme analysis, require large amounts of cultured parasites and are difficult to perform, especially under conditions of limited resources. Species characterization using monoclonal antibodies is complicated by antigenic variation of *Leishmania* in distinct geographical areas. PCR is a sensitive and rapid technique that can be adapted for low-cost routine application (Belli et al., 1998; Harris et al., 1996). Important genetic information can be obtained from the same procedure used for detection of the parasite. Another advantage is that less-invasive clinical samples are suitable for PCR diagnosis because of the high sensitivity of the assay.

3.4 Intraregional Cooperation

The establishment of intraregional cooperation is extremely important in the sustainable transfer of a new technology. The most relevant information for one country considering the implementation of a new technology is the experience of a neighboring country faced with a similar situation. International workshops can serve as a nexus for forming regional contacts, partnerships, and networks. Such venues provide an opportunity for sharing experiences and technical tips, forming potential collaborations, establishing communication, and planning follow-up courses and conferences. It is possible that a colleague in a neighboring country with experience in implementing a given technology can serve as a project consultant. International organizations that promote and facilitate regional collaborations and sponsor international workshops can play an important role; several of these that focus on Latin America are listed below.[10]

Another key element is the promotion of regional expertise and regional sourcing when possible. There are many centers of excellence in less-developed countries, which should be given priority as reference centers, consulting resources, and quality-control monitors. Likewise, when available, equipment and materials should be obtained from commercial enterprises in developing countries in an effort to support intraregional trading links. Collaborations with the more-developed countries are useful for additional technology transfer, scientific guidance, and resource accessibility.

References

Belli, A., Rodriguez, B., Avilés, H., and Harris, E. (1998) Simplified PCR detection of New World *Leishmania* from clinical specimens. *Am. J. Trop. Med. Hyg.* 58:102–109.

Bouare, M., Sangare, D., Bagayoko, M., Toure, A., Toure, Y.T., and Vernick, K.D. (1996) Short report: Simultaneous detection by polymerase chain reaction of mosquito species and *Plasmodium falciparum* infection in *Anopheles gambiae* sensu lato. *Am. J. Trop. Med. Hyg.*, 54:629–631.

---

10. Programa de las Naciones Unidas para el Desarrollo (PNUD); Pan American Health Organization (PAHO); Programa Iberoamericano de Ciencia y Tecnología para el Desarrollo (Cyted); Programa Regional de Biotecnología PNUD/UNESCO/ONUDI para America Latina; Red Regional de Intercambio de Investigadores para el Desarrollo de America Latina y el Caribe (RIDALC).

Brown, A.E., Kain, K.C., Pipithkul, J., and Webster, H.K. (1992) Demonstration by the polymerase chain reaction of mixed *Plasmodium falciparum* and *P. vivax* infections undetected by conventional microscopy. *Trans. R. Soc. Trop. Med. Hyg.*, 86:609–612.

Contamin, H., Fandeur, T., Rogier, C., Bonnefoy, S., Konate, L., Trape, J.F., and Mercereau-Puijalon, O. (1996) Different genetic characteristics of *Plasmodium falciparum* isolates collected during successive clinical malaria episodes in Senegalese children. *Am. J. Trop. Med. Hyg.*, 54:632–643.

Edoh, D., Steiger, S., Genton, B., and Beck, H.P. (1997) PCR amplification of DNA from malaria parasites on fixed and stained thick and thin blood films. *Trans. R. Soc. Trop. Med. Hyg.*, 91:361–363.

Eldin de Pecoulas, P., Abdallah, B., Dje, M.K., Basco, L.K., le Bras, J., and Mazabraud, A. (1995a) Use of a semi-nested PCR diagnosis test to evaluate antifolate resistance of *Plasmodium falciparum* isolates. *Mol. Cell. Probes*, 9:391–397.

Eldin de Pecoulas, P., Basco, L.K., Abdallah, B., Dje, M.K., Le Bras, J., and Mazabraud, A. (1995b) *Plasmodium falciparum*: detection of antifolate resistance by mutation-specific restriction enzyme digestion. *Exp. Parasitol.*, 80:483–487.

Embury, S. H., G. L. Kropp, Warren, T. C., Cornett, P. A., and Chehab, F. F. (1990) Detection of the hemoglobin E mutation using the color complementation assay: Application to complex genotyping. *Blood* 76:619–623.

Ferreira, M.M., Ferrazoli, L., Palaci, M., Salles, P.S., Medeiros, L.A., Novoa, P., Kiefer, C.R., Schechtmann, M., Kritski, A.L., Johnson, W.D., Riley, L.W., and Ferreira, O.C., Jr. (1996) Tuberculosis and HIV infection among female inmates in Sao Paulo, Brazil: A prospective cohort study. *J. AIDS Human Retrovirol.*, 13:177–183.

Friedman, C.R., Stoeckle, M.Y., Johnson, W.D., Jr., and Riley, L.W. (1995a) Double-repetitive-element PCR method for subtyping *Mycobacterium tuberculosis* clinical isolates. *J. Clin. Microbiol.*, 33:1383–1384.

Friedman, C.R., Stoeckle, M.Y., Kreiswirth, B.N., Johnson, W.D., Jr., Manoach, S.M., Berger, J., Sathianathan, K., Hafner, A., and Riley, L.W. (1995b) Transmission of multidrug-resistant tuberculosis in a large urban setting. *Am. J. Resp. Crit. Care Med.*, 152:355–359.

Harris, E., Belli, A., and Agabian, N. (1996) Appropriate transfer of molecular technology to Latin America for public health and biomedical sciences. *Biochem. Educ.*, 24:3–12.

Harris, E., Kropp, G., Belli, A., Rodriguez, B., and Agabian, N. (1998a) A single-step multiplex PCR assay for characterization of New World *Leishmania* complexes. *J. Clin. Microbiol.* 36:1989–1995.

Harris, E., Roberts, T.G., Smith, L., Selle, J., Kramer, L.D., Sandoval, E., Valle, S., and Balmaseda, A. (1998b) Typing of dengue viruses in clinical specimens and mosquitoes by single-tube multiplex reverse transcriptase-PCR. *J. Clin. Microbiol.* 36:2634–2639.

Kadokami, Y., Takao, K., and Saigo, K. (1984) An economic power supply using a diode for agarose and polyacrylamide gel electrophoresis. *Anal. Biochem.*, 137:156–160.

Kain, K.C., Brown, A.E., Lanar, D.E., Ballou, W.R., and Webster, H.K. (1993) Response of *Plasmodium vivax* variants to chloroquine as determined by microscopy and quantitative polymerase chain reaction. *Am. J. Trop. Med. Hyg.*, 49:478–484.

Kain, K.C., Craig, A.A., and Ohrt, C. (1996) Single-strand conformational polymorphism analysis differentiates *Plasmodium falciparum* treatment failures from re-infections. *Mol. Biochem. Parasitol.*, 79:167–175.

Kain, K.C., Keystone, J., Franke, E.D., and Lanar, D.E. (1991) Global distribution of a variant of the circumsporozoite gene of *Plasmodium vivax*. *J. Infect. Dis.*, 164:208–210.

Kain, K.C., Kyle, D.E., Wongsrichanalai, C., Brown, A.E., Webster, H.K., Vanijanonta, S., and Looareesuwan, S. (1994) Qualitative and semiquantitative polymerase chain reaction to predict *Plasmodium falciparum* treatment failure. *J. Infect. Dis.*, 170:1626–1630.

Kain, K.C., and Lanar, D.E. (1991) Determination of genetic variation within *Plasmodium falciparum* by using enzymatically amplified DNA from filter paper disks impregnated with whole blood. *J. Clin. Microbiol.*, 29:1171–1174.

Lanciotti, R., Calisher, C., Gubler, D., Chang, G., and Vorndam, A. (1992) Rapid detection and typing of dengue viruses from clinical samples by using reverse transcriptase-polymerase chain reaction. *J. Clin. Microbiol.*, 30:545–551.

Lin, R.-L., Bernard, E.M., Armstrong, D., Chen, C.-H., and Riley, L.W. (1996) Transmission patterns of tuberculosis in Taiwan: Analysis by restriction fragment length polymorphism. *Int. J. Infect. Dis.*, 1:18–21.

Mahoney, J.B., Luinstra, K.E., Tyndall, M., Sellors, J.W., Krepel, J., and Chernesky, M. (1995) Multiplex PCR for detection of *Chlamydia trachomatis* and *Neisseria gonorrheoae* in genitourinary specimens. *J. Clin. Microbiol.*, 33:3049–3053.

Noordhoek, G.T., Kolk, A.H., Bjune, G., Catty, D., Dale, J.W., Fine, P.E., Godfrey-Faussett, P., Cho, S.N., Shinnick, T., Svenson, S.B., Wilson, S., and van Embden, J.D.A. (1994) Sensitivity and specificity of PCR for detection of *Mycobacterium tuberculosis*: A blind comparison study among seven laboratories. *J. Clin. Microbiol.*, 32:277–284.

Noordhoek, G.T., van Embden, J.D., and Kolk, A.H. (1996) Reliability of nucleic acid amplification for detection of *Mycobacterium tuberculosis*: An international collaborative quality control study among 30 laboratories. *J. Clin. Microbiol.*, 34:2522–2525.

Oliveira, D.A., Shi, Y.P., Oloo, A.J., Boriga, D.A., Nahlen, B.L., Hawley, W.A., Holloway, B.P., and Lal, A.A. (1996) Field evaluation of a polymerase chain reaction-based nonisotopic liquid hybridization assay for malaria diagnosis. *J. Infect. Dis.*, 173:1284–1287.

Plowe, C.V., Djimde, A., Bouare, M., Doumbo, O., and Wellems, T.E. (1995) Pyrimethamine and proguanil resistance-conferring mutations in *Plasmodium falciparum* dihydrofolate reductase: Polymerase chain reaction methods for surveillance in Africa. *Am. J. Trop. Med. Hyg.*, 52:565–568.

Riley, L.W., and Harris, E. Double repetitive element-polymerase chain reaction method for subtyping *Mycobacterium tuberculosis* strains. In *Basic Techniques in Mycobacterial and Nocardial Molecular Biology*, R. Ollar and N. Connell, eds., Philadelphia, Raven Publishers, in press.

Schriefer, M.E., Sacci, J.B., Jr., Wirtz, R.A., and Azad, A.F. (1991) Detection of polymerase chain reaction-amplified malarial DNA in infected blood and individual mosquitoes. *Exp. Parasitol.*, 73:311–316.

Sepkowitz, K.A., Friedman, C.R., Hafner, A., Kwok, D., Manoach, S., Floris, M., Martinez, D., Sathianathan, K., Brown, E., Berger, J.J., Segal-Maurer, S., Kreiswirth, B., Riley, L.W., and Stoeckle, M.Y. (1995) Tuberculosis among urban health care workers: A study using restriction length polymorphism typing. *Clin. Infect. Dis.*, 21:1098–1102.

Sethabutr, O., Brown, A.E., Panyim, S., Kain, K.C., Webster, H.K., and Echeverria, P. (1992) Detection of *Plasmodium falciparum* by polymerase chain reaction in a field study. *J. Infect. Dis.*, 166:145–148.

Snounou, G., Viriyakosol, S., Jarra, W., Thaithong, S., and Brown, K.N. (1993) Identification of the four human malaria parasite species in field samples by the polymerase chain reaction and detection of a high prevalence of mixed infections. *Mol. Biochem. Parasitol.*, 58:283–292.

Stoffels, J.A., Docters van Leeuwen, W.M., and Post, R.J. (1995) Detection of *Plasmodium* sporozoites in mosquitoes by polymerase chain reaction and oligonucleotide rDNA probe, without dissection of the salivary glands. *Med. Vet. Entomol.*, 9:433–437.

Stringer, E.T. (1996) *Action Research: A Handbook for Practitioners.* London, Sage Publications.

Suffys, P.N., de Araujo, M.E.I., and Degrave, W.M. (1997) The changing face of the epidemiology of tuberculosis due to molecular strain typing-A review. *Mem. Inst. Oswaldo Cruz*, 92:297–316.

Tassanakajon, A., Boonsaeng, V., Wilairat, P., and Panyim, S. (1993) Polymerase chain reaction detection of *Plasmodium falciparum* in mosquitoes. *Trans. R. Soc. Trop. Med. Hyg.*, 87:273–275.

Tirasophon, W., Rajkulchai, P., Ponglikitmongkol, M., Wilairat, P., Boonsaeng, V., and Panyim, S. (1994) A highly sensitive, rapid, and simple polymerase chain reaction-based method to detect human malaria (*Plasmodium falciparum* and *Plasmodium vivax*) in blood samples. *Am. J. Trop. Med. Hyg.*, 51:308–313.

Tornieporth, N.G., John, J., Salgado, K., de Jesus, P., Latham, E., Melo, M.C., Gunzburg, T., S., and Riley, L.W. (1995) Differentiation of pathogenic *Escherichia coli* strains in Brazilian children by PCR. *J. Clin. Microbiol.*, 33:1371–1374.

Van Embden, J.D., Cave, M.D., Crawford, J.T., Dale, J.W., Eisenach, K.D., Gicquel, B., Hermans, P., Martin, C., McAdam, R., Shinnick, T.M., and Small, P.M. (1993) Strain identification of *Mycobacterium tuberculosis* by DNA fingerprinting: recommendations for a standardized methodology. *J. Clin. Microbiol.*, 31:406–409.

Walsh, P.S., Metzger, D.A., and Higushi, R. (1991) Chelex 100 as a medium for simple extraction of DNA for PCR-based typing from forensic material. *BioTechniques*, 10:506–513.

Wang, P., Brooks, D.R., Sims, P.F., and Hyde, J.E. (1995) A mutation-specific PCR system to detect sequence variation in the dihydropteroate synthetase gene of *Plasmodium falciparum*. *Mol. Biochem. Parasitol.*, 71:115–125.

Wilson, S., McNerney, R., Nye, P., Godfrey-Faussett, P., Stoker, N., and Voller, A. (1993) Progress toward a simplified polymerase chain reaction and its application to diagnosis of tuberculosis. *J. Clin. Microbiol.*, 31:776–782.

4

Case Study: The AMB/ATT Program

4.1   Introduction

The Applied Molecular Biology/Appropriate Technology Transfer (AMB/ATT) Program presented in this chapter is an example of the approach outlined previously. Much of the information contained in this book was gained from experience while developing this progam over the past ten years. The following chapter describes this technology transfer approach in practice and summarizes the resulting projects and their impact.

4.2   Program Description

4.2.1   Objectives

The overall goal of the AMB/ATT Program is to effect the appropriate transfer of molecular biological techniques to developing countries for use in public health and biomedical sciences. The objectives are (1) to *introduce* appropriate molecular techniques for diagnosis, environmental surveillance, and epidemiology of infectious diseases prevalent in the host country; (2) to oversee the *application* of these techniques in molecular diagnostic and epidemiological studies; and (3) to foster the continued *implementation* of molecular biology to address relevant public health and biomedical objectives.

The program consists of a series of hands-on workshops conducted in less-developed countries with the following specific aims:

- To present molecular biological approaches in a manner that enables local investigators to employ the techniques themselves.

- To conduct the workshops on-site to adapt the techniques to available resources.

- To stage the courses in local institutions in order to establish routine use and resident expertise in molecular biological techniques for both the applied and basic research objectives of each host country.

- To provide theoretical and practical knowledge to a broad range of scientists and health providers in each country and to disseminate knowledge and expertise as widely as possible. The goal is to create a national base for the use of molecular biological techniques and to abrogate the trend of reserving advanced scientific training for isolated cases or for the socioeconomically privileged. In addition, this approach aims to minimize the emigration of scientists from the country of origin (brain drain) and to develop a format for their long-term participation in country-specific activities.

- To design the courses to reflect local interest in specific uses of molecular biological techniques and to emphasize local participation, in keeping with the principles of sustainable transfer of appropriate technology.

- To provide training throughout the program, not only in the implementation of new technologies but also in the design of research strategies and the development of funding applications.

- To limit the role of the outside instructors to the training of local scientists, subsequent consulting on appropriate applications, and professional collaborations.

4.2.2   Format

Workshops, including lectures, laboratory sessions, and course materials, are conducted in the language of each host country. The courses are participatory in nature and serve as a vehicle for the transfer of molecular biology tools to local scientists and physicians; often many of these participants have never worked with DNA prior to the first workshop. A low-cost, do-it-yourself approach to implementing the techniques is stressed, with an emphasis on having a solid understanding of the procedures and reagents. Simple, effective methods are taught to avoid sample cross-contamination problems, and innovative solutions are sought to overcome the material constraints when resources are limited. Participants are provided with training not only in molecular biology techniques but also in good laboratory practices and in the scientific method. They are taught how to organize and equip a PCR laboratory and solve technical problems as well as formulate research questions and design projects.

The sustainability of the AMB/ATT Program derives in part from its three-phase structure. Progressively more complex courses are incorporated into Phases I, II, and III, from the introduction of molecular biological techniques to their implementation by local scientists. The techniques are introduced in Phase I. Phase II facilitates the application of the techniques to health problems identified by local scientists and provides assistance in developing funding applications; in addition, long-term projects are defined and important professional contacts established. Phase III supports the sustained implementation of these techniques by assisting in the design of additional projects and preparation of scientific manuscripts and funding applications. Ongoing communication and consulting as well as collaborations between laboratories (intraregional and international) ensure the continued application of molecular biology techniques to health problems and scientific research in each host country.

Long-term support is provided through the creation of networks of communication and shared resources at the national, regional, and international levels. An international network of instructors, participants, and consultants acts as a continuous resource for the resolution of technical problems, advice on study design and development, and assistance in the preparation of grant applications. The inclusion of instructors from the host country and from countries in the region also helps to build and sustain these networks. Local scientists are trained to teach new courses, to supervise the routine use of PCR in local institutions, and to maintain quality control. Instructional materials are produced to aid in this process, including a manual containing laboratory protocols (in the relevant language), a current bibliography, and audio/visual aids (e.g., slides and overheads).

To date, the flexible format of these workshops has been applied successfully in a number of countries and under different constraints. Table 4.1 lists the countries in which Phase I AMB/ATT workshops have been executed and the pathogens selected for these courses. International courses modeled on the AMB/ATT format are shown in Table 4.3. The AMB/ATT Program has generated interest among scientists in both developing and developed countries as well as among the general public (Barinaga, 1994). The program was initiated in Latin America, and scientists from other regions of the world, including Africa, Southeast Asia, India, and the Middle East continue to inquire about the possibility of setting up similar programs. The information compiled in this book should facilitate such efforts.

4.3   Program Structure

The key concept behind the AMB/ATT Program is the continuity of the scientific and educational process as a whole. This process can be broken down into its component parts, including introduction to molecular biology techniques, evaluation of

Table 4.1. Phase I AMB/ATT Workshops to Date

Course Title	Country/Date	No. Partic. Institutions*	Pathogens Detected
First Nicaraguan Applied Biotechnology Workshop	Nicaragua June 1991	7	Human D-loop, *Leishmania*
Second Nicaraguan Molecular Diagnostics Workshop	Nicaragua July 1992	7	*M. tuberculosis, Vibrio cholerae, P. falciparum, Shigella,* Enterotoxigenic *E. coli*
First Ecuadorian Applied Molecular Biology Workshop	Ecuador April 1994	14	*M. tuberculosis, Vibrio cholerae,* Dengue virus
Transfer of Molecular Technology for the Diagnosis and Epidemiology of Infectious Diseases of Great Importance in Bolivia	Bolivia June 1998	7	*Leishmania, M. tuberculosis, Trypanosoma cruzi*

*Within each institution, several departments were represented.

local public health needs, design of a pilot study, sample collection and processing, and pilot study analysis. This is followed by design of a larger project, proposal development, preparation and submission of funding applications, execution of the larger study, data analysis, preparation and submission of final reports and scientific manuscripts, and application of the results to address public health needs. In order to devise a comprehensive and workable strategy to incorporate these various elements into a series of workshops, they were divided into three general phases (I-III) as shown in the Flowchart (Figure 4.1). These phases should be considered as part of a flexible framework for facilitating the sustainable transfer of relevant knowledge and technology. Within this framework, each group defines its own pace. Representative photographs of the workshops are shown in Figures 4.2–4.7.

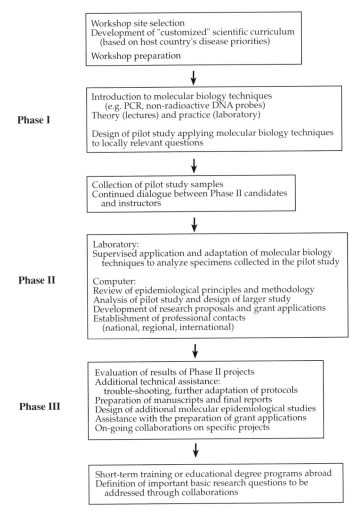

Fig. 4.1. Flowchart of the progression of the AMB/ATT Program (Phases I-III).

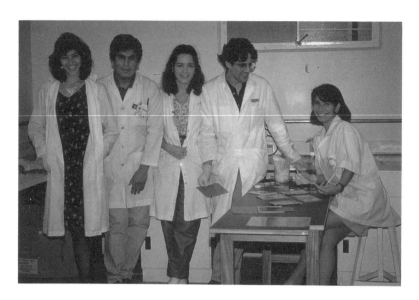

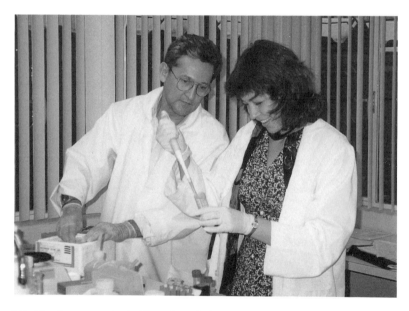

Fig. 4.2. *Top*, instructors in the Phase I workshop in Ecuador, from left to right: Eva Harris (U.S.), Wilson Paredes (Ecuador); Josefina Coloma (Ecuador); Alejandro Belli (Nicaragua); and Eugenia Rojas (Costa Rica). *Bottom*, the author preparing samples for amplification in the Phase I Ecuador workshop with course participant Dr. Luis Enrique Plaza.

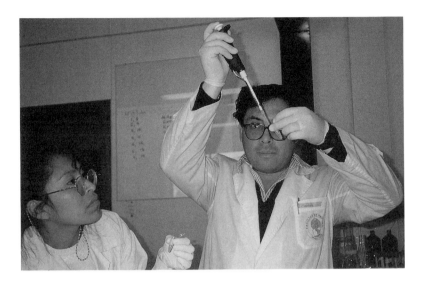

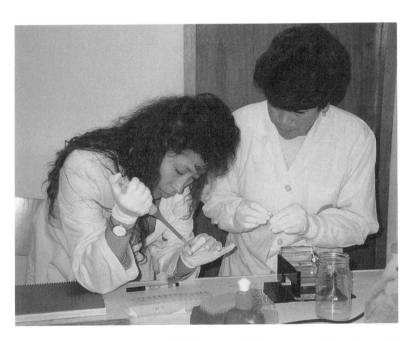

Fig. 4.3. *Top*, participants extracting DNA prior to PCR during the Phase I workshop in Bolivia. *Bottom*, participants preparing PCR products for application to agarose gels.

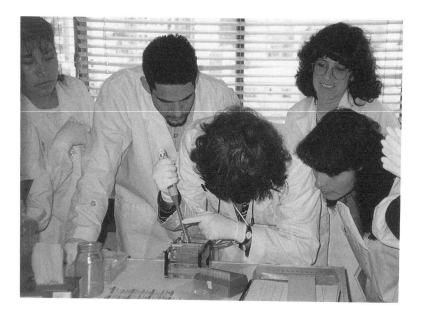

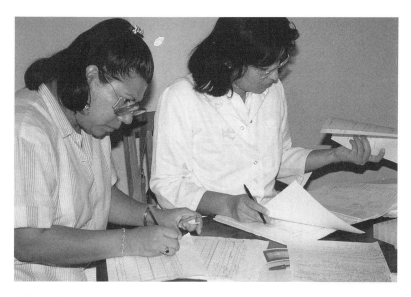

Fig. 4.4. *Top*, instructor Alejandro Belli supervising the application of PCR products to agarose gels for electrophoresis. *Bottom*, participants in the 1992 workshop in Nicaragua analyzing the results of gel electrophoresis.

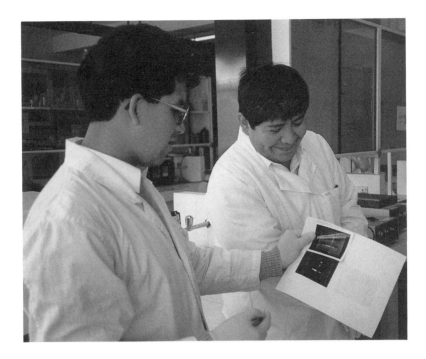

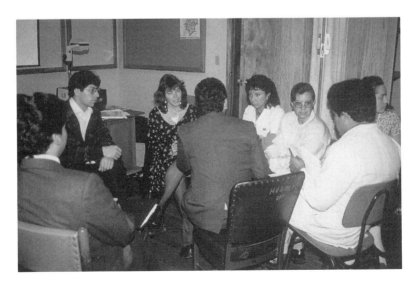

Fig. 4.5. *Top*, instructor Giovanni Garcia and course participant Nataniel Mamani discussing data during the Phase I course in Bolivia. *Bottom*, group discussion at the end of the Phase I Ecuadorian workshop with participants proposing a pilot study on tuberculosis for the Phase II workshop.

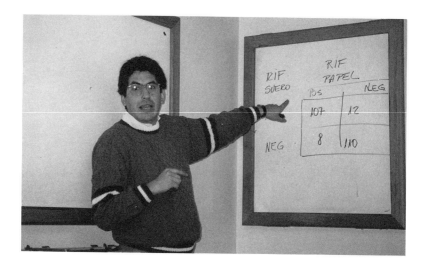

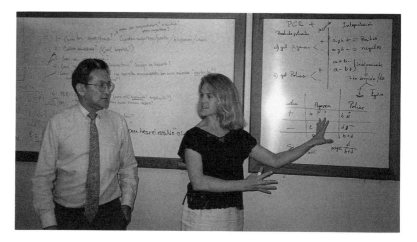

Fig. 4.6. *Top*, Ecuadorian professor Marcelo Aguilar giving a lecture on calculating the sensitivity and specificity of a diagnostic test during the Phase II workshop. *Bottom*, course instructor Elinor Fanning discussing study design with a Phase II team during the second week of the workshop in Ecuador (shown here with one member of the team).

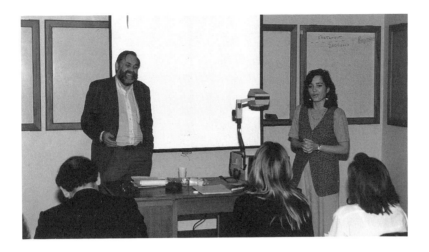

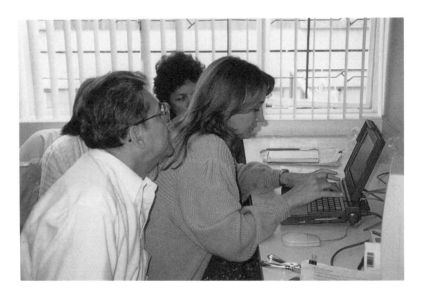

Fig. 4.7. *Top*, course instructor Professor Richard Cash presenting a lecture on proposal development and grant application preparation during the Phase II workshop in Ecuador, with course instructor Josefina Coloma providing translation. *Bottom*, a Phase II team writing a proposal for a grant application on PCR identification of malarial parasites.

4.3.1   Phase I

Workshop Format

The first workshop (Phase I) in a host country serves as a theoretical and practical introduction to molecular techniques, providing an overview of their application to diagnostic, epidemiologic, and basic research objectives. The Phase I courses are typically 5 days of intensive study, consisting of morning lectures followed by a hands-on laboratory workshop during the afternoon. Theoretical aspects of the molecular technique of interest in addition to the epidemiology and classical methods of diagnosis of the organisms under study are presented in lectures. In the laboratory sessions, the participants are divided into four work groups, and all perform the techniques discussed in the morning.

Prior to the workshop, pathogens prevalent in each particular country are chosen in consultation with local health care professionals and scientists. The techniques relevant to the interests of the participants, the participants' technical background, and the availability of resources are all assessed. Taking these country-specific issues into consideration, a "customized" course is then prepared. The necessary equipment and reagents required to supplement existing materials are obtained, and course manuals are assembled. Each experimental protocol is tested on-site beforehand to assure efficiency and accuracy in its application and to minimize the risk of unforeseen problems during the workshop. Five or more course instructors are chosen, including the course organizer, instructors who have been trained in previous courses in another country, local scientists with the necessary preparation, and interested outside instructors. The local contacts, who serve as course organizers on-site, choose approximately 20 scientists, physicians, medical technicians, and professors from national universities and institutions as participants in the first workshop.

Selection of Phase II Participants

In the Phase II workshop, new techniques introduced in the first workshop are applied in a pilot study where participants analyze samples collected during the interval between the Phase I and II workshops. During Phase I, candidates for the second workshop are identified as follows.

1. An announcement is made at the beginning of the first workshop introducing the goal of the Phase II workshop.

2. Potentially interested Phase I participants are encouraged to think about possible applications of molecular biology techniques to their work and to select an epidemiological or clinical question that can be addressed using molecular methods.

3. Course instructors then meet with the interested participants to discuss potential projects and to evaluate the level of commitment of the candidates.

Based on previous experience, it is expected that the most motivated participants will distinguish themselves of their own accord, resulting in a process of "autoselection." Those most interested will stand out not only on the basis of their per-

formance in the Phase I workshop but also by demonstrating initiative and participating in further discussion. Thus, by the end of the first workshop, several proposals for pilot studies are drawn up, where the topics for the proposals are chosen
by local scientists. For example, five such proposals emerged from the first
Ecuadorian workshop, each based in a different region of the country, and five arose
from the Phase I workshop in Bolivia (Table 4.2). With the advice of instructors, the
organism of interest is defined and the methodology of sample collection is determined (which clinical subjects, what type of specimens, how many, and so forth).
The second course is scheduled for a date that is mutually accepted by all participants, approximately 12 months after the Phase I workshop. During the intervening
period, Phase II candidates collect the relevant samples for analysis and, if possible,
begin to analyze the specimens on their own using the molecular techniques learned
in Phase I. A continuous dialog is maintained between instructors and course participants via electronic mail, regular mail, and fax.

4.3.2   Phase II

The objective of the second phase is to oversee the application of molecular biology
techniques to local projects and to provide further training in study design and proposal development. The Phase II workshop is 2 weeks long and consists of two main
sections. The first section involves the molecular biological analysis of samples collected by the participants between the Phase I and II workshops. The second section
entails the design of a larger molecular diagnostic or epidemiological study and the
development of a proposal that forms the basis for funding applications. The four to
five Phase II teams are assembled from individuals or groups of participants selected
from the Phase I workshop plus colleagues from their respective work units.
Collaborations between local institutions are strongly encouraged, in addition to the
inclusion of an epidemiologist in each team.

Section I: Molecular Biological Analysis of Pilot Study Samples

The first week of Phase II concerns the molecular biological aspect of the pilot project.
In order to determine the most effective procedures, a number of sample preparation
methods are investigated, along with different PCR primers and protocols selected
from the literature. This section also serves as a test phase for the project under development, whereby it is determined whether the molecular biology techniques can be
adequately performed under the existing laboratory conditions, whether the techniques
are appropriate for the chosen application, and whether the initial results (when the
specimens were analyzed by participants on their own) are reproducible. The project
leaders consist of returning Phase I instructors and international scientists with expertise in the particular project areas. The objective is to provide sufficient training in this
first section for local participants to (1) decide how to incorporate the techniques into
their studies; (2) determine which applications are the most appropriate; (3) design
their own experiments; (4) modify the techniques to better adapt them to the existing
circumstances; and (5) troubleshoot technical problems that may arise.

Section II: Study Design and Development of Funding Applications

The second section of Phase II provides participants with training in the design and execution of the epidemiological aspect of a research study. It also provides the tools necessary to develop a grant application. A number of outside experts in the fields of epidemiology, grant application preparation, scientific research, and technology transfer participate in this second section. The application of molecular biology techniques to basic science questions is expected to follow, most likely in the context of ensuing collaborations and subsequent technology transfer.

Again, the approach of the AMB/ATT Program emphasizes experiential learning. While basic principles of epidemiology and study design as well as guidelines for grant application development are discussed during the theoretical portion, participants spend the majority of the time in teams, working at a computer actually preparing a proposal. The products of each day's work are submitted to the instructors and reviewed for discussion the following day. The results of the pilot study are also analyzed in order to determine whether the research question is appropriate; whether enough subjects can be enrolled; whether the methodology of sample collection, processing, and analysis is suitable; and whether a larger study is even appropriate. Supporting materials are drawn from the "Proposal Development Workbook" compiled by the Applied Diarrheal Disease Research Project at the Harvard Institute for International Development (ADDR, 1992).

The proposal generated in Phase II should outline a study that is well designed, short-term, simple, low-budget, and well defined. The research question posed must be interesting, relevant, and "do-able" within a reasonable period of time. In the preparation of the grant application, emphasis is placed on the need for carefully following instructions, defining the Objectives and Experimental Design before proceeding to the other sections, and making sure that the answers specifically correspond to the questions. A rough draft of the grant application, consisting of the customary sections (Objectives, Background and Significance, Rationale, Experimental Design, Budget, and Budget Justification), is submitted to the instructors at the end of the second week. Potential funding agencies are identified and evaluated to determine possible sources of funding for each project. After the workshop, participants continue to work together to complete the applications and submit them to Phase II instructors, who continue to serve as advisors. A number of research scientists with relevant expertise are selected to review the grant applications generated by the Phase II workgroups and to suggest improvements, if necessary. Finally, the most promising funding sources are selected by the participants, and the applications are submitted.

Emphasis is placed on collaborations between local research teams or between laboratories in different countries. Throughout the progression of the courses, the formation of "horizontal" connections is emphasized in order to create a regional network of scientists to facilitate shared resources and experience, communication, and common standards. Vertical links between interested parties in more-developed and less-developed countries are also established, in order to provide continued support for resources, information, consulting, and (perhaps) funding.

As an illustration, the projects included in the Phase II workshop in Ecuador (May 1995) and proposed for the Phase II workshop in Bolivia (scheduled for October 1998) are listed in Table 4.2. These projects were proposed by teams assembled as a result of the Phase I course, and each involved interinstitutional and/or international collaborations. Scientists from different countries supervised the projects and maintained communication with participants after completion of the workshop.

Table 4.2. Phase II Projects in Ecuador and Bolivia

Phase II Projects	Participating Institutions
Ecuador	
Molecular characterization of *Leishmania* in an endemic region of Ecuador	Universidad Central del Ecuador, Quito; Universidad de Loja; Instituto Nacional de Higiene, Quito; Universidad Católica, Quito; U.C. San Francisco
RT-PCR detection and typing of dengue virus in the mosquito vector *Aedes aegypti*	Instituto Juan César García, Quito; U.C. San Francisco
Validation of PCR detection of *Mycobacterium tuberculosis* in sputum	Hospital Regional de Zumbahua; Hospital Vozandes, Quito; Universidad Católica, Quito; U.C. San Francisco
Molecular detection of *Plasmodium falciparum* and *Plasmodium vivax* in blood	Laboratorio de Inmunopatología del Instituto Ecuatoriano de Seguro Social (IESS), Guayaquil; Servicio Nacional Ecuatoriano de Malaria; U.C. San Francisco
Assessment of toxigenicity of Ecuadorian *Vibrio cholerae* strains by PCR	Instituto Nacional de Higiene Isquieta Perez (INH), Quito; U.C. San Francisco
Bolivia	
Evaluation of treatment efficacy of Bolivian patients with leishmaniasis using molecular and immunological tools	Insituto SELADIS, Universidad Mayor de San Andrés (UMSA), La Paz; Centro Nacional de Diagnóstico y Referencia, Managua, Nicaragua; U.C. San Francisco
Molecular epidemiology of tuberculosis in Bolivia	Instituto Nacional de Laboratorios de Salud (INLASA), La Paz; Instituto SELADIS, UMSA, La Paz; Hospital Thorax, La Paz; U.C. San Francisco; U.C. Berkeley School of Public Health
RT-PCR typing of dengue virus in patient serum and mosquitoes	Centro Nacional de Enferemedades Tropicales (CENETROP), Santa Cruz; U.C. San Francisco
PCR analysis of strains of *Trypanosoma cruzi* circulating in Bolivian patients with megasyndrome or cardiac symptoms	Centro de Investigación y Diagnóstico de la Enfermedad de Chagas, Sucre; Insituto SELADIS, Universidad Mayor de San Andrés, La Paz; U.C. San Francisco
Characterization of cytokines produced by T cells, macrophages, and natural killer cells in human *T. cruzi* infection	Instituto Boliviano de Biología de las Alturas, La Paz; U.C. San Francisco

4.3.3   Phase III

Phase III can be organized less formally through continued communication and site visits by instructors or, alternatively, as a workshop. In this phase, the same groups that participated in the Phase II workshop continue to work with instructors to evaluate their progress on the projects defined in Phase II, and each group participates according to its current level of progress. Instructors provide technical assistance, if necessary, troubleshooting problems or further adapting the techniques to improve their suitability to the conditions on-site. Phase III also includes more rigorous training in epidemiological study design and statistical data analysis, and each group's experimental results are analyzed. Assistance is provided with the preparation of final reports and scientific manuscripts based on completed Phase II projects. Finally, subsequent projects are designed to address molecular epidemiological or basic research questions through international collaborations, and the corresponding grant applications are developed. Individual relationships continue after the workshops end, with instructors acting as direct research consultants to local scientists.

4.4   Program Development

The initial workshops were held in Nicaragua in 1991–1992 (Harris et al., 1993). Since then, workshops have been conducted in Bolivia, Ecuador, Guatemala, Cuba, and the United States. A number of follow-up projects on diseases such as dengue fever, leishmaniasis, and tuberculosis are underway in Nicaragua, Bolivia, Ecuador, and Guatemala.

The First Nicaraguan Applied Biotechnology Workshop, given in June 1991, provided an introduction to classical molecular biology and molecular diagnostics (PCR), using the detection of the parasite *Leishmania* as an example of a host-country-identified disease project. The success of the first course resulted in a second Molecular Diagnostics Workshop held in Managua, Nicaragua in July 1992. Pathogens responsible for the most serious health problems in Nicaragua were identified by participants in the first course and selected for study in the second workshop. These included *Vibrio cholerae, Mycobacterium tuberculosis, Shigella,* and enterotoxigenic *E. coli* (detected by PCR), as well as the malarial parasite *Plasmodium falciparum* (detected with non-radioactive DNA probes). Twenty scientists and professors from various academic and governmental institutions throughout the country were selected by Nicaraguan course organizers to participate in each workshop.

A number of projects were developed as a result of the Nicaraguan workshops and are on-going at the Centro Nacional de Diagnóstico y Referencia (CNDR), Ministry of Health, Managua. Because of the importance of leishmaniasis as a significant health problem and the limitations of classical methods for parasite identification, detection and genetic characterization of *Leishmania* parasites by PCR has been a priority of the Department of Parasitology at the CNDR since 1991. Simplified methods have been developed for the routine diagnosis of leishmaniasis by PCR (Belli et al., 1998). This work was presented in international conferences and received funding from the European Economic Community. The head of the

Department of Parasitology completed a Masters degree in the Applied Molecular Biology of Infectious Diseases Program at the London School of Hygiene and Tropical Medicine and focused his thesis work on the molecular characterization of putative Nicaraguan hybrid strains of *Leishmania* (Belli et al., 1994). A novel multiplex PCR protocol for single-tube identification of the three complexes of New World *Leishmania* was developed and was field-tested at the CNDR (Harris et al., 1998a). In 1997, these PCR techniques were used to identify an apparent epidemic of atypical cutaneous leishmaniasis (non-ulcerative leishmaniasis) and to implicate *L. chagasi* as the causative agent (Belli et al., submitted for publication).

Other projects include a study initiated at the CNDR in February of 1994 to assess PCR-based diagnosis of tuberculosis. In July 1995, detection and typing of dengue virus in patient serum by reverse transcriptase-PCR (RT-PCR) was introduced (Harris et al., 1998b). This technique was used by Nicaraguan scientists in October 1995 to investigate an outbreak of hemorrhagic fever in Northern Nicaragua, which was initially thought to be caused by dengue virus. Much international interest was generated when scientists at the CNDR used RT-PCR and other techniques to rapidly demonstrate that dengue was in fact *not* the cause, and teams from various countries soon discovered that the etiological agent was *Leptospira* (U.S. Centers for Disease Control [CDC], 1995b). The CNDR now has access to PCR-based techniques for the detection and genetic characterization of *Leptospira* and is using these techniques to investigate the current status of leptospirosis in Nicaragua. The CNDR continues to use RT-PCR for epidemiological surveillance of dengue virus to identify the circulating serotypes and to enable a more rapid response by the mosquito control program. A comprehensive database combining demographic, clinical, and laboratory information about confirmed dengue cases is being created for future epidemiological studies. A study is underway using RT-PCR to screen pools of mosquitoes reared from field-collected eggs and larvae for evidence of vertical transmission of dengue virus in *Aedes aegypti*. In February 1996, the standardization of PCR protocols for detection of *Chlamydia trachomatis* and *Neisseria gonorrhoeae* (Mahoney et al., 1995) was initiated. This technique was used to monitor both of these pathogens in a study of prostitutes in Managua and in a study of rural health clinics in the province of Estelí.[1] A molecular epidemiological study investigating *C. trachomatis* genotypes circulating among prostitutes in Managua is currently under way.[2] In 1997, the Department of Virology began using PCR for detection of Hepatitis B virus, yellow fever, herpesvirus, and enteroviruses. PCR has become a standard technique for diagnostic and investigative work at the CNDR.

Based on the work in Nicaragua and on presentations at international conferences, a number of Latin American scientists expressed interest in hosting Applied Molecular Biology workshops in Ecuador, Bolivia, Guatemala, Honduras, Colombia, Venezuela, Argentina, Paraguay, Mexico, and Brazil. In response, a Phase I workshop was organized in Ecuador with funding from the American Society of Biochemistry

---

1. A. Belli, E. Flores, B. Rodriguez, and E. Harris, unpublished results.
2. D. Dean, A. Belli, B. Rodriguez, A. Gorter, and E. Harris, unpublished results.

and Molecular Biology. The course was designed in collaboration with Ecuadorian scientists and conducted in Quito, Ecuador, in April 1994. The curriculum included detection of *Leishmania braziliensis* and *Mycobacterium tuberculosis* by PCR and typing of dengue virus using RT-PCR and nonradioactive DNA probes. The participants represented 14 institutions from eight Ecuadorian cities. Five groups proposed pilot projects (Table 4.2) for the subsequent Phase II workshop, which was held in Quito in May 1995, with participants from 11 institutions across Ecuador. Several of these projects have continued (notably those involving leishmaniasis, tuberculosis, and malaria), have received funding from national and international sources, and have resulted in manuscripts for publication (Avilés et al., submitted for publication; Moleón-Borodowsky et al., manuscript in preparation).

The third site for the AMB/ATT courses is in Bolivia, and the first workshop was given in 1997 in La Paz. Twenty scientists and graduate students from the five major scientific institutes in La Paz as well as from the cities of Cochabamba and Sucre participated. The course curriculum consisted of detection and identification of *L. braziliensis* from clinical samples, characterization of the New World complexes of *Leishmania* by multiplex PCR, fingerprinting of individual strains of *M. tuberculosis* using double repetitive element (DRE)-PCR, and genetic characterization of *Trypanosoma cruzi* using random amplified polymorphic DNA (RAPD)-PCR. Phase II projects proposed by the participants are listed in Table 4.2. Grant applications to seek funding for some of these projects have been written through collaborative efforts facilitated by electronic mail and have been submitted to international agencies.

4.5 Examples of Projects

A number of on-going collaborative projects have arisen from the AMB/ATT courses in various institutions in Nicaragua, Bolivia, Ecuador, and Guatemala. A description of several of these projects is presented below.

4.5.1 Molecular Characterization of *Leishmania* (Nicaragua/Bolivia)

Leishmaniasis is an important public health problem in tropical and subtropical countries worldwide, involving 400,000 new cases annually, with 12 million people infected and 350 million at risk (Ashford et al., 1992). The disease is associated with a variety of clinical manifestations, depending on the species of the parasite, the host immune response, and factors in the saliva of the sandfly vector. In the Americas, 13 species of New World *Leishmania* are grouped into three complexes, which are responsible for (1) a self-curing ulcerative disease and diffuse cutaneous leishmaniasis (typically caused by the *L. mexicana* complex), (2) persistent cutaneous and often disfiguring mucocutaneous lesions (*L. braziliensis* complex), and (3) the potentially fatal visceral disease attributed to *L. chagasi* (*L. donovani* complex) (Grimaldi and Tesh, 1993). Parasitological confirmation of leishmaniasis is critical, because the wide spectrum of symptoms can be caused by a number of other etiological agents, leading to potential misdiagnosis. In addition, the treatment for leishmaniasis is expensive, lengthy, and associated with toxic side effects (Pearson et al., 1995). Further, species identification is important because different species can require distinct treatment regimens (Grimaldi and Tesh, 1993; Navin et al., 1990). Existing microbiological and biochemical techniques for identification of *Leishmania* are often inadequate, and PCR is a rapid, sensitive, and specific alternative technique.

Since the first course in Nicaragua in 1991, molecular methods have been employed in the detection and characterization of *Leishmania* strains in the Department of Parasitology at the CNDR in Managua (Belli et al., 1992). Simplified methods of sample preparation have been developed for rapid PCR analysis directly from clinical specimens and cultured strains; for instance, PCR from boiled dermal scrapings was shown to be more sensitive than microscopy and is able to replace the more invasive skin biopsies often used as PCR specimens (Belli et al., 1998). These techniques are being used to characterize clinical samples from Nicaragua and are also being employed to analyze *Leishmania* strains as part of a Central America-wide project (Zeledon et al., 1993). In addition, a novel multiplex PCR has been developed which yields products of different sizes for the three New World complexes of *Leishmania* (Harris et al., 1998a) and was tested with field isolates and specimens. These methods have been used to identify *L. chagasi* as the etiological agent of atypical cutaneous leishmaniasis (ACL) during a recent upsurge in the number of reported ACL cases. This is important since the disease had been misdiagnosed as cutaneous tuberculosis or lupus vulgaris and thus was refractory to the treatment applied. Another area of interest is the application of PCR techniques to the detection of *Leishmania* in its sandfly vector *Lutzomyia* (Pérez et al., 1994) for use in vector incrimination studies and development of behavioral control strategies.

In another study, Nicaraguan strains of *Leishmania* were characterized by both isoenzyme electrophoresis at the protein level and restriction fragment length polymorphism at the DNA level. Characterization of Nicaraguan strains of *Leishmania* by both isoenzyme analysis (Darce et al., 1991) and DNA fingerprinting (Belli et al., 1994) revealed heterozygous patterns consistent with a naturally occurring *L. panamensis/L. braziliensis* hybrid strain. These results, which imply the possibility of genetic exchange during reproduction of *Leishmania*, are interesting in view of the commonly held belief that *Leishmania* reproduce asexually.

In Bolivia, PCR has been used to detect and characterize *Leishmania* in clinical samples.[3] A study has been proposed to evaluate the efficacy of treatment for leishmaniasis in Bolivian patients, using molecular and immunological tools. Objectives are (1) to evaluate a panel of PCR-based tools for the diagnosis, characterization and therapeutic evaluation of leishmaniasis patients, (2) to investigate the frequency in which *Leishmania* DNA can be detected in peripheral blood mononuclear cells and serum of Bolivian patients with active leishmanial lesions, and (3) to evaluate PCR as a new tool for monitoring treatment of leishmaniasis and as a predictor of relapse.

---

3. E. Harris, A. Belli, and S. Revollo, unpublished results.

4.5.2   Epidemiological Surveillance of Dengue Virus in Clinical Specimens by RT-PCR (Nicaragua/Guatemala/Bolivia)

During the last 15 years, dengue fever and the more severe form of Dengue Hemorrhagic Fever/Dengue Shock Syndrome (DHF/DSS) have spread throughout Latin America at an alarming rate (Pan American Health Organization, 1994). Since previous infection with one of the four dengue serotypes may be an important risk factor for developing DHF/DSS upon infection with a heterotypic serotype (Halstead, 1988; Morens, 1994), it is crucial to determine which serotypes of dengue virus are circulating where and when. The current reference method or "gold standard" for typing dengue by isolation of the virus in cultured cells followed by typing using indirect immunofluorescence is a lengthy and expensive procedure. Nicaragua has experienced several epidemics of dengue in recent years, and all four serotypes have been reported recently (Kouri et al., 1991; U.S. CDC, 1995a). However, the Nicaraguan Ministry of Health had been unable to type circulating dengue virus due to the expense of classical viral isolation procedures and the requirement for cell culture facilities. Dengue epidemics have also occurred in the low-lying region of Santa Cruz, Bolivia, but health officials did not have access to techniques that allow on-site typing of dengue virus.[4] In both instances, only a small percentage of serum samples had been typed by sending them to laboratories outside the country, which is a costly and extremely lengthy process. RT-PCR detection and typing of dengue offers a sensitive, specific, rapid, and low-cost alternative.

An RT-PCR protocol for detecting and typing dengue virus was adapted for field application, combining all steps into a single tube and thereby reducing the risk of sample cross-contamination (Harris et al., 1998b). In this protocol, the viral RNA is reverse-transcribed, and the resulting cDNA is immediately amplified to yield a product of a different size for each dengue serotype. This modified RT-PCR technique was introduced in the CNDR at the Ministry of Health in Managua in July 1995 and used to detect and type dengue virus directly from patient serum samples during Nicaraguan dengue outbreaks in 1995 and 1997-8 (Figure 4.8). As stated in section 4.4, this technique was used by Nicaraguan scientists to rapidly rule out dengue as the cause of a recent epidemic of hemorrhagic fever, which turned out to be caused by *Leptospira* (U.S. CDC, 1995b). This differential diagnosis is crucial because leptospirosis is a bacterial infection that is treatable with antibiotics. The modified dengue RT-PCR has been used in Ecuador[5] and in Guatemala[6] to type circulating dengue strains. In August 1997, Bolivian scientists at the Centro Nacional de Enfermedades Tropicales (CENETROP) were able to type dengue virus in Bolivia for the first time and to identify dengue-2 as the serotype responsible for the 1997 epidemic in Santa Cruz, corroborating results reported by the CDC (Peredo et al., submitted for publication).

---

4. C. Peredo and A. Gianella, personal communication.
5. I. Moleon and L. E. Plaza, personal communication.
6. O. Torres, personal communication.

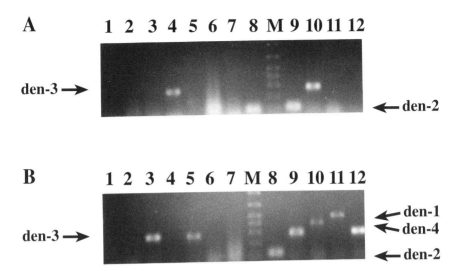

Fig. 4.8. RT-PCR detection and typing of dengue virus in patient serum during the 1995 epidemic in Nicaragua. RNA was extracted from the samples and amplified using a single-tube RT-PCR assay; products were analyzed by gel electrophoresis. Panel A, lane 1, negative control (water); lanes 2-8, 11, and 12, patient samples from the Atlantic coast of Nicaragua (Bluefields); lane M, Amplisize DNA Size Standards (*see* Appendix C; lowest band shown, 100 bp); lane 9, dengue-2 RNA (positive control); lane 10, dengue-3 RNA (positive control). Panel B, lanes 1-7, patient samples from the Atlantic coast of Nicaragua (Bluefields); lane M, Amplisize DNA Size Standards (*see* Appendix C; lowest band shown, 100 bp); lane 8, dengue-2 RNA (positive control); lane 9, dengue-3 RNA (positive control); lane 10, dengue-4 RNA (positive control); lane 11, dengue-1 RNA (positive control); lane 12, patient sample from central Nicaragua (Chontales). Expected product sizes: dengue-2, 119 bp; dengue-3, 290 bp; dengue-4, 389 bp; dengue-1, 482 bp.

The single-tube RT-PCR technique will be used as an epidemiological surveillance tool to monitor the movement of dengue serotypes in Nicaragua, Bolivia, and Guatemala, while routine diagnosis will be maintained by IgM-ELISA. A small viral isolation laboratory will be maintained to isolate dengue virus from RT-PCR-positive serum samples in order to create a bank of local strains for future molecular epidemiological studies.

Distinct genetic subtypes have been identified within each dengue serotype (Lanciotti et al., 1998; Lanciotti et al., 1994; Lewis et al., 1993; Rico-Hesse, 1990), some of which may be associated with more severe epidemics correlated with greater incidence of DHF (Rico-Hesse et al., 1997; Deubel, 1992). A PCR-based fingerprinting technique, restriction site specific (RSS)-PCR, has been developed to make molecular genotyping techniques accessible for on-site implementation, thereby increasing the scope of analysis (Harris et al., in press). The strains isolated in collaborating countries will be analyzed using this technique to identify the circulating dengue subtypes.

4.5.3   RT-PCR Detection and Typing of Dengue Virus in the Mosquito Vector (Nicaragua)

Dengue virus is transmitted to humans by the mosquitoes *Aedes aegypti* and *Aedes albopictus*. Information about dengue virus infection of mosquitoes is essential to the understanding and control of the virus, especially since no animal reservoirs are known—implying that the transmission cycle includes only humans and mosquitoes. Rapid identification and typing of dengue virus in mosquitoes can furnish critical information about the infection rate of *Ae. aegypti* during and between epidemics (Chow et al., 1998); the potential for prediction and prevention of dengue outbreaks through detection of the virus in field-caught mosquitoes; validation of existing mathematical simulation models describing dengue epidemics (Focks, 1995; Jetten and Focks, 1997); and vertical transmission of dengue virus in *Ae. aegypti* in nature. While detection of dengue virus in pools of mosquitoes can be accomplished by viral isolation and indirect immunofluorescence, it is a costly and time-consuming technique. RT-PCR combined with an appropriate RNA extraction technique is an attractive alternative, due to the rapidity, sensitivity, and specificity of the assay.

To prepare mosquito samples for the RT-PCR amplification, a suitable RNA extraction procedure is required to isolate viral RNA from pools of mosquitoes without degradation of the RNA or inhibition of the PCR amplification. Using a combination of a guanidine-based lysis buffer, organic solvents, and silica particles, a protocol was developed that reproducibly isolates very small quantities of viral RNA (equivalent to less than 100 viral particles) without PCR inhibitors, even in the presence of up to 50 *Ae. aegypti* mosquitoes (Harris et al., 1998b). Dengue virus can be detected in laboratory-infected mosquitoes as early as one day postinoculation using this protocol (Figure 4.9). This approach is being used to examine mosquitoes captured in dengue-endemic areas of Nicaragua in order to test its efficacy in the field.

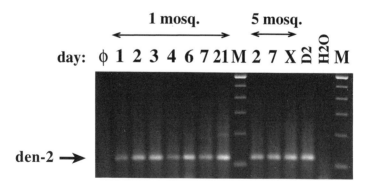

Fig. 4.9. Detection of dengue virus in infected mosquitoes by RT-PCR. Mosquitoes were inoculated with dengue-2 (strain 16681) and frozen at $-70°C$ at the indicated times. RNA was extracted and amplified by RT-PCR (RAV-2 reverse transcriptase/*Taq* polymerase), and the products were analyzed by gel electrophoresis. Legend: day, number of days postinoculation; ϕ, five uninfected mosquitoes; X, five mosquitoes frozen 1 day after natural death; D2, dengue-2 RNA (positive control); H_2O, negative control; M, 100-bp ladder (*see* Appendix C; lowest band shown, 100 bp). Expected product size: dengue-2, 119 bp.

Persistence of dengue virus in the environment and survival of the virus during dry seasons is poorly understood. The rate of vertical transmission of dengue virus in *Ae. aegypti* in laboratory experiments is reportedly low, and relatively little information has been published on this topic based on field data. In Nicaragua, the RNA extraction protocol and RT-PCR assay previously described is being applied to the study of vertical transmission of dengue virus in nature by analysis of pools of mosquitoes reared from eggs and larvae collected in areas reporting dengue fever.

4.5.4 Molecular Epidemiology of Tuberculosis (Bolivia)

Tuberculosis (TB) is the leading cause of death due to infectious disease among adults worldwide, with 95% of cases occurring in developing countries (Haas and Des Prez, 1995). The estimated annual incidence of TB in Latin America and the Caribbean was 120 per 100,000 inhabitants in 1990 (Sudre et al., 1992). One of the highest reported rates in the region is in Bolivia, and the incidence has been increasing over the past several years. In rural areas of Bolivia, diagnosis of TB relies on clinical symptoms, and when possible, microscopy of acid-fast bacilli (AFB) smears. Reference hospitals and the National Institute for Health Laboratories (INLASA) perform cultures of *M. tuberculosis* as well. Anti-tuberculosis drugs are provided free of charge by the government, but ensuring proper treatment has been a problem. Thus, the primary public health issues are timely detection of smear-positive cases and assurance of proper treatment in order to reduce transmission.

It also important to fully understand the transmission patterns and risk factors of TB in various communities so that appropriate interventions can be designed. DNA-based typing methods have proven to be extremely useful in molecular epidemiological studies aimed at analyzing outbreaks and community transmission, contact tracing, identifying laboratory cross-contamination and mixed infections, and conducting geographical studies on global transmission (Suffys et al., 1997). RFLP based on the repetitive element IS*6110* is the standard method for identifying individual *M. tuberculosis* strains (Van Embden et al., 1993). However, recently described fingerprinting techniques based entirely on PCR are much quicker, easier, and cheaper than the standard RFLP procedure (Friedman et al., 1995; Groenen et al., 1993). These methods make molecular epidemiological studies more accessible, since *M. tuberculosis* isolates can be typed on-site in minimally equipped laboratories.

To this end, a project was initiated in La Paz, Bolivia as a collaboration among the Molecular Biology Unit at the SELADIS Institute (Universidad Mayor de San Andrés), the Tuberculosis Laboratory at INLASA, the Thorax Hospital in La Paz, the University of California, San Francisco, and the School of Public Health at the University of California, Berkeley. The objective is to conduct molecular epidemiological studies of TB in Bolivian communities by using the DRE-PCR technique. DRE-PCR is based on two sets of primers, each of which targets a repetitive *M. tuberculosis* element; namely, IS*6110* and the polymorphic GC-rich sequence (PGRS). The primers hybridize to the ends of the repetitive sequences pointing outward, so that the amplified products that are generated consist of the regions between the repetitive elements (Friedman et al., 1995; Riley and Harris, in press). Since these elements are found in different chromosomal locations in different strains, distinct patterns are generated by DRE-PCR for each strain.

In La Paz, the DRE-PCR technique has been standardized using Bolivian isolates of *M. tuberculosis* and has been used to analyze strains from local hospitals. A study currently underway involves genetic analysis of *M. tuberculosis* isolates collected prospectively in clinics in La Paz and in Santa Cruz, representing up to 10% of the cases in each geographical area. The data will be examined for the appearance of cluster strains (isolates with identical patterns). Cluster strains may have unique biological characteristics that correlate with widespread dissemination of tuberculosis in a particular community (Ehrt et al., 1997; Friedman et al., 1997). This increase in incidence could be due to more rapid progression from the infection to disease stages. It is therefore particularly important to control transmission of these strains. If such strains are identified among the Bolivian isolates, epidemiological analyses will be conducted using the information obtained in the questionnaires administered at the time of sample collection. This will help identify risk factors associated with transmission of these cluster strains, so that control measures can be designed. The biological properties of these Bolivian strains will be investigated as part of future collaborations. In addition, the DRE-PCR technique will be used to conduct similar studies in specific Bolivian communities and to investigate *M. tuberculosis* strains in contacts of particular index cases when appropriate.

4.6   International Courses

The format of the AMB/ATT workshops has also been adapted to international courses, where the main focus is on regional networking and collaborations instead of country-specific problems. International Phase I workshops have been given both in Latin America and in the United States (Table 4.3). An International Postgraduate Course was given in December 1994 in Havana, with scientists from 10 Latin American countries participating. In addition to illustrating the application of PCR to molecular diagnostics, this workshop contained a section on the use of PCR in the research laboratory, including its use in sequence modification, cloning and sequencing, and heteroduplex analysis (Delwart et al., 1993). In July 1995, a workshop was conducted in Guatemala, which included participants from Guatemala, Nicaragua, El Salvador, Costa Rica, Honduras, Mexico, Panama, and Colombia. A Phase II workshop in Guatemala is planned for 1998. These courses require more complex organization and higher cost, but they provide unique opportunities for interchange of experiences at the international level and often result in long-term regional collaborations. Communication with course participants from Mexico, Guatemala, Costa Rica, and Panama for technical advice and consulting still continues.

The format of the Phase I introductory AMB/ATT workshop has also been adapted for sites in the United States. In October 1992, an international laboratory workshop was held in conjunction with the Rockefeller Foundation North/South Institutional Strengthening Network conference at Stanford University, Palo Alto, California. This workshop included members of each of the eight network laboratories in the United States, Mexico, Brazil, and India.

Table 4.3. International Courses Modeled on the AMB/ATT Phase I Format

Course Title, Country, Date	Participating Countries	Pathogens Detected
Linking Molecular Epidemiology, Field Investigations, and Health Services Research, United States, October 1992	Mexico, Brazil, India, China, United States	*Vibrio cholerae, Salmonella typhi,* Enterotoxigenic *E. coli, Entamoeba histolytica,* Rotavirus
PCR in Basic Research, Biomedical Diagnostics, and Environmental Surveillance, Cuba, December 1994	Guatemala, Nicaragua, Costa Rica, Colombia, Mexico, Venezuela, Bolivia, Ecuador, Cuba	*M. tuberculosis, Vibrio cholerae,* Dengue virus, HIV
PCR '95: PCR and Nonradioactive Probes for the Diagnosis of Tropical Infectious Diseases, Guatemala, July 1995	Guatemala, Nicaragua, El Salvador, Costa Rica, Honduras, Panama, Colombia, Mexico	*M. tuberculosis, Leishmania, Vibrio cholerae,* Dengue virus
Biotechnology on a Shoestring, United States, September 1995	United States, Ecuador, Kenya, Dominican Republic, India	*Vibrio cholerae,* Dengue virus

In September 1995, a workshop was given at the University of Florida, Gainesville, for international graduate students and high school teachers. One of the workshop's outreach goals was to provide high school teachers with both teacher training and potential high school course material. Another objective was to offer students from less-developed countries who were receiving training in the United States a concrete example of how to transfer advanced technologies when they return to their home countries. While this course was directed to students and educators, rather than health care professionals and scientists, the emphasis was the same as in all of the AMB/ATT workshops; namely, a low-cost, do-it-yourself approach to the practical application of advanced molecular biology techniques. This workshop was enthusiastically received, and subsequently partnerships were established between course instructors at the University of Florida and local high school teachers. These linkages provide educational and material resources to help support the transfer of knowledge and skills learned in the workshop to other high school teachers and students.

References

The Applied Diarrheal Disease Research Project (1992) *Proposal Development Workshop.* Cambridge, Massachusetts, Harvard Institute for International Development.

Ashford, R.W., Desjeux, P., and Deraadt, P. (1992) Estimation of populations at risk of infection with leishmaniasis. *Parasit. Today,* 8:104–105.

Avilés, H., Belli, A., Armijos, R., Monroy, F.P., and Harris, E. PCR detection and identification of *Leishmania* parasites in clinical specimens in Ecuador: A comparison with classical diagnostic methods. Submitted for publication.

Barinaga, M. (1994) A personal technology transfer effort in DNA diagnostics. *Science*, 266:1317–1318.

Belli, A., Moran, J., and Harris, E. (1992). Adaptation of PCR for field studies of leishmaniasis in Nicaragua. In *Biotechnología '92*. Havana, Cuba, Centro de Ingeniería Genética y Biotecnología.

Belli, A., Rodriguez, B., Avilés, H., and Harris, E. (1998) Simplified PCR detection of New World *Leishmania* from clinical specimens. *Am. J. Trop. Med. Hyg.* 58:102–109.

Belli, A., Garcia, D., Palacios, X., Rodriguez, B., Videa, E., Valle, S., Tinoco, E., Marin, F., and Harris, E. *Leishmania chagasi* causes visceral disease and widespread atypical cutaneous leishmaniasis. Submitted for publication.

Belli, A.A., Miles, M.A., and Kelly, J.M. (1994) A putative *Leishmania panamensis/Leishmania braziliensis* hybrid is a causative agent of human cutaneous leishmaniasis in Nicaragua. *Parasitology*, 109:435–442.

Chow, V.T.K., Chan, Y.C., Yong, R., Lee, K.M., Lim, L.K., Chung, Y.K., Lam-Phua, S.G., and Tan, B.T. (1998) Monitoring of dengue viruses in field-caught *Aedes aegypti* and *Aedes albopictus* mosquitoes by a type-specific polymerase chain reaction and cycle sequencing. *Am. J. Trop. Med. Hyg.*, 58:578–586.

Darce, M., Moran, J., Palacios, X., Belli, A., Gomez-Urcuyo, F., Valle, S., Gantier, J.C., Momen, H., and Grimaldi, G. (1991) Etiology of human cutaneous leishmaniasis in Nicaragua. *Trans. R. Soc. Trop. Med. Hyg.*, 85:58–59.

Delwart, E.L., Shpaer, E.G., Louwagie, J., McCutchan, F.E., Grez, M., Rübsamen-Waigmann, H., and Mullins, J.I. (1993) Genetic relationships determined by a DNA heteroduplex mobility assay: Analysis of HIV-1 *env* genes. *Science*, 262:1257–1261.

Deubel, V. (1992) Recent advances and prospective researches on molecular epidemiology of dengue viruses. *Mem. Inst. Oswaldo Cruz*, 87:133–136.

Ehrt, S., Shiloh, M.U., Ruan, J., Choi, M., Gunzburg, S., Nathan, C., Xie, Q.-W., and Riley, L.W. (1997) A novel antioxidant gene from *Mycobacterium tuberculosis*. *J. Exp. Med.* 186:1885–1896.

Focks, D.A. (1995) A simulation model of the epidemiology of urban dengue fever: Literature analysis, model development, preliminary validation, and samples of simulation results. *Am. J. Trop. Med. Hyg.*, 53:489–506.

Friedman, C.R., Quinn, G.C., Kreiswirth, B.N., Perlman, D.C., Salomon, N., Schluger, N., Lutfey, M., Berger, J., Poltoratskaia, N., and Riley, L.W. (1997) Widespread dissemination of a drug-susceptible strain of *Mycobacterium tuberculosis*. *J. Infect. Dis.*, 176:478–484.

Friedman, C.R., Stoeckle, M.Y., Johnson, W.D., Jr., and Riley, L.W. (1995) Double-repetitive-element PCR method for subtyping *Mycobacterium tuberculosis* clinical isolates. *J. Clin. Microbiol.*, 33:1383–1384.

Grimaldi, G., Jr., and Tesh, R.B. (1993) Leishmaniasis of the New World: Current concepts and implications for future research. *Clin. Microbiol. Rev.*, 6:230–250.

Groenen, P.M., Bunschoten, A.E., van Soolingen, D., and van Embden, J.D. (1993) Nature of DNA polymorphism in the direct repeat cluster of *Mycobacterium tuberculosis*; application for strain differentiation by a novel typing method. *Mol. Microbiol.*, 10:1057–1065.

Haas, D.W., and Des Prez, R.M. (1995) Mycobacterium tuberculosis. In *Principles and Practice of Infectious Diseases*, G. L. Mandell, J. E. Bennett, and R. Dolin, eds., New York, Churchill Livingstone.

Halstead, S.B. (1988) Pathogenesis of dengue: Challenges to molecular biology. *Science*, 239:476–481.

Harris, E., Kropp, G., Rodriguez, B., Belli, A., and Agabian, N. (1998a) Single-step multiplex PCR assay for characterization of New World *Leishmania* complexes. *J. Clin. Microbiol.*, 36:1989–1995.

Harris, E., López, M., Arévalo, J., Bellatin, J., Belli, A., Moran, J., and Orrego, O. (1993)

Short courses on DNA detection and amplification in Central and South America: The democratization of molecular biology. *Biochem. Educ.*, 21:16–22.

Harris, E., Roberts, T.G., Smith, L., Selle, J., Kramer, L.D., Valle, S., Sandoval, E., and Balmaseda, A. (1998b) Typing of dengue viruses in clinical specimens and mosquitoes by single-tube multiplex reverse transcriptase-PCR. *J. Clin. Microbiol.*, 36:2634–2639.

Harris, E., Sandoval, E., Xet-Mull, A.M., Johnson, M., and Riley, L.W. Rapid subtyping of dengue viruses by restriction site specific (RSS)-PCR. In press.

Jetten, T.H., and Focks, D.A. (1997) Potential changes in the distribution of dengue transmission under climate warming. *Am. J. Trop. Med. Hyg.*, 56:285–297.

Kouri, G., Valdez, M., Arguello, L., Guzman, M.G., Valdes, L., Soler, M., and Bravo, J. (1991) Dengue epidemic in Nicaragua, 1985. *Revista do Instituto de Medicina Tropical de Sao Paulo*, 33:365–71.

Lanciotti, R.S., Lewis, J.G., Gubler, D.J., and Trent, D.W. (1994) Molecular evolution and epidemiology of dengue-3 viruses. *J. Gen. Virol.*, 75:65–75.

Lewis, J.G., Chang, G.-J., Lanciotti, R.S., Kinney, R.M., Mayer, L.M., and Trent, D.W. (1993) Phylogenetic relationships of dengue-2 viruses. *Virology*, 197:216–224.

Mahoney, J.B., Luinstra, K.E., Tyndall, M., Sellors, J.W., Krepel, J., and Chernesky, M. (1995) Multiplex PCR for detection of *Chlamydia trachomatis* and *Neisseria gonorrheoae* in genitourinary specimens. *J. Clin. Microbiol.*, 33:3049–3053.

Moleón-Borodowsky, I., Altamirano, F., Plaza, L.E., Mite, P., Jurado, H., and Harris, E. Utilización de la técnica de la reacción en cadena de la polimerasa para la detección de *P. falciparum* y *P. vivax* en el Servicio Nacional de Control de la Malaria del Ecuador. Manuscript in preparation.

Morens, D.M. (1994) Antibody-dependent enhancement of infection and the pathogenesis of viral disease. *Clin. Infect. Dis.*, 19:500–512.

Navin, T.R., Arana, B.A., Arana, F.E., de Merida, A.M., Castillo, A.L., and Pozuelos, J.L. (1990) Placebo-controlled clinical trial of Meglumine antimoniate (Glucantime) vs. localized controlled heat in the treatment of cutaneous leishmaniasis in Guatemala. *Am. J. Trop. Med. Hyg.*, 42:43–50.

Pan American Health Organization (1994) *Dengue and Dengue Hemorrhagic Fever in the Americas: Guidelines for Prevention and Control.* Scientific Publication #548.

Pearson, R.D., and de Querez Sousa, A. (1995) *Leishmania* species: Visceral (kala-azar), cutaneous, and mucosal leishmaniasis. In *Principles and Practice of Infectious Diseases*, G. L. Mandell, J. E. Bennett, and R. Dolin, eds., New York, Churchill Livingstone.

Peredo, C., Garron, T., Pellegrino, J.L., Harris, E., and Gianella, A. Detection and identification of dengue 2 virus from Santa Cruz, Bolivia, by a one-step RT-PCR method. Submitted for publication.

Pérez, J.E., Ogusuku, E., Inga, R., López, M., Monje, J., Paz, L., Nieto, E., and Arévalo, J. (1994) Natural *Leishmania* infection of *Lutzomyia* spp. in Peru. *Trans. R. Soc. Trop. Med. Hyg.*, 88:161–164.

Rico-Hesse, R. (1990) Molecular evolution and distribution of dengue viruses type 1 and 2 in nature. *Virology*, 174:479–493.

Rico-Hesse, R., Harrison, L.M., Alba Salas, R., Tovar, D., Nisalak, A., Ramos, C., Boshell, J., De Mesa, M.T.R., Nogueira, R.M.R., and Travassos Da Rosa, A. (1997) Origins of dengue type 2 viruses associated with increased pathogenicity in the Americas. *Virology*, 230:244–251.

Riley, L.W., and Harris, E. Double Repetitive Element-Polymerase Chain Reaction method for subtyping *Mycobacterium tuberculosis* strains. In *Basic Techniques in Mycobacterial and Nocardial Molecular Biology*, R. Ollar and N. Connell, eds., Philadelphia, Raven Publishers, in press.

Sudre, P., ten Dam, G., and Kochi, A. (1992) Tuberculosis: A global overview of the situation today. *Bull. WHO*, 70:149–159.

Suffys, P.N., de Araujo, M.E.I., and Degrave, W.M. (1997) The changing face of the epidemiology of tuberculosis due to molecular strain typing—A review. *Mem. Inst. Oswaldo Cruz*, 92:297–316.

U.S. Centers for Disease Control and Prevention (1995a) Dengue type 3 infection—Nicaragua and Panama, October–November, 1994. *Morbidity Mortality Weekly Rep.*, 44:21–24.

U.S. Centers for Disease Control and Prevention (1995b) Leptospirosis identified in Nicaragua. *Weekly Epidemiol. Rec.* 70:322.

Van Embden, J.D., Cave, M.D., Crawford, J.T., Dale, J.W., Eisenach, K.D., Gicquel, B., Hermans, P., Martin, C., McAdam, R., Shinnick, T.M., and Small, P.M. (1993) Strain identification of *Mycobacterium tuberculosis* by DNA fingerprinting: Recommendations for a standardized methodology. *J. Clin. Microbiol.*, 31:406–409.

Zeledon, R., Maingon, R., Ward, R., Arana, B., Belli, A., de Carreira, P., and Ponce, C. (1993) The characterization of *Leishmania* parasites and their vectors from Central America using molecular techniques. *Arch. Inst. Pasteur Tunis*, 70:325–329.

II

Selected Protocols

5

Infectious Disease Protocols

5.1 PCR Protocols

5.1.1 Overview

The second part of this book contains a number of protocols for the PCR amplification of nucleic acids from selected pathogenic organisms, each of which has been developed, tested, and applied in the field during workshops and collaborative projects over the past 10 years. Each protocol is preceded by an introduction to the clinical manifestations and epidemiology of the disease caused by the pathogen, classical methods of diagnosis, PCR-based procedures reported to date, and points to consider in using PCR. It is important to keep in mind when reviewing published PCR protocols that some have been assessed only in research laboratories. Therefore, continuous review of the literature for reports of field evaluations of these techniques is recommended.

The protocols are all presented in a similar format, which consists of sample preparation, amplification, and product analysis (gel electrophoresis and visualization). A preferred method for sample preparation is provided for each protocol; additional methods are discussed in section 3.1.3. The amplification step can be accomplished using a thermocycler or by manual cycling; equipment necessary for either procedure is noted at the beginning of the amplification section of each protocol. Section 5.1.2, immediately preceding the protocols, contains a list of equipment and materials, necessary amplification controls, and a standard gel electrophoresis procedure common to all PCR protocols. Any variations and additions to these items as well as all required reagents are noted within each protocol. An inventory of general laboratory equipment and materials to adequately equip a PCR laboratory and recipes for the preparation of common solutions are provided in Appendices B and C. Since the *Taq* polymerase enzyme is central to all PCR protocols, information on obtaining this reagent is also provided in section 5.1.2.

Classical techniques for diagnosis of infectious diseases fall into several categories, and each method has its advantages and limitations. Microscopic examination for morphological identification of pathogenic organisms is rapid and inexpensive but is associated with low sensitivity and specificity. Microbiological techniques that rely on culturing the organism can be specific and sensitive but are often lengthy and are prone to contamination. A variety of serological techniques exist for detection of host antibodies to a particular pathogen, such as Enzyme-Linked Immunoabsorbant Assay (ELISA), Hemagglutination, Immunofluorescent Antibody Test (IFAT), and Western blot. These methods, especially ELISA, are well-suited for screening large numbers of samples but must be properly calibrated to avoid false-negative or false-positive results. In addition, these serological tests are indirect, since they do not detect the pathogen itself but rather an immune response and are thus subject to problems due to antibody cross-reactivity. Antibody-based techniques (ELISA, IFAT) can also detect antigens of the pathogenic microorganism but have limited sensitivity.

PCR-based detection of infectious disease agents is based on the amplification of DNA sequences specific to the particular organism. These techniques can be categorized according to the type of sequence that is targeted:

1. Organism-specific virulence genes, e.g., *Vibrio cholerae, Shigella*, and diarrheagenic *E. coli*.

2. Organism-specific structural genes, e.g., dengue virus.

3. Repetitive chromosomal sequences, e.g., *Leishmania* species, *Mycobacterium tuberculosis, Plasmodium* species, *Trypanosoma cruzi*.

4. Extrachromosomal elements, e.g., *Leishmania* species, *Trypanosoma cruzi, Chlamydia trachomatis, Neisseria gonorrhoeae*.

This section contains detailed protocols for the amplification of each of these types of target sequences in the infectious agents listed above.

PCR assays can also be categorized according to the amount of genetic information obtained from the amplification; in other words, whether the primers are designed to identify the genus, the species, or individual strains. Thus, the PCR technique can serve for (1) detecting the presence of a pathogen at the genus level; (2) characterizing the species, complex, or serotype of the organism in addition to detecting its presence in a given sample; or (3) identifying individual isolates. The protocols that are presented in the following section provide examples of each of these categories. For three infectious agents (*Leishmania, M. tuberculosis*, and *T. cruzi*), two protocols each are provided, one for detection of the organism in clinical samples and one for genetic characterization of the pathogen.

5.1.2   Equipment, Materials, Controls, and Procedures Common to All PCR Protocols

Note 1: A complete inventory for a PCR laboratory is provided in Appendix C. Recipes for common solutions can be found in Appendix B.

Note 2: A beaker with bleach is required in every work area for disposal of used pipet tips and microcentrifuge tubes. The top of the beaker containing the bleach should be covered with a paper towel, which is secured to the perimeter of the beaker with a rubber band. A hole is then made in the center of the paper towel through which the items are disposed of. This prevents the spread of aerosolized DNA that can occur during the process of pipet tip disposal or due to splashing of the contents of the beaker.

Note 3: In several protocols, 1.5-mL screw-cap microcentrifuge tubes with O-rings are called for. These tubes are preferred for boiling samples and for manual amplification, because a tight seal is formed and because there is no risk of the cap exploding from the pressure created as a result of the heating process. However, if such tubes are not available, standard 1.5-mL microcentrifuge tubes may be used, with the precaution that the caps may pop open from pressure at high temperature.

A.   Common Equipment and Materials

I. Sample Preparation in the Grey Area

EQUIPMENT
Refrigerator (4°C)
Freezer (−20°C)
Vortex
Microcentrifuge
Adjustable pipettors (1000 µL, 200 µL, and 20 µL)

MATERIALS
Beaker with bleach
Sterile yellow and blue pipet tips
Sterile 1.5-mL and 0.5-mL microcentrifuge tubes
Plastic racks for microcentrifuge tubes
Timer
Colored laboratory tape
Scissors or razor blade
Paper towels
Permanent markers (indelible ink)
Gloves (disposable latex or vinyl)
Parafilm®
Ice buckets with ice

II. Preparation of PCR Master Mix and Reaction Tubes in the White Area

EQUIPMENT
Microcentrifuge
Pipettors: 1000 µL, 200 µL, and 20 µL; (0.5–10 µL, if possible)

MATERIALS
Sterile yellow and blue pipet tips
Sterile 1.5-mL and 0.5-mL tubes (or 0.2-mL tubes)
Floating rack for microcentrifuge tubes (plastic or Styrofoam)
Plastic racks for microcentrifuge tubes
Timer
Colored laboratory tape
Scissors or razor blade
Paper towels
Permanent markers
Gloves (disposable latex or vinyl)
Ice buckets with ice
Beaker filled with bleach (1.5% sodium hypochlorite final concentration)

III. Amplification in the Black Area

EQUIPMENT
Thermocycler or water baths set at the appropriate temperatures
Microcentrifuge

The amplification profiles in the following protocols are optimized for 0.5-mL tubes, unless otherwise indicated. As mentioned in section 2.2.2, cycling parameters may need to be adjusted when 0.2-mL tubes are used.

B. Amplification Controls

In order to control for potential problems with contamination of PCR reactions (false-positive results) or inhibition of amplification (false-negative results), the following controls should be included in each amplification, in the order listed:

- **"White Area" negative control**—consisting of "white" ddH_2O as a control for the PCR reagents in the White Area.
- **"Grey Area" negative control**—consisting of "grey" ddH_2O as a control for the water and pipettor used for preparation of the DNA or RNA template in the Grey Area.
- **Negative extraction control**—consisting of ddH_2O, used instead of a specimen during the extraction procedure as a control for contamination during the DNA or RNA preparation process.
- **Negative specimen**—as a control for specificity.
- **Interspersed negative control**—consisting of ddH_2O, used as a control every 15 to 20 test samples when analyzing large numbers of samples.
- **Inhibition control**—consisting of a representative sample(s) to which purified DNA or RNA has been added. If this control does not yield the expected product whereas the purified DNA or RNA (positive control) does, this indicates that the sample may be inhibiting the amplification.
- **Positive control**—consisting of purified DNA/RNA or a crude lysate of the organism of interest.
- **"Final" negative control**—consisting of ddH_2O added as the final sample in an amplification run, as a control for the process of sample addition.

C. *Taq Polymerase and PCR*

Taq polymerase can be purchased for research use from the following suppliers: Perkin-Elmer Corp., Boehringer Mannheim, Amersham Corp., Sigma Chemical Co., Pharmacia Biotech, Promega Corp., among others. *Taq* polymerase can also be obtained by using published purification procedures, e.g., Desai et al. (1995); Engelke et al. (1990); Grimm et al. (1995); Pluthero (1993). Note that PCR methods and materials are covered by various U.S. Patents, e.g., U.S. Patent Nos. 4,683,202, 4,683,195, 4,800,159, 4,965,188, 4,889,818, 5,079,352, owned by Hoffman-La Roche Inc., as well as by other patents that may have been issued in countries outside the United States. For information on obtaining licenses to perform PCR for commercial services, the user is advised to contact the Director of Licensing at Roche Molecular Systems, Inc., 1145 Atlantic Ave., Alameda, CA, USA 94501.

D. *Agarose Gel Electrophoresis*

III. Product Analysis: Gel Electrophoresis: Black Area

EQUIPMENT
Microcentrifuge
Balance (for weighing ~1 g)
Microwave or Bunsen burner to melt the agarose
Power supply
UV transilluminator
Camera (preferably Polaroid)
Orange filter
Hood or darkroom
Pipettors (200 µL, 20 µL)

MATERIALS
Gel tray
Gel box
Combs
Erlenmeyer flask (250 mL)
Graduated cyclinders (100 mL, 250 mL, and 1 L)
Weighing paper
Sterile yellow pipet tips
Plastic microcentrifuge tube racks
Colored laboratory tape (or masking tape)
Gloves (disposable latex or vinyl)
Permanent markers
Parafilm®
UV protective eyewear (goggles or face shield)
Polaroid 667 film

REAGENTS
1X TBE (Tris Borate EDTA Running Buffer)
Agarose
Sample loading buffer
Standard DNA size markers
Ethidium bromide (10 mg/mL)

Wear gloves at all times when handling the carcinogen ethidium bromide.

*A. Gel Electrophoresis: **Black Area***

Procedure 1: Gel and Running Buffer containing ethidium bromide (no post-electrophoresis staining step is necessary).

1. For each gel, prepare a solution of 1.5% agarose in 1X TBE and heat it until the agarose melts.
2. Let the solution cool until it reaches ~55°C. Add 10 mg/mL ethidium bromide to a final concentration of 0.5 μg/mL (1/20,000 dilution). Prepare the gel tray with the combs and pour the melted agarose into the tray, moving the bubbles to the sides with a pipet tip.
3. Prepare 1X TBE buffer with ethidium bromide at a final concentration of 0.5 μg/mL.
4. Prepare a Gel Chart showing the order of the samples in the gel.
5. Cover a microcentrifuge tube rack with a piece of Parafilm.® Make shallow wells in the Parafilm over the holes in the rack. With a permanent marker, label the wells with the number of the PCR reactions in the predetermined order.
6. Transfer 2 μL of sample loading buffer to each well in the Parafilm.
7. Transfer 10 μL of each PCR reaction to the appropriately labeled well in the Parafilm and mix with the loading buffer.
8. Prepare 5 μL of the DNA size marker plus 2 μL of loading buffer and 3 μL of distilled water in one well.
9. Place the gel in the gel box and cover it with 1X TBE Running Buffer.
10. Load the entire volume of each sample into the wells in the gel in the predetermined order.
11. Run the gel at ~100 V until the bromophenol blue (dark blue dye) has migrated approximately 70–80% of the length of the gel.

Procedure 2: Gel and Running Buffer without ethidium bromide (post-electrophoresis staining with ethidium bromide). This procedure minimizes the use of the hazardous reagent ethidium bromide and is therefore safer and better for the environment.

1. For each gel, prepare a solution of 1.5% agarose in 1X TBE and heat it until the agarose melts.
2. Let the solution cool until it reaches ~55°C. Prepare the gel tray with the combs and pour the melted agarose into the tray, moving the bubbles to the sides with a pipet tip.
3. Prepare 1X TBE buffer from the 10X stock.

Steps 4 through 11 are as in Procedure 1.

12. After electrophoresis, incubate the gel with gentle rocking for 20–30 minutes in a Staining Solution that consists of distilled water with ethidium bromide at a final concentration of 0.5 μg/mL (1/20,000 dilution of a stock 10 mg/mL solution).
13. Incubate the gel with gentle rocking in distilled water for 15–20 minutes to destain it.

*B. Visualization: **Black Area/Darkroom***

Appropriate eye protection must be worn in the presence of UV light.

1. Place the gel on a UV transilluminator and turn the transilluminator on to visualize the DNA fragments, which should appear orange in color. Expose the gel to UV light for as short a time as possible, since the UV light nicks the DNA, gradually destroying it. UV light is dangerous to the viewer as well.

2. If no camera is available, manually draw the size of the observed bands on the Gel Chart.

3. If a camera is available, take a photograph using the UV transilluminator and the camera with an orange filter. A Polaroid camera with Polaroid 667 film is preferable; first try 1/2 second with an 5.6 or 8 aperture and adjust as necessary. If an instant Polaroid is not available, use a 35-mm camera with standard settings.

4. Dispose of the gel in an ethidium bromide solid waste container.

Note 1: The TBE Running Buffer can be re-used approximately 5–8 times.

Note 2: Since ethidium bromide is light-sensitive, the ethidium bromide stock solution and Staining Solution should be stored in a dark place, in a dark bottle, or covered with aluminum foil.

Note 3: To dispose of the ethidium bromide-containing running buffer or Staining Solution, the solution should be treated with activated charcoal. Briefly, powdered activated charcoal is added to the solution to a final concentration of 1 mg/mL, the solution is incubated for 1 hour at ambient temperature with intermittent shaking and then filtered through a Whatman No. 1 filter. The filtrate can be discarded and the filter and activated charcoal sealed in a plastic bag and placed in the hazardous waste container. Since ethidium bromide decomposes at 262°C, standard incineration procedures should destroy it. For further information, the reader is referred to Sambrook et al. (1989).

5.1.3 Dengue Virus

Clinical Manifestations and Epidemiology

In recent years, dengue viruses have spread alarmingly thoughout Latin America and tropical regions worldwide, with an annual estimate of up to 100 million cases of classic dengue fever (DF) and approximately 250,000 cases of the more severe form of the disease, dengue hemorrhagic fever/dengue shock syndrome (DHF/DSS) (Monath, 1994). Dengue fever is caused by four distinct serotypes of dengue virus, an enveloped single-stranded RNA flavivirus, which is transmitted to humans by the domestic mosquitoes *Aedes aegypti* and *Ae. albopictus*. Classic DF, also known as "breakbone fever," is an acute debilitating febrile illness with rapid onset and symptoms of fever, headache, malaise, retro-orbital and lumbrosacral aching, and joint or bone pain. DF is self-limiting and nonfatal, although it can be associated with prolonged convalescence. DHF/DSS is characterized by hemorrhagic manifestations and concurrent low platelet count and hemoconcentration. In severe cases, circulatory failure and shock may occur, with up to 50% mortality if untreated (Monath, 1994). DHF/DSS is more common in young children, although cases are being reported in adults with greater frequency (Pan American Health Organization [PAHO], 1994). The exact mechanism of DHF/DSS is poorly understood, but it may involve immunopathological processes associated with sequential infections with different dengue serotypes (Halstead, 1988; Morens, 1994). Viral virulence factors as well as genetic and acquired host factors may also be determinants of disease severity. In the human host, dengue virus replicates preferentially within mononuclear phagocytes. Two to seven days after being bitten by an infected mosquito, the host develops high titers of virus in the blood, accompanied by the symptoms of the disease. When antibody titers begin to rise after 5–7 days, viremia decreases and symptoms wane.

Classical Methods of Diagnosis

Classical methods of diagnosis include serological techniques and viral isolation. Serological diagnosis involves the demonstration of a rise in antibody titer in acute and convalescent paired sera using IgM-ELISA, Hemagglutination Inhibition, Plaque Neutralization, or Complement Fixation. However, in endemic countries with limited resources, a single serum sample positive by IgM-ELISA is often recorded as a probable case of dengue, even though WHO guidelines require demonstration of seroconversion for confirmatory diagnosis (PAHO, 1994). The most rapid serological techniques, such as IgM-ELISA with a single sample, do not furnish information about the serotype of the virus, and other methods that allow typing are time-consuming and can be hampered by antibody cross-reactivity. Virological isolation of dengue is commonly achieved by inoculation of mosquito cell lines or intrathoracic inoculation of mosquitoes followed by indirect immunofluorescence for typing. While it is critical to maintain viral stocks for future analysis, virological methods are time-consuming and expensive for routine diagnosis.

PCR-Based Procedures

More recently, molecular approaches based on the detection and characterization of dengue viral RNA have been described. Identification of the four serotypes can be achieved by (1) nested amplification of a primary product generated with universal dengue virus primers (Lanciotti et al., 1992; Meiyu et al., 1997; Yenchitsomanus et al., 1996), (2) simultaneous amplification with four sets of type-specific primers (Morita et al., 1991), or (3) use of a single 5' universal primer and four type-specific 3' primers (Harris et al., 1998b; Lanciotti et al., 1992; Seah et al., 1995), to generate different-sized products for each serotype. Other protocols require hybridization with type-specific probes (Deubel et al., 1990; Henchal et al., 1991; Pierre et al., 1994). RT-PCR can be used to detect dengue viral RNA in clinical samples (Chan et al., 1994; Chungue et al., 1993; Harris et al., 1998b; Henchal et al., 1991; Lanciotti et al., 1992; Morita et al., 1994) or in the mosquito vector (Chungue et al., 1993; Harris et al., 1998b; Lanciotti et al., 1992).

Distinct genetic subgroups (subtypes) have been identified within each dengue serotype by sequence analysis and oligonucleotide fingerprinting, some of which may be associated with more severe epidemics. One technique for subtype identification that does not require sequencing involves RT-PCR amplification of a 2.4 kilobase fragment of the viral genome followed by restriction enzyme digestion and agarose gel electrophoresis (Vorndam et al., 1994); another combines RT-PCR with SSCP analysis (Farfan et al., 1997). A much simpler technique, restriction site specific (RSS)-PCR, is based solely on RT-PCR without the requirement for restriction enzyme analysis or complicated electrophoresis. The results of this simple fingerprinting method correlate with previously defined genetic subgroups (Harris et al., in press).

Points to Consider in Using PCR

RT-PCR of dengue virus is reported to be as sensitive as viral isolation (Chan et al., 1994; Deubel et al., 1990). If implemented using a low-budget approach, RT-PCR compares favorably to viral isolation in cost (approximately US\$1 versus US\$10). The process, from sample extraction through amplification and detection, can be done in 24 hours, as opposed to the 7–14 days required for isolation of the virus. Because of their genetic specificity, nucleic acid-based techniques allow detection and typing of dengue virus in the same procedure. Another advantage is that cases can be diagnosed from a single serum sample in the first days of illness during the viremic stage, whereas serological methods are not effective until antibody levels begin to rise in the second week. When combined with the rapidity of the RT-PCR technique, this early diagnosis allows for the possibility of mounting a rapid response to focus mosquito control measures on locations surrounding confirmed cases in the hope of reducing transmission.

Single-Tube RT-PCR Detection and Typing of Dengue Virus

In this protocol, reverse transcription of dengue viral RNA and amplification of the resulting cDNA are combined and performed in one tube. The use of one 5′ primer, complementary to sequences conserved in all four dengue serotypes and four 3′ primers, each of which hybridizes to sequences specific to each of the four serotypes, allows the detection of all four serotypes simultaneously. The primer sites are designed to generate products of distinct sizes for each serotype, which can be easily distinguished by agarose gel electrophoresis (Lanciotti et al., 1992). In this manner, the dengue virus detection and serotype identification can be achieved in a single tube, starting with viral RNA (Harris et al., 1998b). Two versions of the combined protocol are presented; Version 1 utilizes a labile but effective reverse transcriptase (RAV-2, Amersham Corp.) to convert the viral RNA to cDNA for subsequent amplification with *Taq* polymerase. In Version 2, the bifunctional, thermostable r*Tth* (Perkin-Elmer Corp.) carries out both the reverse transcriptase and polymerase activities. Detailed protocols are provided for extraction of dengue viral RNA from serum or infected cell culture supernatant as well as from infected mosquitoes (Harris et al., 1998b).

I. Sample Preparation: Grey Area

A. Extraction of Dengue Viral RNA from Serum Specimens or Cell Culture Supernatant

ADDITIONAL EQUIPMENT AND MATERIALS
15-mL polypropylene tubes

REAGENTS
Sterile RNase-free ddH$_2$0 (commercial or in-house DEPC-treated ddH$_2$0)
RNA GITC Lysis Buffer (6 M GITC, 50 mM sodium citrate, 1% Sarkosyl, 20 μg/mL tRNA, 100 mM β-mercaptoethanol[1])
2 M sodium acetate, pH 4.0
Water-equilibrated phenol[2]
Chloroform[2]
Isopropanol
75% ethanol (made with RNase-free ddH$_2$0)

1. Calculate the amount of each reagent required for the number of samples to be processed, add approximately 10% extra volume, and aliquot the appropriate amount of each reagent into 15-mL polypropylene tubes or 1.5-mL microcentrifuge tubes.
2. Aliquot 300 μL of supernatant fluid or human serum samples into sterile microcentrifuge tubes (if the sample volume is less than 300 μL, bring the volume to 300 μL with sterile RNase-free ddH$_2$O). Use 300 μL of ddH$_2$O as a negative control. Label the tubes without completely wrapping the tube with tape. Label the top of the tubes as well. Keep the samples on ice.

---

1. The β-mercaptoethanol should be added immediately before use. Therefore, it is recommended to calculate the approximate amount of RNA GITC Lysis Buffer required for the samples to be processed, aliquot this amount to a new tube, and add the appropriate volume of β-mercaptoethanol.
2. Phenol and chloroform waste should be collected in a separate container and transferred to the organic waste container stored in the chemical fume hood.

Between manipulation of each sample, clean the tip of the pipet barrel with a paper towel soaked in bleach and dry thoroughly with a clean paper towel.

3. To each sample, add 300 μL (equal volume) of RNA GITC Lysis Buffer at ambient temperature. Mix by inversion and keep tubes at ambient temperature.
4. Sequentially add the following reagents to each tube and mix by inversion *after each addition*:
   60 μL 2 *M* sodium acetate, pH 4.0 (1/10 volume of the sample plus lysis buffer)
   600 μL water-equilibrated phenol
   240 μL chloroform
5. Centrifuge the tubes at 12,000g for 15 minutes in a microcentrifuge at ambient temperature.
6. Transfer the aqueous upper phase to a new tube and place on ice. Clean the tip of the pipet barrel between each sample. Discard the organic lower phase into the organic waste.
7. Add an equal volume of isopropanol (approximately 600 μL) and mix by inversion.
8. Centrifuge the tubes at 12,000g for 15 minutes at 4°C, with the hinge between the tube and the cap pointing outward.
9. Remove the supernatant, being very careful not to lose the tiny pellet. First use a 1000-μL pipettor with a blue tip to remove most of the supernatant, followed by a 200-μL pipettor with a yellow tip to remove the remaining liquid.
10. Add 500 μL of 75% ethanol (must be made with RNase-free ddH$_2$O) to the RNA pellet.
11. Centrifuge the tubes at 12,000g for 10 minutes at 4°C.
12. Remove the supernatant, being very careful not to lose the pellet, which may become detached from the wall of the tube.
13. Air-dry the pellet for 10 minutes in a horizontal position.
14. Resuspend the pellet in 20 μL of sterile RNase-free ddH$_2$O.
15. Store the RNA at $-70°C$ (or $-20°C$ if a $-70°C$ freezer is not available).

B. Extraction of Dengue Viral RNA from Mosquitoes

ADDITIONAL EQUIPMENT AND MATERIALS
Water bath at 50–55°C
Handmade "pestles" to grind up the mosquitoes (prepared by heating blue pipet tips and molding them to the shape of an Eppendorf tube; these work best with a fairly small smooth tip)
or blue plastic pestles with hand-held motor (Kontes #K749540–0000)

REAGENTS
PBS (10X)
RNA GITC buffer (*see* Appendix B)
Phenol[3] (water-saturated)
Chloroform[3]
2 *M* sodium acetate, pH 4.0
Sodium-ethanol wash (50% EtOH, 10 m*M* Tris pH 7.4, 1 m*M* EDTA, 50 m*M* NaCl in RNase-free ddH$_2$O)
Silica particles (*see* Appendix B)
RNase-free ddH$_2$O

---

3. Phenol and chloroform waste should be collected in a separate container and transferred to the organic waste container stored in the chemical fume hood.

1. Label four sets of 1.5-mL microcentrifuge tubes; mark the level of 100 μL on the first three sets.

Perform steps 2–10 on ice.

2. Aliquot mosquitoes into the tubes and *keep on ice*.
3. Centrifuge the tubes for 15 seconds in a microcentrifuge to collect the mosquitoes at the bottom of the tubes.
4. Compress and macerate the mosquitoes using a 1000-μL pipettor with a homemade "blue tip pestle" or with sterile plastic pestles and hand-held motor. As a positive control, add 10 μL of dengue-infected cell culture supernatant to one tube of mosquitoes.
5. Add ice-cold 1X PBS to 100 μL and continue to macerate the mosquitoes in PBS *on ice* until the bodies are fully mashed.
6. Centrifuge the tubes for 30–60 seconds at 4°C in a microcentrifuge at 12,000g.
7. Transfer the supernatant to a fresh labeled tube and centrifuge again for 30–60 seconds at 4°C at 12,000g.
8. Transfer the supernatant to a fresh labeled tube.
9. Add 1X PBS so that the samples contain 100-μL total volume and place the tubes on ice.
10. If needed, remove a 10-μL aliquot for plaque assays at this time. Store this aliquot at −70°C if it is not used immediately.
11. Add 100 μL of RNA GITC lysis buffer (with β-mercaptoethanol added to a final concentration of 100 m*M* immediately before use).
12. Add 200 μL of water-saturated phenol and vortex thoroughly.
13. Add 20 μL of 2 *M* sodium acetate (1/10 volume of the aqueous phase).
14. Add 200 μL of chloroform and vortex thoroughly.
15. Centrifuge the tubes for 10 min at 12,000g.
16. Transfer the aqueous upper phase to a fresh tube and place on ice. A second extraction with 200 μL of chloroform (steps 14–16) is optional.
17. Add 5 μL of fully resuspended silica particle suspension.
18. Mix well and incubate for 5 minutes at ambient temperature or on ice, mixing every 1–2 minutes by inversion.
19. Centrifuge the tubes for 1 minute.
20. Pipet off and discard the supernatant, taking care not to remove the silica particles.
21. Add 100 μL of sodium-ethanol wash and resuspend completely, using the point of the pipet tip to break up the pellet if necessary.
22. Centrifuge for 5–10 seconds only and discard the supernatant.
23. Repeat steps 21 and 22.
24. Resuspend the pellet in 15 μL of RNase-free ddH$_2$O.
25. Incubate the tubes at 50–55°C for 5 minutes to elute the RNA from the silica particles.
26. Use 2.5 μL of the fully resuspended slurry for each PCR reaction.

II. Amplification

*A. Preparation of PCR Master Mix and Reaction Tubes: **White Area***

Version 1: Reverse Transcription (RAV-2) and Amplification (*Taq* polymerase)

REAGENTS
10X Dengue RT-PCR Buffer (500 m*M* KCl, 100 m*M* Tris [pH 8.5], 15 m*M* MgCl$_2$, 0.1% gelatin)
dNTPs (5 m*M* each dATP, dCTP, dGTP, dTTP; 20 m*M* total dNTPs)
Primers (10 μ*M*):
    D1:   5′-TCA ATA TGC TGA AAC GCG CGA GAA ACC G

TS1:   5'-CGT CTC AGT TGA TCC GGG GG
TS2:   5'-CGC CAC AAG GGC CAT GAA CAG
TS3:   5'-TAA CAT CAT CAT GAG ACA GAG C
DEN4: 5'-TGT TGT CTT AAA CAA GAG AGG TC

ddH$_2$0
Taq polymerase (5 U/µL)
DTT (100 m*M*)
Reverse transcriptase RAV-2 (Amersham Corp.)
RAV-2 reverse transcriptase storage buffer (*see* Appendix B)
Tetramethylammonium chloride (TMAC; 1 *M*)
Betaine (4 *M*; Sigma Chemical Co., B-2629)
Mineral oil
Positive control (dengue viral RNA from serotypes 1–4)

Note: Before preparing the PCR Master Mix, go to the **Black Area** to enter the appropriate program in the thermocycler. If the program has already been entered, review it to ensure no changes have been inadvertently introduced; if so, correct the program and store it for later use. If the PCR will be manually amplified, prepare three water baths at the following temperatures: 42°C, 55°C, 72°C, and 94°C, and ensure that these temperatures are stably maintained.

1. Calculate the amount of PCR Master Mix that will be necessary for the desired number of reactions, each containing 20 µL of Master Mix. For every 10 reactions, add 1 extra volume of Master Mix to compensate for volume lost during pipetting.
2. Fill out the PCR Worksheet according to the following table.

3.

Ingredient	Description	Stock conc.	Vol/25 µL rxn	Final conc.
Buffer 10X	Dengue RT-PCR	10X	2.5 µL	1X
dNTPs	20 m*M* total dNTPs	5 m*M* A,C,G,T	1.0 µL	0.2 m*M* A,C,G,T
Primer 1	D1	10 µ*M*	2.5 µL	1.0 µ*M*
Primer 2	TS1	10 µ*M*	2.5 µL	1.0 µ*M*
Primer 3	TS2	10 µ*M*	1.25 µL	0.5 µ*M*
Primer 4	TS3	10 µ*M*	1.25 µL	0.5 µ*M*
Primer 5	DEN4	10 µ*M*	1.25 µL	0.5 µ*M*
DTT		100 m*M*	1.25 µL	5 m*M*
TMAC[4]		1 *M*	0.75 µL	30 m*M*
Betaine[4]		4 *M*	3.125 µL	0.5 M
ddH$_2$0	RNase-free ddH$_2$O		2.375 µL	
Taq	*Taq*	5 U/µL	0.125 µL	0.025 U/µL
Reverse Transcriptase	RAV-2[5]	0.3–5 U/µL	0.125 µL	0.025 U/µL

Vol. of Master Mix	20 µL
Vol. of sample (to be added in step 13)	5 µL
Total reaction volume	25 µL

4. TMAC and betaine are not essential, but they improve the sensitivity of the assay.
5. The concentration of the RAV-2 reverse transcriptase varies with each lot and is indicated on each tube (usually 10–25 U/µL). Due to the high concentration of enzyme, each RT-PCR amplification requires minute volumes that are difficult to manipulate accurately. Therefore, it is advisable to prepare a working stock of 1–5 U/µL, to be used within several weeks. To prepare this stock, the enzyme should be diluted in storage buffer (*see* Appendix B).

4. Label the appropriate tubes (0.5-mL or 0.2-mL tubes for thermocyclers; 1.5-mL screw-cap tubes for manual amplification).
5. Thaw aliquot(s) of each reagent. Vortex each thawed solution well and briefly spin the tubes (pulse spin) in a microcentrifuge to collect all the liquid at the bottom of the tubes.

Keep all the ingredients and tubes on ice at all times.

6. In the **White Area**, using a **white** color-coded pipettor, prepare the PCR Master Mix with all the ingredients except the *Taq* polymerase and the reverse transcriptase. Check off each ingredient on the Worksheet after adding it to the Master Mix.
7. Mix well using a vortex or a large pipettor.
8. Add both of the enzymes and mix by pipetting carefully with a pipettor set at half the total volume of the PCR Master Mix. Be careful not to create bubbles.
9. Distribute 20 μL of the PCR Master Mix into each labeled tube.
10. Add 1 drop of mineral oil to each tube using a 1000-μL pipettor.
11. Add 5 μL of ddH$_2$O to prepare a "white area" negative control across the layer of mineral oil.
12. Transfer the tubes from the **white** ice bucket to a **grey** ice bucket.

Version 2: Reverse Transcription and Amplification (r*Tth*)

REAGENTS

10X Dengue r*Tth* Buffer (115 m*M* potassium acetate, 8% glycerol, 50 m*M* bicine [pH 8.2])
dNTPs (5 m*M* each dATP, dCTP, dGTP, dTTP; 20 m*M* total dNTPs)
Primers (10 μ*M*):

D1:   5'-TCA ATA TGC TGA AAC GCG CGA GAA ACC G
TS1:   5'-CGT CTC AGT TGA TCC GGG GG
TS2:   5'-CGC CAC AAG GGC CAT GAA CAG
TS3:   5'-TAA CAT CAT CAT GAG ACA GAG C
DEN4: 5'-TGT TGT CTT AAA CAA GAG AGG TC

ddH$_2$0
r*Tth* reverse transcriptase-polymerase (2.5 U/μL; Perkin-Elmer Corp.)
Manganese acetate (25 m*M*)
Mineral oil
Positive control (dengue viral RNA from serotypes 1–4)

Note: Before preparing the PCR Master Mix, go to the **Black Area** to enter the appropriate program in the thermocycler. If the program has already been entered, review it to ensure no changes have been inadvertently introduced; if so, correct the program and store it for later use. If the PCR will be manually amplified, prepare three water baths at the following temperatures: 50°C, 60°C, and 94°C, and ensure that these temperatures are stably maintained.

1. Calculate the amount of PCR Master Mix that will be necessary for the desired number of reactions, each containing 20 μL of Master Mix. For every 10 reactions, add 1 extra volume of Master Mix to compensate for volume lost during pipetting.
2. Fill out the PCR Worksheet according to the following table.

3.

Ingredient	Description	Stock conc.	Vol/25 µL rxn	Final conc.
Buffer 10X	Dengue r*Tth*	5X	5 µL	1X
dNTPs	20 m*M* total dNTPs	5 m*M* A,C,G,T	1.0 µL	0.2 m*M* A,C,G,T
Primer 1	D1	10 µ*M*	1.25 µL	0.5 µ*M*
Primer 2	TS1	10 µ*M*	1.25 µL	0.5 µ*M*
Primer 3	TS2	10 µ*M*	0.625 µL	0.25 µ*M*
Primer 4	TS3	10 µ*M*	0.625 µL	0.25 µ*M*
Primer 5	DEN4	10 µ*M*	0.625 µL	0.25 µ*M*
Mn(OAc)$_2$	Manganese acetate	25 m*M*	21 µL	2 µ*M*
ddH$_2$0	RNase-free ddH$_2$O		7.125 µL	
r*Tth*	r*Tth*	2.5 U/µL	0.5 µL	0.05 U/µL

Vol. of Master Mix	20 µL
Vol. of sample (to be added in step 13)	5 µL
Total reaction volume	25 µL

4. Label the appropriate tubes (0.5-mL or 0.2-mL tubes for thermocyclers; 1.5-mL screw-cap tubes for manual amplification).
5. Thaw aliquot(s) of each reagent. Vortex each thawed solution well and briefly spin the tubes (pulse spin) in a microcentrifuge to collect all the liquid at the bottom of the tubes.

Keep all the ingredients and tubes on ice at all times.

6. In the **White Area**, using a **white** color-coded pipettor, prepare the PCR Master Mix with all the ingredients except the *Taq* polymerase and the reverse transcriptase. Check off each ingredient on the Worksheet after adding it to the Master Mix.
7. Mix well using a vortex or a large pipettor.
8. Add both of the enzymes and mix by pipetting carefully with a pipettor set at half the total volume of the PCR Master Mix. Be careful not to create bubbles.
9. Distribute 20 µL of the PCR Master Mix into each labeled tube.
10. Add 1 drop of mineral oil to each tube using a 1000-µL pipettor.
11. Add 5 µL of ddH$_2$O to prepare a "white area" negative control across the layer of mineral oil.
12. Transfer the tubes from the **white** ice bucket to a **grey** ice bucket.

*B. Sample Addition: **Grey Area***

13. In the **Grey Area**, using a **grey** color-coded pipettor, add 5 µL of the sample[6] or control to the appropriate tube, *across* the layer of mineral oil. The controls should be added in the order of the most negative to the most positive. Use a new pipet tip for each sample. Remember to include a negative control consisting of the Grey Area water.

Between manipulation of each sample, clean the tip of the pipet barrel with a paper towel soaked in bleach and dry thoroughly with a clean paper towel.

---

6. When analyzing clinical specimens, 5 µL of each sample should be used as template; however, when amplifying purified DNA or lysates of cultured strains, 1–2.5 µL is sufficient template for each PCR reaction. In the latter case, the volume can be adjusted to 5 µL with ddH$_2$O.

*C. Amplification Procedure: **Black Area***

EQUIPMENT
Thermocycler
Microcentrifuge

14. Amplification profile: Version 1 (RAV-2 reverse transcriptase + *Taq* polymerase)

42°C	1 hour	1 cycle	Reverse transcription

94°C	30 sec		
55°C	1 min	40 cycles	Amplification
72°C	2 min		

72°C	5 min	1 cycle	Final extension

Amplification profile: Version 2 (r*Tth* reverse transcriptase-polymerase)

60°C	30 min	1 cycle	Reverse transcription

94°C	2 min	1 cycle	Initial denaturation

94°C	45 sec		
50°C	1 min	40 cycles	Amplification
60°C	1 min		

60°C	7 min	1 cycle	Final extension

Product sizes: Both versions of the RT-PCR protocol generate a 482-bp dengue-1-specific product (D1–TS1), a 119-bp dengue-2-specific product (D1–TS2), a 290-bp dengue-3-specific product (D1–TS3), and a 389-bp dengue-4-specific product (D1–DEN4) (Figure 5.1).

III. Product Analysis

Use a 1.5% agarose gel and the procedure in section 5.1.2.

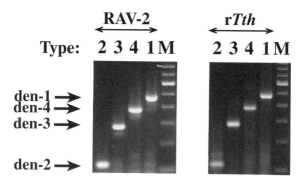

Fig. 5.1. Detection and typing of dengue virus using two versions of the RT-PCR assay followed by gel electrophoresis. *Left panel*, reverse transcription using RAV-2 reverse transcriptase and amplification with *Taq* DNA polymerase. *Right panel*, reverse transcriptase and amplification using the bifunctional enzyme r*Tth*. Dengue serotypes as indicated; M, 100-bp ladder (*see* Appendix C; lowest band shown, 100 bp). Expected product sizes: dengue-2, 119 bp; dengue-3, 290 bp; dengue-4, 389 bp; dengue-1, 482 bp.

5.1.4   New World *Leishmania*

Clinical Manifestations and Epidemiology

Leishmaniasis is an important public health problem in tropical and subtropical countries worldwide, involving 400,000 new cases annually, with 12 million people infected and 350 million at risk (Ashford et al., 1992). It is a zoonosis caused by the transmission of the kinetoplastid parasite *Leishmania* to accidental human hosts by certain species of sandflies. In the Americas, human leishmaniasis occurs from Mexico to Argentina and is caused by 13 distinct species grouped into three complexes. These New World *Leishmania* produce several forms of disease, depending on the species of the parasite, the immune status of the host, and possibly factors deriving from its sandfly vector. Symptoms range from self-curing cutaneous lesions (*L. mexicana* complex), to persistent and disfiguring cutaneous and mucocutaneous manifestations (*L. braziliensis* complex), to the potentially fatal visceral disease (*L. chagasi*, of the *L. donovani* complex) (Grimaldi and Tesh, 1993). In addition, atypical infections have been reported, which constitute exceptions to these rules (Barral et al., 1986, 1991; Belli et al., submitted for publication; Hernandez et al., 1991; Ponce et al., 1991).

Classical Methods of Diagnosis

Microscopic examination of skin scrapings of cutaneous leishmanial lesions, though rapid and low-cost, has limited sensitivity and is not adequate for species identification due to the morphological similarity of the different species (Neva and Sacks, 1990). In vitro culture techniques, while more sensitive, are susceptible to microbiological contamination and are hampered by the particular growth requirements of different strains of *Leishmania*; in addition, since certain strains grow better than others in vitro, "dominant" strains can be inadvertently selected when culturing mixed infections (Armijos et al., 1990). The Montenegro skin test detects specific cutaneous delayed-type hypersensitivity but cannot distinguish between current and past infection. Serological diagnostic techniques present drawbacks that include the cross-reactivity of leishmanial antigens with antibodies induced by other kinetoplastids, such as *Trypanosoma cruzi* (Badaro et al., 1986; Camargo and Rebonato, 1969), as well as poor sensitivity due to the low antibody titer characteristic of cutaneous leishmaniasis (Grimaldi and Tesh, 1993).

   Species identification has been conventionally achieved using isoenzyme electrophoresis (zymodeme analysis)[7] (Kreutzer and Christensen, 1980), immunological approaches using monoclonal antibodies (serodeme analysis) (Grimaldi et al., 1987), and classical molecular biological techniques involving restriction analysis of kinetoplast DNA (schizodeme analysis). Zymodeme and schizodeme analyses involve lengthy, complicated, and expensive procedures that require large-scale cultivation

---

7. Certain enzymes have different isoforms in different species of parasites, and this polymorphism can
    be exploited to differentiate species based on variations in the electrophoretic mobility of these
    enzymes.

of parasites and a sophisticated laboratory setting. While certain monoclonal anti-bodies appear promising for species identification by serodeme analysis, the reactivity patterns of some species vary significantly depending on the geographical origin of the parasites (Grimaldi and McMahon-Pratt, 1996).

PCR-Based Procedures

A number of PCR assays have been described for identification of *Leishmania* at the genus level (Bhattacharyya et al., 1996; Mathis and Deplazes, 1995; Rodgers et al., 1990) and for characterization of individual complexes of *L. braziliensis* (de Brujin and Barker, 1992; Guevara et al., 1992; López et al., 1993; Meredith et al., 1993), *L. mexicana* (Eresh et al., 1994; Meredith et al., 1993), or *L. donovani* (Costa et al., 1996; Hassan et al., 1993; Meredith et al., 1993; Ravel et al., 1995; Smyth et al., 1992). One method allows the single-step identification of all three New World complexes by generating different-sized fragments for each complex (Harris et al., 1998a). Random amplified polymorphic DNA (RAPD) analysis has been reported for species-level identification of *Leishmania* but requires highly standardized conditions and results in a much lower sensitivity than standard PCR (Noyes et al., 1996). Other molecular biological approaches involve identification of the *Leishmania* complexes by PCR coupled with DNA probe hybridization (Bozza et al., 1995; Nuzum et al., 1995; Qiao et al., 1995; Ramos et al., 1996; Uliana et al., 1994), restriction enzyme analysis, or single-strand conformation polymorphism (SSCP) (van Eys et al., 1992). DNA probes have been developed for speciation of *Leishmania*, but they are substantially more time-consuming and less sensitive than PCR amplification (Wilson, 1995).

Points to Consider in Using PCR

Confirmation of diagnosis by identification of the parasite is critical because of the potential for misdiagnosis and because the treatment for leishmaniasis is expensive, lengthy, and can induce toxic side effects.[8] It is also important to identify the species of *Leishmania* for both clinical and epidemiological purposes. Both detection and characterization of the parasite can be accomplished simultaneously using PCR. This is particularly useful for the investigation of atypical *Leishmania* infections, such as atypical cutaneous leishmaniasis (ACL) caused by *L. chagasi* in Central America (Ponce et al., 1991; Belli et al., submitted for publication). In addition, the sensitivity of PCR allows detection of *Leishmania* in less-invasive samples. For example, dermal scrapings are sufficient for diagnosis of cutaneous leishmaniasis, instead of punch biopsies (Belli et al., 1998) (Figures 5.2 and 5.3), and venous blood is an adequate specimen for PCR diagnosis of visceral disease, instead of a bone marrow sample (Adhya et al., 1995; Nuzum et al., 1995; Ravel et al., 1995). PCR can also be applied to the identification of *Leishmania* in sandflies and animal reservoirs to obtain important epidemiological information for design of control measures.

---

8. The commonly prescribed antimony-based treatments (e.g., Glucantime® or Penstostam®) can induce cardiologic and hepatic complications.

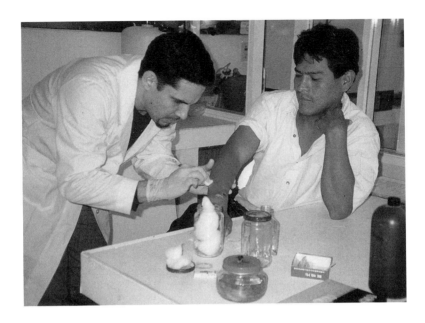

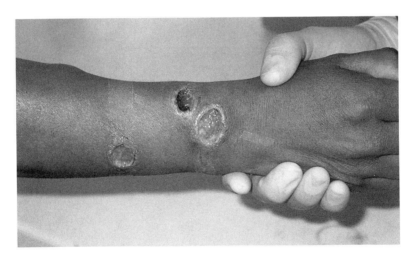

Fig. 5.2. *Top*, Alejandro Belli cleaning the area around presumptive leishmanial lesions on the arm of a Bolivian patient. *Bottom*, lesions characteristic of cutaneous leishmaniasis caused by *L. braziliensis*.

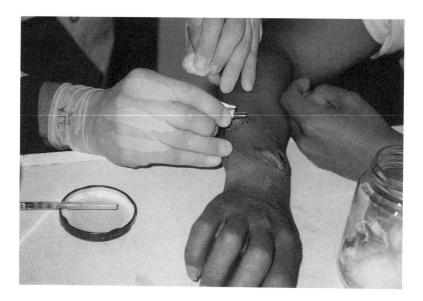

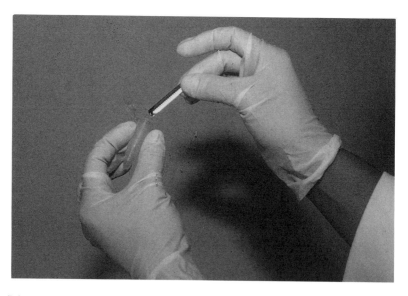

Fig. 5.3. *Top*, taking a dermal scraping from the border of the lesion using a sterile lancet. *Bottom*, transferring the lesion scraping from the lancet to a sterile microcentrifuge tube containing 5% Chelex® 100 prior to boiling.

PCR Detection of the *Leishmania braziliensis* Complex

This amplification protocol, adapted from López et al. (1993), uses a single pair of primers to amplify a 70-bp product from the kinetoplast DNA (kDNA) minicircles of members of the New World *Leishmania braziliensis* complex. Since there are approximately 10,000 copies of these minicircles per parasite, this PCR amplification is very sensitive and can be used to reliably detect parasites directly from clinical samples (Belli et al., 1998).

I. Sample Preparation: Grey Area

ADDITIONAL EQUIPMENT AND MATERIALS
Boiling water bath (100°C)
Sterile Pasteur pipets and bulbs
Sterile wooden toothpicks or sterile lancets
Sterile 1.5-mL screw-cap microcentrifuge tubes
Cotton balls

REAGENTS
Sterile ddH$_2$0 (double-distilled water)
5% Chelex® 100 (Bio-Rad Laboratories, #143–2832) in ddH$_2$0 or
Sterile Tris-EDTA (TE; 10 mM Tris-HCl [pH 8.0], 1 mM EDTA)
70% ethanol
Leishmania cultures

A. Lysis of Parasite Cultures

1. Label sterile 1.5-mL screw-cap microcentrifuge tubes by writing the appropriate number on the tube *and* on the cap with a permanent marker.
2. Transfer 200 μL of sterile ddH$_2$0 to each labeled tube.
3. Using a sterile Pasteur pipet, transfer two drops of the *Leishmania* culture to the appropriately labeled tube containing 200 μL of sterile ddH$_2$0. Remember to include a negative control for the lysis procedure, which consists of 2 drops of ddH$_2$0 added to an appropriately labeled tube containing 200 μL of sterile ddH$_2$0, as above.
4. Incubate the tubes at 100°C in the boiling water bath for 5 minutes using a floating rack.
5. Centrifuge the tubes for 2 minutes in a microcentrifuge at ambient temperature.
6. Transfer the supernatant to a sterile microcentrifuge tube. Proceed directly to the Amplification step or store the tubes at −20°C until further use. If the supernatant is not promptly transferred to a new tube, be sure to repeat the centrifugation in step 5 after thawing the samples and before proceeding to the Amplification.
7. Use 5 μL of the supernatant for PCR amplification.

B. Collection and Preparation of Skin Scrapings from Cutaneous Lesions

1. Prepare 1.5-mL centrifuge tubes containing 100 μL of 5% Chelex® 100 or 100 μL of TE buffer (chelating agent).
2. Clean the area around the lesion with 70% ethanol and, using a sterile wooden toothpick or a sterile lancet, take a skin scraping from the border of the presumptive leishmanial lesion. Probe deeply below the surface layer so as to obtain material that includes tissue and not only dead skin cells.

3. Immerse the toothpick or lancet tip in the Chelex or TE solution and agitate it so as to dislodge the lesion material into the solution.
4. Incubate the tubes at 100°C in the boiling water bath for 10 minutes using a floating rack.
5. Centrifuge the tubes for 2 minutes in a microcentrifuge at ambient temperature.
6. Transfer the supernatant to a sterile microcentrifuge tube. Proceed directly to the Amplification step or store the tubes at $-20°C$ until further use. If the supernatant is not promptly transferred to a new tube, be sure to repeat the centrifugation in step 5 after thawing the samples and before proceeding to the Amplification.
7. Use 5 μL of the supernatant for PCR amplification.

II. Amplification

A. Preparation of PCR Master Mix and Reaction Tubes: **White Area**

REAGENTS
10X Buffer B (100 mM Tris [pH 8.3], 500 mM KCl)
dNTPs (5 mM each dATP, dCTP, dGTP, dTTP; 20 mM total dNTPs)
Primers (10 μM)
  MP1L: 5'-TAC TCC CCG ACA TGC CTC TG
  MP3H: 5'-GAA CGG GGT TTC TGT ATG C
MgCl$_2$ (25 mM)
Dithiothreitol (DTT; 100 mM)
ddH$_2$0
Taq polymerase (5 U/μL)
Mineral oil
Positive control (purified *Leishmania* DNA or boiled lysate of reference parasites)

Note: Before preparing the PCR Master Mix, go to the **Black Area** to enter the appropriate program in the thermocycler. If the program has already been entered, review it to ensure no changes have been inadvertently introduced; if so, correct the program and store it for later use. If the PCR will be manually amplified, prepare three water baths at the following temperatures: 54°C, 72°C, and 94°C, and ensure that these temperatures are stably maintained.

1. Calculate the amount of PCR Master Mix that will be necessary for the desired number of reactions, each containing 20 μL of Master Mix. For every 10 reactions, add 1 extra volume of Master Mix to compensate for volume lost during pipetting.
2. Fill out the PCR Worksheet according to the following table.
3.

Ingredient	Description	Stock conc.	Vol/25 μL rxn	Final conc.
Buffer 10X	Buffer B	10X	2.5 μL	1X
dNTPs	20 mM total dNTPs	5 mM A,C,G,T	1.0 μL	0.2 mM A,C,G,T
Primer 1	MP1L	10 μM	2.5 μL	1.0 μM
Primer 2	MP3H	10 μM	2.5 μL	1.0 μM
MgCl$_2$		25 mM	2.0 μL	2.0 mM
DTT		100 mM	0.25 μL	1 mM
H$_2$0	ddH$_2$0		9.125 μL	
Taq	*Taq*	5 U/μL	0.125 μL	0.025 U/μL
Vol. of Master Mix			20 μL	
Vol. of sample (to be added in step 13)			5 μL	
Total reaction volume			25 μL	

4. Label the appropriate tubes (0.5-mL or 0.2-mL tubes for thermocyclers; 1.5-mL screw-cap tubes for manual amplification).

5. Thaw aliquot(s) of each reagent. Vortex each thawed solution well and briefly spin the tubes (pulse spin) in a microcentrifuge to collect all the liquid at the bottom of the tubes.

Keep all the ingredients and tubes on ice at all times.

6. In the **White Area**, using a **white** color-coded pipettor, prepare the PCR Master Mix with all the ingredients except the *Taq* polymerase. Check off each ingredient on the Worksheet after adding it to the Master Mix.
7. Mix well using a vortex or a large pipettor.
8. Add the *Taq* polymerase and mix by pipetting carefully with a pipettor set at half the total volume of the PCR Master Mix. Be careful not to create bubbles.
9. Distribute 20 µL of the PCR Master Mix into each labeled tube.
10. Add 1 drop of mineral oil to each tube using a 1000-µL pipettor.
11. Add 5 µL of ddH$_2$O to prepare a "white area" negative control across the layer of mineral oil.
12. Transfer the tubes from the **white** ice bucket to a **grey** ice bucket.

B. Sample Addition: **Grey Area**

13. In the **Grey Area**, using a **grey** color-coded pipettor, add 5 µL of the sample[9] or control to the appropriate tube, *across* the layer of mineral oil. The controls should be added in the order of the most negative to the most positive. Use a new pipet tip for each sample. Remember to include a negative control consisting of the Grey Area water.

C. Amplification Procedure: **Black Area**

EQUIPMENT
Thermocycler or water baths at 54°C, 72°C, and 94°C
Microcentrifuge

14. Amplification profile:

94°C	3 min	1 cycle	Initial denaturation
94°C	1 min		
54°C	1 min	35 cycles	Amplification
72°C	1 min		
72°C	2 min	1 cycle	Final extension

Product size: A 70-bp fragment is generated from the kDNA minicircles of members of only the *L. braziliensis* complex (Figure 5.4).

III. Product Analysis

Use a 1.8% agarose gel and the procedure in section 5.1.2.

---

9. When analyzing clinical specimens, 5 µL of each sample should be used as template; however, when amplifying purified DNA or lysates of cultured strains, 1–2.5 µL is sufficient template for each PCR reaction. In the latter case, the volume can be adjusted to 5 µL with ddH$_2$O.

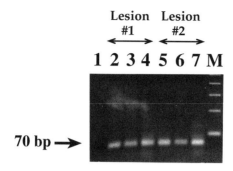

Fig. 5.4. Amplification of *Leishmania braziliensis* kDNA in clinical specimens. Dermal scrapings were taken from the border of leishmanial lesions with a sterile toothpick, placed in 200 µL Tris-EDTA buffer, and boiled for 10 minutes prior to amplification. Products were analyzed by gel electrophoresis. Lane 1, negative control (water); lanes 2 and 5, extract plus purified *L. braziliensis* DNA (inhibition control); lanes 3 and 6, undiluted extract; lanes 4 and 7, extract diluted five-fold; lane M, 100-bp ladder (*see* Appendix C; lowest band shown, 100 bp).

Multiplex PCR Characterization of New World *Leishmania* Complexes

This amplification protocol can be used to identify all three complexes of New World *Leishmania* (*L. mexicana*, *L. braziliensis*, and *L. donovani*) in a single reaction by generating different-sized products for each complex (Harris et al., 1998a). This is achieved by using four primers in the same reaction: one 5′ primer, complementary to a sequence conserved in all *Leishmania* species, and three distinct 3′ primers, specific to a variable region in each of the three New World *Leishmania* complexes. The target sequence is the spliced leader RNA (or mini-exon) gene repeat, with 200–400 copies per parasite genome, which contains a highly conserved transcribed region and a nontranscribed region that is variable in both sequence and size.

I. Sample Preparation: Grey Area

ADDITIONAL EQUIPMENT AND MATERIALS
Boiling water bath (100°C)
Sterile Pasteur pipets and bulbs
Sterile wooden toothpicks or sterile lancets
Sterile 1.5-mL screw-cap microcentrifuge tubes
Cotton balls

REAGENTS
Sterile ddH$_2$0 (double-distilled water)
5% Chelex® 100 (Bio-Rad Laboratories) in ddH$_2$0 or
Sterile Tris-EDTA (TE; 10 m*M* Tris-HCl [pH 8.0], 1 m*M* EDTA)
70% ethanol
Leishmania cultures

A. Lysis of Parasite Cultures

1. Label sterile 1.5-mL screw-cap microcentrifuge tubes by writing the appropriate number on the tube *and* on the cap with a permanent marker.
2. Transfer 200 µL of sterile ddH$_2$0 to each labeled tube.
3. Using a sterile Pasteur pipet, transfer two drops of the *Leishmania* culture to the appropriately labeled tube containing 200 µL of sterile ddH$_2$0. Remember to include a negative control for the lysis procedure, which consists 2 drops of ddH$_2$0 added to an appropriately labeled tube containing 200 µL of sterile ddH$_2$0, as above.
4. Incubate the tubes at 100°C in the boiling water bath for 5 minutes, using a floating rack.
5. Centrifuge the tubes for 2 minutes in a microcentrifuge at ambient temperature.
6. Transfer the supernatant to a sterile microcentrifuge tube. Proceed directly to the Amplification step or store the tubes at −20°C until further use. If the supernatant is not promptly transferred to a new tube, be sure to repeat the centrifugation in step 5 after thawing the samples and before proceeding to the Amplification.
7. Use 5 µL of the supernatant for PCR amplification.

B. Collection and Preparation of Skin Scrapings from Cutaneous Lesions

1. Prepare 1.5-mL centrifuge tubes containing 100 µL of 5% Chelex® 100 or 100 µL of TE buffer.
2. Clean the area around the lesion with 70% ethanol and, using a sterile wooden toothpick or a sterile lancet, take a skin scraping from the border of the presumptive leish-

manial lesion. Probe deeply below the surface layer so as to obtain material that includes tissue and not only dead skin cells.

3. Immerse the toothpick or lancet tip in the Chelex or TE solution and agitate it so as to dislodge the lesion material into the solution.
4. Incubate the tubes at 100°C in the boiling water bath for 10 minutes using a floating rack.
5. Centrifuge the tubes for 2 minutes in a microcentrifuge at ambient temperature.
6. Transfer the supernatant to a sterile microcentrifuge tube. Proceed directly to the Amplification step or store the tubes at −20°C until further use. If the supernatant is not promptly transferred to a new tube, be sure to repeat the centrifugation in step 5 after thawing the samples and before proceeding to the Amplification.
7. Use 5 μL of the supernatant for PCR amplification.

II. Amplification

A. *Preparation of PCR Master Mix and Reaction Tubes:* **White Area**

REAGENTS

10X Buffer B (100 mM Tris [pH 8.3], 500 mM KCl)
dNTPs (5 mM each dATP, dCTP, dGTP, dTTP; 20 mM total dNTPs)
Primers (10 μM)
  LU-5A: 5′-TTT ATT GGT ATG CGA AAC TTC
  LB-3C: 5′-CGT SCC GAA CCC CGT GTC (where S = C/G)
  LM-3A-17: 5′-GCA CCG CAC CGG RCC AC (where R = A/G)
  LC-3L-19: 5′- GCC CGC GYG TCA CCA CCA T (where Y = C/T)
MgCl$_2$ (25 mM)
Dithiothreitol (DTT; 100 mM)
Dimethyl sulfoxide (DMSO)
Tetramethylammonium chloride (TMAC; 1 M)
Betaine (4 M; Sigma Chemical Co., B-2629)
ddH$_2$0
Taq polymerase (5 U/μL)
Mineral oil
Positive control (purified *Leishmania* DNA or boiled lysate of reference parasites)

Note: Before preparing the PCR Master Mix, go to the **Black Area** to enter the appropriate program in the thermocycler. If the program has already been entered, review it to ensure no changes have been inadvertently introduced; if so, correct the program and store it for later use. If the PCR will be manually amplified, prepare three water baths at the following temperatures: 54°C, 72°C, and 95°C, and ensure that these temperatures are stably maintained.

1. Calculate the amount of PCR Master Mix that will be necessary for the desired number of reactions, each containing 45 μL of Master Mix. For every 20 reactions, add 1 extra volume of Master Mix to compensate for volume lost during pipetting.
2. Fill out the PCR Worksheet according to the following table.

3.

Ingredient	Description	Stock conc.	Vol/50 µL rxn	Final conc.
Buffer 10X	Buffer B	10X	5.0 µL	1X
dNTPs	20 mM total dNTPs	5 mM A,C,G,T	2.0 µL	0.2 mM A,C,G,T
Primer 1	LU-5A	10 µM	2.0 µL	0.4 µM
Primer 2	LB-3C	10 µM	1.0 µL	0.2 µM
Primer 3	LC-3L-19	10 µM	1.0 µL	0.2 µM
Primer 4	LM-3A-17	10 µM	1.0 µL	0.2 µM
MgCl$_2$		25 mM	3.0 µL	1.5 mM
DTT		100 mM	0.5 µL	1 mM
DMSO		100%	5.25 µL	10.5%
TMAC		1 M	2.5 µL	50 mM
Betaine		4 M	7.5 µL	0.6 M
H$_2$0	ddH$_2$0		14.05 µL	
Taq	*Taq*	5 U/µL	0.4 µL	0.04 U/µL

Vol. of Master Mix	45 µL
Vol. of sample (to be added in step 13)	5 µL
Total reaction volume	50 µL

4. Label the appropriate tubes (0.5-mL or 0.2-mL tubes for thermocyclers; 1.5-mL screw-cap tubes for manual amplification).
5. Thaw aliquot(s) of each reagent. Vortex each thawed solution well and briefly spin the tubes (pulse spin) in a microcentrifuge to collect all the liquid at the bottom of the tubes.

Keep all the ingredients and tubes on ice at all times.

6. In the **White Area**, using a **white** color-coded pipettor, prepare the PCR Master Mix with all the ingredients except the *Taq* polymerase. Check off each ingredient on the Worksheet after adding it to the Master Mix.
7. Mix well using a vortex or a large pipettor.
8. Add the *Taq* polymerase and mix by pipetting carefully with a pipettor set at half the total volume of the PCR Master Mix. Be careful not to create bubbles.
9. Distribute 45 µL of the PCR Master Mix into each labeled tube.
10. Add 2 drops of mineral oil to each tube using a 1000-µL pipettor.
11. Add 5 µL of ddH$_2$O to prepare a "white area" negative control across the layer of mineral oil.
12. Transfer the tubes from the **white** ice bucket to a **grey** ice bucket.

B. Sample Addition: Grey Area

13. In the **Grey Area**, using a **grey** color-coded pipettor, add 5 µL of the sample[10] or control to the appropriate tube, *across* the layer of mineral oil. The controls should be added in the order of the most negative to the most positive. Use a new pipet tip for each sample. Remember to include a negative control consisting of the Grey Area water.

---

10. When analyzing clinical specimens, 5 µL of each sample should be used as template; however, when amplifying purified DNA or lysates of cultured strains, 1–2.5 µL is sufficient template for each PCR reaction. In the latter case, the volume can be adjusted to 5 µL with ddH$_2$O.

*C. Amplification Procedure: **Black Area***

EQUIPMENT
Thermocycler or water baths at 54°C, 72°C, and 95°C
Microcentrifuge

14. Amplification profile:
    Thermal cycler for 0.5-mL tubes

94°C	5 min	1 cycle	Initial denaturation
95°C	30 sec		
54°C	45 sec	35 cycles	Amplification
72°C	30 sec		
72°C	5 min	1 cycle	Final extension

Thermal Cycler for 0.2-mL tubes

94°C	5 min	1 cycle	Initial denaturation
95°C	15 sec		
Ramp	1 min		
52°C	45 sec	35 cycles	Amplification
Ramp	1 min		
72°C	30 sec		
Ramp	1 min		
72°C	5 min	1 cycle	Final extension

Product size: Products indicative of members of the *L. braziliensis* complex range from 146 to 149 base pairs (LU-5A/LB-3C); those of the *L. mexicana* complex range from 218 to 240 base pairs, and those of *L. chagasi* (*L. donovani* complex) range from 351 to 397 base pairs (LU5A/LC-3L-19) (Figure 5.5).

III. Product Analysis

Use a 1.5% agarose gel and the procedure in section 5.1.2.

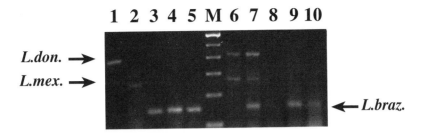

Fig. 5.5. Identification of New World *Leishmania* complexes in cultures and clinical material using the Multiplex PCR assay. Two drops of cultured parasites were diluted in sterile water and boiled for 10 minutes. Boiled dermal scrapings were prepared as described in Fig. 5.2. One microliter of the boiled culture or 5 µL of the boiled clinical specimen were amplified and analyzed by gel electrophoresis. Lane 1, *L. chagasi*; lane 2, *L. mexicana*; lane 3, *L. panamensis*; lane 4, *L. braziliensis*; lane 5, *L. panamensis*; lane M, 100-bp ladder (*see* Appendix C; lowest band shown, 100 bp); lane 6, *L. mexicana* and *L. chagasi*; lane 7, *L. braziliensis*, *L. mexicana*, and *L. chagasi*, lane 8, water (negative control); lane 9, Patient lesion 1; lane 10, Patient lesion 2. Expected product sizes: *L. braziliensis*, 146–149 bp; *L. mexicana*, 218–240 bp; *L. donovani*, 351–397 bp.

5.1.5 *Mycobacterium tuberculosis*

Clinical Manifestations and Epidemiology

Tuberculosis (TB) is presently the leading cause of adult mortality from infectious diseases worldwide. Approximately one-third of the world's population is infected with the tuberculous bacillus (1.8 billion people), with 8 million new cases and 3 million deaths occurring per year (Haas and Des Prez, 1995; Sepkowitz et al., 1995). While 95% of cases are in developing countries, TB is a major public health problem in developed countries as well. In nineteenth century Europe, TB was responsible for more than 30% of all adult deaths (Haas and Des Prez, 1995). Though there is evidence of TB since neolithic times, TB did not become a major problem until the Industrial Revolution, due to urbanization and overcrowded living conditions in Europe. A major step toward the control of TB was the introduction of streptomycin (1946), isoniazid (1952), and rifampin (1972) for treatment of disease and prophylaxis (Sepkowitz et al., 1995). However, the situation has worsened considerably in recent years due to the AIDS epidemic[11] and the emergence of drug-resistant *Mycobacterium tuberculosis*, brought about by the inaccessibility or misuse of drugs. In the United States, the annual rate of TB has risen since 1984, due to drug resistance, AIDS, deterioration of public health infrastructure, and increases in the numbers of homeless, intravenous drug users, and prison populations.

Tuberculosis in humans is primarily caused by *M. tuberculosis* and to a lesser extent by *M. bovis* and *M. africanum* (the *M. tuberculosis* complex). In immuno-compromised patients, *M. avium-intracellulare* complex (MAC) infections can also occur. *M. tuberculosis* is an aerobic nonmotile bacillus with a waxy cell wall that protects it from dessication. It is slow-growing, with a generation time of 15–20 hours (Haas and Des Prez, 1995). The major route of transmission is through inhalation of airborne droplet nuclei containing *M. tuberculosis* that are aerosolized by coughing, sneezing, or talking. Minor transmission routes include ingestion of contaminated food (e.g., unpasteurized milk) or direct inoculation (e.g., health care workers). Key determinants of infection are the closeness of contact and the infectiousness of the source; an acid-fast bacilli (AFB) smear-positive index case infects around 30% of contacts, while a smear-negative, culture-positive case infects less than 10% of contacts. Approximately 10% of immunocompetent individuals infected with *M. tuberculosis* will progress to full-blown tuberculosis in their lifetime, 5% in the first 2 years and 5% over the remainder of their life. In HIV-positive hosts, active disease develops at 10% per year, with rates up to 37% in the first 2 years (Sepkowitz et al., 1995). The three periods when infection is most likely to progress to disease are infancy, young adulthood (15–25 years) and old age.

M. tuberculosis most often causes pulmonary disease, but extrapulmonary TB occurs as well, including tuberculous meningitis (infection of the central nervous system), miliary (disseminated) TB, genitourinary (especially renal) TB, gastroin-

---

11. HIV+ individuals who become infected with *M. tuberculosis* progress to active tuberculosis at a much faster rate than do HIV- people.

testinal TB, hepatic TB, cutaneous TB, tuberculous pericarditis, and skeletal TB. The primary infection is usually through the lungs, where *M. tuberculosis* infects and replicates within alveolar macrophages; infected macrophages also carry the bacilli throughout the host's body. After development of acquired immunity by the host, macrophages are activated by T lymphocytes to kill intracellular bacilli and regulate further multiplication of *M. tuberculosis*. In the pulmonary lesion or at any site to which the bacilli have spread, a characteristic tuberculoid granuloma forms that may progress to form caseous necrosis. The primary tuberculous lesion usually heals with fibrosis and calcification, but reactivation may occur later in life. Pulmonary TB is associated with a productive cough, fever, fatigue, and severe weight loss, but other forms of TB present a wide array of symptoms (Fox, 1991; Haas and Des Prez, 1995).

Classical Methods of Diagnosis

Clinical diagnosis of pulmonary TB is based on characteristic symptoms and a chest X-ray (roentgenogram), which is critical for determination of the extent of the disease and later, for evaluation of response to therapy. The tuberculin skin test, which consists of an injection of purified protein derivative (PPD), is often used to identify individuals with TB infection or disease. In order to detect the bacillus itself, the first step in preparing clinical material usually involves treatment of the sputum specimen with a mucolytic agent (*N*-acetyl-L-cysteine), to free mycobacteria from proteinaceous material, and with sodium hydroxide, to kill non-acid-fast organisms. Standard diagnosis is the Acid-Fast Bacilli (AFB) smear, in which fuchsin stain (Ziehl-Neelsen or Kinyoun method) or fluorochrome dyes (e.g., auramine-rhodamine) are used to identify the mycobacteria. The slides are examined by microscopy, and this technique usually results in 30–70% sensitivity as compared with culture. While AFB smears are rapid and low-cost, they have fairly low sensitivity (requiring 10,000 organisms/mL) and cannot distinguish *M. tuberculosis* from the other types of mycobacteria. In addition, microscopy cannot provide information about drug susceptibility.

The reference method or "gold standard" remains culture of the bacilli in solid medium (Löwenstein-Jensen or Middlebrook 7H10 and 7H11) or liquid medium (Middlebrook 7H9). This technique is selective for *M. tuberculosis*; however, since *M. tuberculosis* is so slow-growing, this procedure requires 3–6 weeks to generate mycobacterial colonies and an additional 3–6 weeks to obtain drug susceptibility information. Another liquid culture technique is the radiometric BACTEC assay (Becton-Dickinsen, Sparks, MD), which is faster than standard culture but much more expensive. Serological methods exist for measurement of IgG antibody, using specific antigens in an ELISA format. These tests generally have a fairly high specificity but lower sensitivity; new antigens are currently under evaluation (Daniel, 1996). A novel method for rapid evaluation of the drug sensitivity of *M. tuberculosis* isolates has been devised using firefly luciferase as a reporter for live mycobacteria (Jacobs et al., 1993).

PCR-Based Protocols

Most amplification strategies for detection of *M. tuberculosis* target the repetitive element IS*6110* (Andersen et al., 1993; Eisenach et al., 1992; Forbes and Hicks, 1993; Hermans et al., 1990; Kaltwasser et al., 1993; Nolte et al., 1993; Thierry et al., 1990; Wilson et al., 1993). Other targets include another repetitive chromosomal element (De Wit et al., 1990), the *M. tuberculosis*-specific *mtp40* gene (Del Portillo et al., 1991), the 65 kD heat shock protein (Brisson-Noel et al., 1989; Pao et al., 1990), and the protein antigen B (PAB) gene (Forbes and Hicks, 1993). Commercial PCR kits are available with primers directed to IS*6110* (AMPLICOR MTB, Roche Diagnostic Systems, Inc., Branchburg, NJ), *M. tuberculosis* rRNA (Amplified Mycobacterium Tuberculosis Direct Test, Gen-Probe Inc., San Diego, CA), and *mtp40* (Digene PT1 and PT2 Primer-Probe Kit and SHARP Signal System, Digene Diagnostic Inc, Silver Spring, MD). Many reports have been published evaluating the sensitivity and specificity as well as the positive and negative predictive value of these kits.

While sputum is the most common specimen for diagnosis of pulmonary tuberculosis by PCR, many other clinical specimens have been evaluated for PCR diagnosis of pulmonary and extrapulmonary tuberculosis, with varying sensitivities. These include gastric aspirate, bronchoalveolar lavage fluid, blood, cerebrospinal fluid, urine, pleural fluid, and tissues (fresh or paraffin-embedded) (Del Portillo et al., 1991; Kaltwasser et al., 1993; Schluger et al., 1994; Tan et al., 1997; van Vollenhoven et al., 1996). Sample preparation is a critical step, because first, the waxy coat of the mycobacterium makes the bacillus resistant to simple lysis procedures, and second, the clinical specimens (especially sputum and blood) are known to contain inhibitors of amplification. Sample preparation techniques include DNA purification (phenol-chloroform extraction followed by ethanol precipitation) and cruder methods such as treatment with heat, proteinase K, Tris/chloroform, silica particles, and sodium iodide. Several techniques have been described for removal of inhibitors from clinical material, including the use of silica particles, capture resins, and bovine serum albumin (Amicosante et al., 1995; Forbes and Hicks, 1996).

PCR approaches have been used to monitor treatment of TB by detection of *M. tuberculosis* DNA (Afghani and Stutman, 1997; Kennedy et al., 1994; Levee et al., 1994; Scarpellini et al., 1995; Yuen et al., 1997) or RNA (Jou et al., 1997). The problem with this approach is that DNA from dead as well as live mycobacteria can be amplified; RT-PCR amplification of *M. tuberculosis* RNA is more likely to detect only viable bacilli.

PCR methods are useful for distinguishing *M. tuberculosis* from other mycobacteria, such as *M. avium* and *M. intracellulare* (Cormican et al., 1995; Cousins et al., 1996; Oggioni et al., 1995). Several multiplex assays have been described that amplify a certain-size fragment from the *Mycobacterium* genus, a different-size fragment from the *M. tuberculosis* complex (Mustafa et al., 1995), and a third specific fragment from only the *M. tuberculosis* species (Del Portillo et al., 1996).

Reports have been published describing the use of PCR for detection of drug-resistant *M. tuberculosis*, but a problem inherent with this approach is that resistance can be due to a number of genetic defects. A phenotypic method (such as the luciferase assay previously mentioned) will identify all strains that are resistant to a particular drug, whereas a genotypic method such as PCR must identify each mutation separately. Telenti et al. (1993) describe a method combining PCR and single-strand conformation polymorphism (SSCP) to detect all of the different rifampin-resistant mutations reported at the date of publication. A kit is now commercially available for detection of point mutations in the *rpoB* gene associated with rifampicin resistance (Inno-Lipa RifTB; Innogenetics, Belgium). A similar approach has been used to identify mutations in the catalase (*katG*) gene associated with isoniazid resistance (Temesgen et al., 1997) and likewise with pyrazinamide and floroquinolone resistance (Scorpio et al., 1997; Sougakoff et al., 1997). However, it is unlikely that these difficult and costly approaches will be widely used for clinical management or large-scale epidemiological studies. Plikaytis et al. (1994) reported a PCR method for identification of the New York City multidrug-resistant (MDR) strain W by generating a genetic fingerprint characteristic of this particular MDR strain and not by the identification of mutations that cause drug resistance.

Genetic fingerprinting methods based on restriction fragment length polymorphism (RFLP) of IS*6110* have been standardized for typing *M. tuberculosis* strains worldwide (Van Embden et al., 1993). PCR-based typing methods have been developed as an easier alternative, with variable success, as reviewed in Suffys et al. (1997). Some techniques involve PCR alone (Friedman et al., 1995; Groenen et al., 1993), whereas others require additional hybridization or restriction analysis (Haas et al., 1993; Kamerbeek et al., 1997). A number of typing methods are based on repetitive elements: either IS*6110* alone (Neimark et al., 1996; Ross and Dwyer, 1993) or IS*6110* in combination with another sequence, such as the polymorphic GC-rich repetitive sequence (PGRS) (Friedman et al., 1995), the major polymorphic tandem repeat (MPTR) sequence (Plikaytis et al., 1993), the direct repeat (DR) cluster (Groenen et al., 1993), a linker ligated to digested genomic DNA (Haas et al., 1993), or the restriction site itself (*Bsr*FI) (Patel et al., 1996). Another typing technique amplifies the spacer region between the genes coding for 16S and 23S rRNA, while still others are based on arbitrary primers, using RAPD analysis (Linton et al., 1994) or arbitrary primed (AP)-PCR (Lee et al., 1994). Lastly, spacer oligonucleotide typing (spoligotyping) combines amplification of the DR region with differential hybridization of the products with membrane-bound oligonucleotides (Kamerbeek et al., 1997).

Points to Consider in Using PCR

PCR for diagnosis of TB is more sensitive than microscopy and, if done under controlled circumstances, can detect a fair number of smear-negative, culture-positive samples (Clarridge et al., 1993). However, there have been a number of reproducibility problems among laboratories using PCR (Noordhoek et al., 1994; Noordhoek et al., 1996), and the decision to apply this technique must be carefully considered (Forbes, 1997). As currently marketed in commercial kits, PCR for diagnosis of TB is prohibitively expensive. It is preferable to reserve PCR detection of *M. tuberculosis* for particular situations where rapid and sensitive diagnosis is critical; for example, in HIV⁺ patients suspected of having TB. Other specific diagnostic uses of PCR for TB include: distinguishing *M. tuberculosis* from *M. avium*-complexes, diagnosing TB in patients already initiated on anti-TB treatment, and

PCR Detection of *Mycobacterium tuberculosis*

The following protocol is a one-tube nested PCR procedure that amplifies the IS*6110* repetitive element from the *Mycobacterium tuberculosis* complex (Wilson et al., 1993). The nested technique improves the sensitivity and specificity of the PCR assay. Although both the primary and the nested amplifications are performed in the same tube, the product of the second PCR is preferentially amplified because of its small size (181 base pairs) and because the primers for this second reaction are present at higher concentrations than are those for the first amplification. When labeled with the appropriate molecules (e.g., biotin, digoxigenin), the 181-bp product can be detected by various capture techniques; however, the most straightforward and reliable method is still agarose gel electrophoresis. This PCR assay can be conducted according to the standard procedure (Version 1) or using a "hot start" technique for increased specificity, whereby the primers are separated from the rest of the PCR ingredients by a wax layer until the first denaturation step when the wax melts, allowing all of the reagents to mix and the amplification to begin (Version 2).

I. Sample Preparation: Grey Area

ADDITIONAL EQUIPMENT AND MATERIALS
Water bath at 80°C
Sterile 1.5-mL screw-cap microcentrifuge tubes
Floating racks for microcentrifuge tubes
Sterile Pasteur pipets or plastic pastettes
Pasteur pipet bulbs

REAGENTS
Bleach (1.5% sodium hypochlorite final concentration)
Sterile ddH$_2$0 (double-distilled water)
1.5 *M* NaOH/2.5% N-acetyl cysteine
Sterile 50 m*M* Tris-HCl, pH 8.3
Cloroform
Silica particles; *see* Appendix B
Sodium-ethanol wash (10 m*M* Tris-HCl [pH 7.4], 50 m*M* NaCl, 0.5 m*M* EDTA, 50% ethanol), stored at -20°C
Tris-EDTA (TE; 10 m*M* Tris-HCl [pH 8.0], 1 m*M* EDTA)

1. For each sputum specimen, label three sterile 1.5-mL screw-cap microcentrifuge tubes by writing the appropriate number on the tube *and* on the cap with a permanent marker.

Perform steps 2–4 in a laminar flow hood with adequate biosafety protection.

2. To each sputum specimen, add 1/5 volume of a solution consisting of 1.5 *M* NaOH/2.5% N-acetyl cysteine to decontaminate the sample and break up the mucus.
3. Divide the sample into three aliquots of 0.5 mL in the sterile labeled 1.5-mL screw-cap microcentrifuge tubes. Freeze one aliquot. The remainder of the specimen will be used for microscopy and culture.
4. Incubate the other two 0.5-mL aliquots for 20 minutes at 80°C to inactivate the mycobacteria.

5. Centrifuge the tubes for 5 minutes at 12,000g in a microcentrifuge and, using a sterile Pasteur pipet, discard the supernatant into a beaker containing 1.5% hypochlorite (bleach).
6. Add 500 µL of 50 m*M* Tris-HCl to each tube.
7. Mix thoroughly using a vortex until the pellet is completely resuspended. Verify visually that the pellet has been completely resuspended.
8. Centrifuge the tubes for 5 minutes at 12,000g and, using a sterile Pasteur pipet, discard the supernatant into a beaker containing 1.5% hypochlorite (bleach).
9. Add 50 µL of chloroform to each tube. Mix thoroughly using a vortex until the pellet is completely resuspended.
10. Add 50 µL of ddH$_2$O and mix thoroughly using a vortex.
11. Centrifuge the tubes for 2 minutes at 12,000g.
12. Transfer the aqueous phase to a sterile microcentrifuge tube and use 5 µL for the PCR amplification. These samples can be stored at −20°C, but the DNA may be degraded over time.

To remove potential inhibitors of the PCR reaction and to obtain DNA of higher purity suitable for long-term storage, the samples above can be further purified using silica particles. Add 5 µL of silica particle slurry to each sample and proceed with step 5 of protocol 6.2.3.

II. Amplification

A. *Preparation of PCR Master Mix and Reaction Tubes:* **White Area**

Version 1: Standard Procedure

REAGENTS
10X Buffer B (100 m*M* Tris [pH 8.3], 500 m*M* KCl)
dNTPs (5 m*M* each dATP, dCTP, dGTP, dTTP; 20 m*M* total dNTPs)
Primers (10 µ*M*)
   Tb294: 5'-GGA CAA CGC CGA ATT GCG AAG GGC-3' (exterior)
   Tb850: 5'-TAG GCG TCG GTG ACA AAG GCC ACG-3' (exterior)
   Tb505: 5'-ACG ACC ACA TCA ACC-3' (interior)
   Tb670: 5'-AGT TTG GTC ATC AGC C-3' (interior)
MgCl$_2$ (25 m*M*)
Dimethyl sulfoxide (DMSO)
ddH$_2$0
Taq polymerase (5 U/µL)
Mineral oil
Positive control (reference strain of *M. tuberculosis*)

Note: Before preparing the PCR Master Mix, go to the **Black Area** to enter the appropriate program in the thermocycler. If the program has already been entered, review it to ensure no changes have been inadvertently introduced; if so, correct the program and store it for later use. If the PCR will be manually amplified, prepare three water baths at the following temperatures: 48°C, 65°C, 72°C, and 93°C, and ensure that these temperatures are stably maintained.

1. Calculate the amount of PCR Master Mix that will be necessary for the desired number of reactions, each containing 15 µL of Master Mix. For every 10 reactions, add 1 extra volume of Master Mix to compensate for volume lost during pipetting.
2. Fill out the PCR Worksheet according to the following table.

3.

Ingredient	Description	Stock conc.	Vol/20 µL rxn	final conc.
Buffer 10X	Buffer B	10X	2.0 µL	1X
dNTPs	20 mM total dNTPs	5 mM A,C,G,T	0.8 µL	0.2 mM A,C,G,T
Primer 1	Tb294	1 µM[12]	0.6 µL	0.03 µM
Primer 2	Tb850	1 µM[12]	0.6 µL	0.03 µM
Primer 3	Tb670	10 µM	1.0 µL	0.5 µM
Primer 4	Tb505	10 µM	1.0 µL	0.5 µM
MgCl$_2$		25 mM	1.2 µL	1.5 mM
DMSO		100%	1.0 µL	5%
H$_2$0	ddH$_2$0		6.6 µL	
Taq	*Taq*	5 U/µuL	0.2 µL	0.05 U/µL

Vol. of Master Mix	15 µL
Vol. of sample (to be added in step 13)	5 µL
Total reaction volume	20 µL

4. Label the appropriate tubes (0.5-mL or 0.2-mL tubes for thermocyclers; 1.5-mL screw-cap tubes for manual amplification).

5. Thaw aliquot(s) of each reagent. Vortex each thawed solution well and briefly spin the tubes (pulse spin) in a microcentrifuge to collect all the liquid at the bottom of the tubes.

Keep all the ingredients and tubes on ice at all times.

6. In the **White Area**, using a **white** color-coded pipettor, prepare the PCR Master Mix with all the ingredients except the *Taq* polymerase. Check off each ingredient on the Worksheet after adding it to the Master Mix.

7. Mix well using a vortex or a large pipettor.

8. Add the *Taq* polymerase and mix by pipetting carefully with a pipettor set at half the total volume of the PCR Master Mix. Be careful not to create bubbles.

9. Distribute 15 µL of the PCR Master Mix into each labeled tube.

10. Add 1 drop of mineral oil to each tube using a 1000-µL pipettor.

11. Add 5 µL of ddH$_2$O to prepare a "white room" negative control across the layer of mineral oil.

12. Transfer the tubes from the **white** ice bucket to a **grey** ice bucket.

B. Sample Addition: Grey Area

13. In the **Grey Area**, using a **grey** color-coded pipettor, add 5 µL of the sample[13] or control to the appropriate tube, *across* the layer of mineral oil. The controls should be added in the order of the most negative to the most positive. Use a new pipet tip for each sample. Remember to include a negative control consisting of the Grey Area water.

---

12. Note that the stock concentration of primers Tb294 and Tb850 is 1 µM, not 10 µM.

13. When analyzing clinical specimens, 5 µL of each sample should be used as template; however, when amplifying purified DNA, 1–2.5 µL is sufficient template for each PCR reaction. In the latter case, the volume can be adjusted to 5 µL with ddH$_2$O.

Version 2: Hot-Start

ADDITIONAL EQUIPMENT AND MATERIALS
Water bath at 80°C
Small spatula
Floating rack for PCR tubes (0.5 mL or 0.2 mL)

REAGENTS
10X Buffer B (100 mM Tris [pH 8.3], 500 mM KCl)
dNTPs (5 mM each dATP, dCTP, dGTP, dTTP; 20 mM total dNTPs)
Primers (10 μM)
   Tb294:   5'-GGA CAA CGC CGA ATT GCG AAG GGC-3' (exterior)
   Tb850   5'-TAG GCG TCG GTG ACA AAG GCC ACG-3' (exterior)
   Tb505:   5'-ACG ACC ACA TCA ACC-3' (interior)
   Tb670:   5'-AGT TTG GTC ATC AGC C-3' (interior)
   MgCl$_2$ (25 mM)
Dimethyl sulfoxide (DMSO)
ddH$_2$0
Taq polymerase (5 U/μL)
Mineral oil
Positive control (reference strain of *M. tuberculosis*)
Wax beads (50 μL)

Note: Before preparing the PCR Master Mix, go to the **Black Area** to enter the appropriate program in the thermocycler. If the program has already been entered, review it to ensure no changes have been inadvertently introduced; if so, correct the program and store it for later use. If the PCR will be manually amplified, prepare three water baths at the following temperatures: 48°C, 65°C, 72°C, and 93°C, and ensure that these temperatures are stably maintained.

1. Make a stock of 4X Primer Mix according to the following table.

Primer		4X Primer Mix conc.	Final conc.
Exterior primers	Tb294	120 nM	30 nM
	Tb850	120 nM	30 nM
Interior primers	Tb505	2 μM	500 nM
	Tb670	2 μM	500 nM

2. Calculate the amount of PCR Master Mix that will be necessary for the desired number of reactions, each containing 15 μL of Master Mix. For every 10 reactions, add 1 extra volume of Master Mix to compensate for volume lost during pipetting.
3. Fill out the PCR Worksheet according to the following table.

4.

Ingredient	Description	Stock conc.	Vol/20 μL rxn	Final conc.
Buffer 10X	Buffer B	10X	2.0 μL	1X
dNTPs	20 mM total dNTPs	5 mM A,C,G,T	0.8 μL	0.2 mM A,C,G,T
MgCl$_2$		25 mM	1.2 μL	1.5 mM
DMSO		100%	1.0 μL	5%
H$_2$0	ddH$_2$0	4.8 μL		
Taq	*Taq*	5 U/μuL	0.2 μL	0.05 U/μL
Vol. of Master Mix		15 μL		
Vol. of sample (to be added in step 13)				5 μL
Total reaction volume		20 μL		

5. Label the appropriate tubes (0.5-mL or 0.2-mL tubes for thermocyclers; 1.5-mL screw-cap tubes for manual amplification).
6. Thaw aliquot(s) of each reagent. Vortex each thawed solution well and briefly spin the tubes (pulse spin) in a microcentrifuge to collect all the liquid at the bottom of the tubes.

Keep all the ingredients and tubes on ice at all times.

7. In the **White Area**, using a **white** color-coded pipettor, add 5 µL of the 4X Primer Mix to the bottom of each PCR reaction tube.
8. Add a wax bead using the small spatula and centrifuge the tube for 5 seconds to concentrate the liquid at the bottom of the tube.
9. Incubate the tubes at 80°C until the wax has melted (2–3 minutes). Remove the tubes to allow the wax to harden. The wax forms an impermeable layer above the primers. Keep the tubes on ice while the PCR Master Mix is prepared.
10. In the **White Area**, using a **white** color-coded pipettor, prepare the PCR Master Mix with all the ingredients except the *Taq* polymerase. Check off each ingredient on the Worksheet after adding it to the Master Mix.
11. Mix well using a vortex or a large pipettor.
12. Add the *Taq* polymerase and mix by pipetting carefully with a pipettor set at half the total volume of the PCR Master Mix. Be careful not to create bubbles.
13. Distribute 10 µL of the PCR Master Mix into each labeled tube above the wax layer.
14. Add 5 µL of ddH$_2$O to prepare a "white room" negative control.
15. Transfer the tubes from the **white** ice bucket to a **grey** ice bucket.

B. *Sample Addition:* **Grey Area**

16. In the **Grey Area**, using a **grey** color-coded pipettor, add 5 µL of the sample[14] or control to the appropriate tube in the order of the most negative to the most positive. Use a new pipet tip for each sample. Remember to include a negative control consisting of the Grey Area water.

C. *Amplification Procedure:* **Black Area**

EQUIPMENT
Thermocycler or water baths at 56°C, 72°C, and 95°C
Microcentrifuge

14. When analyzing clinical specimens, 5 µL of each sample should be used as template; however, when amplifying purified DNA, 1–2.5 µL is sufficient template for each PCR reaction. In the latter case, the volume can be adjusted to 5 µL with ddH$_2$O.

17. Amplification profile:

93°C	2 min	1 cycle	Initial denaturation
93°C	45 sec		
65°C	1 min	30 cycles	First amplification
72°C	1 min		
93°C	45 sec		
48°C	1 min	20 cycles	Second (nested) amplification
72°C	30 sec		
72°C	10 min	1 cycle	Final extension

Product size: This nested protocol will preferentially amplify a 181-bp product (Tb505–Tb670). However, when a large amount of template DNA is present, other larger fragments are also generated in addition to the 181-bp product. These fragments result from amplification of the regions between the other primers in the reaction (Tb294–Tb850, Tb294–Tb670, Tb505–Tb850).

III. Product Analysis

Use a 1.5% agarose gel and the procedure in section 5.1.2.

Characterization of *Mycobacterium tuberculosis* by Double Repetitive Element (DRE)-PCR

This protocol can be used to identify individual strains of *Mycobacterium tuberculosis* by generating a unique pattern of amplified fragments, referred to as a "fingerprint." This is achieved by using two pairs of primers. One pair targets the repetitive insertion sequence IS*6110*, while the other is directed to the repetitive polymorphic GC-rich sequence (PGRS) (Friedman et al., 1995). Each primer pair is oriented such that the primers face outward, thereby amplifying the region in between the repetitive elements. Since these elements are distributed differently throughout the bacterial genome of different *M. tuberculosis* strains, a distinct pattern is generated for each strain.

I. Sample Preparation: Grey Area

ADDITIONAL EQUIPMENT AND MATERIALS
Boiling water bath (100°C)
Freezer (-70°C)
Sterile 1.5-mL screw-cap microcentrifuge tubes
Floating racks for microcentrifuge tubes
Sterile Pasteur pipets
Inoculating loop

REAGENTS
Sterile ddH$_2$0 (double-distilled water)
Colonies of *M. tuberculosis* on Lowenstein-Jensen slants

1. Label sterile 1.5-mL screw-cap microcentrifuge tubes by writing the appropriate number on the tube *and* on the cap with a permanent marker.
2. Transfer 1 mL of sterile ddH$_2$0 to each labeled tube.
3. **In a laminar flow hood with adequate biosafety protection**, transfer a colony of *M. tuberculosis* from the Lowenstein-Jensen slant to the water in each tube using an inoculating loop. Agitate the loop to shake free all the bacteria from the loop and deposit them in the water.
4. Close the screw-caps tightly.
5. Incubate the tubes at 100°C in the boiling water bath for 10 minutes using a floating rack.
6. Freeze the samples in a -70°C freezer. If a -70°C freezer is not available, use a -20°C freezer.
7. Thaw the samples and boil the tubes for 10 minutes at 100°C in the boiling water bath.
8. Centrifuge the tubes for 2 minutes in a microcentrifuge at ambient temperature.
9. Transfer the supernatant to a sterile microcentrifuge tube. Proceed directly to the Amplification step or store the tubes at -20°C until further use. If the supernatant is not promptly transferred to a new tube, be sure to repeat the centrifugation in step 8 after thawing the samples and before proceeding to the Amplification.
10. Use 5 µL of the supernatant for each PCR amplification.

II. Amplification

A. Preparation of PCR Master Mix and Reaction Tubes: **White Area**

REAGENTS

10X Buffer B (100 m*M* Tris [pH 8.3], 500 m*M* KCl)

dNTPs (5 m*M* each dATP, dCTP, dGTP, dTTP; 20 m*M* total dNTPs)

Primers (10 µ*M*)

  Ris1:   5′-GGC TGA GGT CTC AGA TCA G
  Ris2:   5′-ACC CCA TCC TTT CCA AGA AC
  Pntb1: 5′-CCG TTG CCG TAC AGC TG
  Pntb2: 5′-CCT AGC CGA ACC CTT TG

MgCl$_2$ (25 m*M*)

ddH$_2$0

Taq polymerase (5 U/µL)

Mineral oil

Positive control (reference strain of *M. tuberculosis* with a DRE-PCR pattern consisting of at least three fragments)

Note: Before preparing the PCR Master Mix, go to the **Black Area** to enter the appropriate program in the thermocycler. If the program has already been entered, review it to ensure no changes have been inadvertently introduced; if so, correct the program and store it for later use. If the PCR will be manually amplified, prepare three water baths at the following temperatures: 56°C, 72°C, and 94°C, and ensure that these temperatures are stably maintained.

1. Calculate the amount of PCR Master Mix that will be necessary for the desired number of reactions, each containing 45 µL of Master Mix. For every 20 reactions, add 1 extra volume of Master Mix to compensate for volume lost during pipetting.
2. Fill out the PCR Worksheet according to the following table.

3. Ingredient	Description	Stock conc.	Vol/50 µL rxn	Final conc.
Buffer 10X	Buffer B	10X	5.0 µL	1X
dNTPs	20 m*M* total dNTPs	5 m*M* A,C,G,T	2.0 µL	0.2 m*M* A,C,G,T
Primer 1	Ris1	10 µ*M*	2.5 µL	0.5 µ*M*
Primer 2	Ris2	10 µ*M*	2.5 µL	0.5 µ*M*
Primer 3	Pntb1	10 µ*M*	2.5 µL	0.5 µ*M*
Primer 4	Pntb2	10 µ*M*	2.5 µL	0.5 µ*M*
MgCl$_2$		25 m*M*	5.0 µL	2.5 m*M*
H$_2$0	ddH$_2$0		22.5 µL	
Taq	*Taq*	5 U/µL	0.5 µL	0.05 U/µL
Vol. of Master Mix			45 µL	
Vol. of sample (to be added in step 13)			5 µL	
Total reaction volume			50 µL	

4. Label the appropriate tubes (0.5-mL or 0.2-mL tubes for thermocyclers; 1.5-mL screw-cap tubes for manual amplification).
5. Thaw aliquot(s) of each reagent. Vortex each thawed solution well and briefly spin the tubes (pulse spin) in a microcentrifuge to collect all the liquid at the bottom of the tubes.

Keep all the ingredients and tubes on ice at all times.

6. In the **White Area**, using a **white** color-coded pipettor, prepare the PCR Master Mix with all the ingredients except the *Taq* polymerase. Check off each ingredient on the Worksheet after adding it to the Master Mix.

7. Mix well using a vortex or a large pipettor.
8. Add the *Taq* polymerase and mix by pipetting carefully with a pipettor set at half the total volume of the PCR Master Mix. Be careful not to create bubbles.
9. Distribute 45 µL of the PCR Master Mix into each labeled tube.
10. Add 2 drops of mineral oil to each tube using a 1000-µL pipettor.
11. Add 5 µL of ddH$_2$O to prepare a "white area" negative control across the layer of mineral oil.
12. Transfer the tubes from the **white** ice bucket to a **grey** ice bucket.

B. Sample Addition: **Grey Area**

13. In the **Grey Area**, using a grey color-coded pipettor, add 5 µL of the sample or control to the appropriate tube, *across* the layer of mineral oil. The controls should be added in the order of the most negative to the most positive. Use a new pipet tip for each sample.

C. Amplification Procedure: **Black Area**

EQUIPMENT
Thermocycler or water baths at 56°C, 72°C, and 95°C
Microcentrifuge

14. Amplification profile:
    Thermocycler for 0.5-mL tubes

94°C	10 min	1 cycle	Initial denaturation
95°C	1 min		
56°C	2 min	35 cycles	Amplification
72°C	2 min		
72°C	5 min	1 cycle	Final extension

Thermocycler for 0.2-mL tubes

94°C	7 min	1 cycle	Initial denaturation
95°C	30 sec		
52°C	1 min	30 cycles	Amplification
72°C	1 min		
72°C	5 min	1 cycle	Final extension

Product size: Products will vary in size, depending on the strain being amplified (Figure 5.6). Informative products range between 100 and 1000 base pairs. To facilitate analysis, patterns should be drawn on graph paper and grouped according to the number of fragments obtained. When two strains appear to have a similar pattern, the PCR products should be compared side by side by agarose gel electrophoresis to confirm identity.

III. Product Analysis

Use a 1.2% agarose gel and the procedure in section 5.1.2.

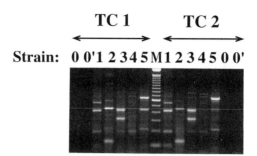

Fig. 5.6. Characterization of individual *M. tuberculosis* strains using DRE-PCR followed by gel electrophoresis. Amplifications were conducted in two different thermocyclers: TC1, PTC-100 thermocycler (MJ Research, Inc.) and TC2, 9600 thermocycler (Perkin-Elmer). 0, "White Area" negative control (water); 0', "Final" negative control (water); 1, strain C; 2, strain H37Ra; 3, strain C3909; 4, strain C696; 5, strain C1; M, 100-bp ladder (*see* Appendix C; lowest band shown, 100 bp).

5.1.6 *Plasmodium falciparum* and *Plasmodium vivax*

Clinical Manifestations and Epidemiology

Malaria is one of the most daunting infectious diseases and has consisitently resisted attempts at eradication and control. The WHO's program of worldwide eradication of malaria, launched in 1957, was based on widespread use of antimalarial drugs (e.g., chloroquine) in humans and the insecticide DDT to control the mosquito vector. However, the program failed to eradicate or even control malaria, which has been steadily increasing in many areas over the last 25 years. Another major complication has been the rise of parasites resistant to chloroquine, pyrimethamine, cycloguanil, proguanil, sulfadoxine, and other antimalarials. Currently, 1.6 billion people are at risk worldwide; 200–300 million cases of malaria with 1–2 million deaths are reported annually (Krogstad, 1995; Strickland, 1991).

Malaria in humans is caused by four different species of the genus *Plasmodium* (*P. falciparum*, *P. vivax*, *P. malariae*, and *P. ovale*). The most serious and life-threatening form of disease is caused by *P. falciparum*, in which drug resistance is widespread. Malarial parasites are transmitted to humans by female *Anopheles* mosquitoes. The life cycle of the parasite includes stages in the human host as well as in the mosquito. Haploid sporozoites injected from the mosquito salivary glands travel through the bloodstream of the human host and enter liver hepatocytes, where they multiply to form large numbers of merozoites in what is called the tissue schizont. Upon rupture of the hepatocytes, the merozoites are released into the bloodstream, where they invade red blood cells (RBCs, or erythrocytes) and mature to ring-, trophozoite-, and schizont-stage asexual intracellular parasites. The schizont-stage parasites rupture the RBCs, releasing more merozoites, which infect more RBCs. Alternatively, some *P. vivax* and *P. ovale* parasites form hypnozoites in the liver, where they remain dormant for 6–11 months before maturing to tissue schizonts and causing a relapse of disease. Some intra-erythrocytic parasites differentiate to form male and female gametocyte sexual forms, which are taken up by mosquitoes. In the midgut of the mosquito, the male gamete fertilizes a female gamete to produce a diploid zygote, which matures to a motile ookinete and invades the midgut epithelium of the mosquito. There it forms an oocyst, which divides to produce sporozoites that migrate to the salivary glands once the oocyst ruptures to begin the cycle again (Krogstad, 1995).

Clinical symptoms of malaria incude high fever with chills, anemia, nausea, dizziness, backache, malaise, fatigue, and splenomegaly. Episodes of fever with characteristic periodicity are associated with *P. vivax* and *P. ovale* (48-hour intervals) and *P. malariae* (72-hour intervals); the symptoms of *P. falciparum* malaria also wax and wane, but with less regularity. These cyclic episodes of fever coincide with waves of parasitemia; thus, during the asymptomatic phase, the blood contains few circulating parasites, whereas a fever episode correlates with high parasitemia. Untreated *P. falciparum* infections in the nonimmune host often lead to serious or fatal complications, such as cerebral malaria, renal failure, pulmonary edema, splenic rupture, gastroenteritis, hypoglycemia, and severe anemia (Strickland, 1991).

Classical Methods of Diagnosis

The classical procedure for diagnosis of malaria is by light microscopy of a Giemsa-stained blood smear. The thick smear is better for detection of parasites, because it concentrates the red blood cells, whereas the thin smear is preferable for species identification. While the technique is low-cost and rapid, adequate processing requires a 15- to 30-minute examination per slide in order to detect low-level parasitemias. It is especially important to detect low levels of circulating parasites because, due to the cyclical nature of the infection, a low parasitemia can convert into a high, life-threatening parasitemia within hours. Morphological differentiation of the different *Plasmodium* species requires an experienced technician, and even so, mixed infections are often overlooked (Brown et al., 1992; Snounou et al., 1993b). Alternative assays concentrate parasites in the blood sample and detect them by staining with acridine orange in the QBC tube test (Rickman et al., 1989) or enhance detection of parasites by staining thick smears with fluorescent dyes (Kawamoto, 1991). A new dipstick technique that shows considerable promise for widespread use is the Parasight F test, based on detection of circulating *P. falciparum* histidine-rich protein-2 antigen (Humar et al., 1997). Serological methods do not distinguish present from past infections, but they can be useful for epidemiologic surveys and screening blood donors. IFAT and ELISA formats using species-specific antigens are the most stardardized but do not distinguish between protective and nonprotective antibodies. IFAT and ELISA assays, as well as the circumsporozoite precipitin reaction, have been developed to detect antisporozoite antibodies (Strickland, 1991).

PCR-Based Protocols

PCR protocols for detection of the four *Plasmodium* species have been described utilizing primers directed to species-specific repetitive sequences (Barker et al., 1992; Sethabutr et al., 1992; Tirasophon et al., 1991, 1994), small subunit ribosomal RNA genes (Snounou et al., 1993b), the circumsporozoite gene (Brown et al., 1992), the dihydrofolate reductase-thymidylate synthase (DHFR-TS) locus (Arai et al., 1994), the 18S rRNA genes (Kimura et al., 1995), and the p126 gene (Zalis et al., 1996). Several assays for the multiplex detection of *P. falciparum* and *P. vivax* have been reported, with primers directed to repetitive sequences (Tirasophon et al., 1994) or the 18S rRNA genes (Das et al., 1995). Most efforts have concentrated on *P. falciparum* and to a lesser extent, *P. vivax*. Note that geographic variability may affect PCR results; therefore, it is advisable to try several PCR assays that target different *Plasmodium* sequences (Jelinek et al., 1996). Many of these procedures involve DNA amplification by PCR and subsequent hybridzation with DNA probes to increase sensitivity and specificity, although a few protocols are based solely on PCR (Snounou et al., 1993b; Tirasophon et al., 1991, 1994).

The simplest sampling techniques involve collection of blood by fingerprick in either capillary tubes or on filter paper. Blood from capillary tubes can be treated with a saponin detergent lysis buffer or lysed by freeze-thaw cycles and blotted onto filter paper (#903, Schleicher and Schull, Keene, NH) (Barker et al., 1992, 1994). DNA from the dried blood spots can be eluted by placing the filter paper in 5% Chelex®

100, then vortexing, boiling, and centrifuging it (Kain and Lanar, 1991; Long et al., 1995; Singh et al., 1996). Alternatively, standard DNA extraction can be performed on peripheral or venous blood (Barker et al., 1994; Snounou et al., 1993b). Detection of *Plasmodium* in mosquitoes by PCR has also been reported (Bouare et al., 1996; Schriefer et al., 1991; Stoffels et al., 1995; Tassanakajon et al., 1993).

PCR assays have been used to monitor the response, if any, of *P. falciparum* (Kain et al., 1994; Sethabutr et al., 1992) and *P. vivax* (Kain et al., 1993a) to treatment and to distinguish re-infection from treatment failure (Kain et al., 1996). Several PCR protocols have been developed to detect specific mutations that confer drug resistance. Mutations in the parasite's dihydrofolate reductase (DHFR) gene that correlate with resistance to pyrimethamine, cycloguanil, and proguanil can be detected by nested PCR (Eldin de Pecoulas et al., 1995a; Plowe et al., 1995), PCR followed by restriction enzyme digestion (Eldin de Pecoulas et al., 1995b; Zindrou et al., 1996), or sequencing of amplified products (Reeder et al., 1996). Sulfadoxine resistance appears to be associated with particular mutations in the dihydropteroate synthase (DHPS) gene, and these can be detected using allele-specific PCR. Likewise, *pfmdr*[15] mutations in chloroquine-resistant parasites can be detected by PCR (Frean et al., 1992). Many of these assays are conducted with DNA obtained from dried blood spots or Giemsa-stained slides.

A number of methods for typing individual strains of *Plasmodium falciparum* have been described. The majority are based on amplification of several polymorphic markers, including the genes coding for merozoite specific proteins (*MSP-1* and *MSP-2*), circumsporozoite protein (*CSP*), ring-infected erythrocyte surface antigen (*RESA*), thrombospondin-related anonymous protein (*TRAP*), glutamate-rich protein (*GLURP*), histidine-rich protein 1 (*HRP1*), and p190 (Contamin et al., 1996; Kaneko et al., 1997; Mercereau-Puijalon et al., 1991; Robert et al., 1996; Viriyakosol et al., 1995; Wooden et al., 1992). Some assays target microsatellite sequences (Su and Wellems, 1997) or multigene families (Carcy et al., 1995). Others involve restriction digestion of amplified polymorphic sequences (Felger et al., 1994) or AP-PCR (Rojas et al., 1996). PCR-based typing methods have also been described for *P. vivax*, targeting the *GAM1* gene, which encodes a transmission-blocking candidate antigen (Snewin et al., 1995). Genetic variability of *P. vivax* has also been assessed by detecting variants of the CS gene (Kain et al., 1991, 1993a).

Points to Consider in Using PCR

The classical thick smear, if properly conducted, is generally adequate for routine diagnosis of malaria. PCR is, however, very useful for the detection of mixed infections, which are often overlooked in conventional microscopy of thick smears (Brown et al., 1992; Oliveira et al., 1996; Snounou et al., 1993b). Thus, it could serve as a tool for quality control of routine diagnostic procedures. Other useful applications of PCR are

---

15. Some investigators believe that the *Plasmodium falciparum* multidrug resistance (*pfmdr*) gene is associated with resistance to chloroquine, although the issue is controversial.

the identification of drug-resistant parasites, the monitoring of treatment response, and the detection of *Plasmodium* in anopheline mosquitoes.

PCR and other DNA-based techniques have been critical for elucidating the genetic structure of the parasite population (Contamin et al., 1996; Kain and Lanar, 1991). For instance, PCR has shown that patients can be infected with a mixture of genetically distinct strains of *P. falciparum* and that *P. falciparum* oocysts in mosquitoes are heterozygous, indicating that cross-mating does occur between clones in the mosquito (Walliker, 1994). Studies using PCR to detect low levels of parasitemia have revealed that the real prevalence of *P. falciparum* infection had been underestimated using classical techniques in Sudan and Guinea Bissau (Roper et al., 1996; Snounou et al., 1993a). Geographical distribution of genetic variants can also be assessed using PCR-based assays (Kain et al., 1991). This body of information is important for the development of vaccine candidates and malaria control strategies.

Multiplex PCR Detection of *Plasmodium falciparum* and *Plasmodium vivax*

This multiplex PCR protocol amplifies repetitive sequences from two human malarial parasites, *P. falciparum* and *P. vivax*. These two species can be distinguished because the products are of different sizes (206 base pairs from *P. falciparum* and 183 base pairs from *P. vivax*) (Tirasophon et al., 1994). The simultaneous detection of the two parasites is particularly useful in identifying mixed infections. The simple saponin lysis procedure (Barker et al., 1992) gives similar results as more elaborate DNA purification methods for preparing PCR samples from whole blood (Moleón-Borodowsky et al., manuscript in preparation).

I. Sample Preparation: Grey Area

ADDITIONAL EQUIPMENT AND MATERIALS
Sterile lancet
Cotton balls

REAGENTS
Sterile ddH_2O (double-distilled water)
Saponin lysis buffer (0.22% NaCl, 0.015% saponin, 1 m*M* EDTA)
70% alcohol

1. Label sterile 1.5-mL microcentrifuge tubes by writing the appropriate number on the tube *and* on the cap with a permanent marker.
2. Transfer 200 µL of saponin lysis buffer to each labeled tube.
3. Clean the patient's finger with cotton soaked in 70% ethanol and prick the finger with a sterile lancet. Before placing blood on a slide for microscopy, allow one drop of blood (approximately 20 µL) to *drip* into an appropriately labeled 1.5-mL microcentrifuge tube containing saponin lysis buffer. It is very important that the patient's finger *does not* touch the tube.
4. Close the tube and immediately mix the blood with the saponin lysis buffer by inversion. The solution should appear red but transparent (the saponin clarifies the blood by lysing red blood cells).
5. Prepare the thick or thin smear for microscopy.
6. If possible, proceed immediately with the following steps. If not, the blood samples in saponin lysis buffer can be stored for up to 24 hours at room temperature before processing.
7. After at least 5 minutes (but no more than 24 hours) at ambient temperature, centrifuge the tubes for 1 minute in a microcentrifuge.
8. Remove the supernatant with a pipettor and discard.
9. Resuspend the pellet *completely* in 500 µL of saponin lysis buffer. Be careful not to lose the pellet, which can may become attached to the inside wall of the pipet tip.
10. Centrifuge the tubes for 1 minute.
11. Remove *all* of the supernatant with a pipettor and discard.
12. Store the pellet at $-20°C$ until ready to amplify.
13. Immediately before preparing the PCR amplification, completely resuspend the pellet (fresh or frozen) in 10 µL of ddH_2O. Use 2.5–5 µL for each reaction. Store the remainder of the sample at $-20°C$.

II. Amplification

A. *Preparation of PCR Master Mix and Reaction Tubes:* **White Area**

REAGENTS
10X Buffer B (100 mM Tris [pH 8.3], 500 mM KCl)
dNTPS (5 mM each dATP, dCTP, dGTP, dTTP; 20 mM total dNTPs)
Primers (10 µM)
   K114-P1: 5′-CGC TAC ATA TGC TAG TTG CCA GAC
   K114-P2: 5′-CGT GTA CCA TAC ATC CTA CCA AC
   PV-1: 5′-GGT GAA AAT CGA AGG TAT CGA
   PV-2: 5′-TCC CTG CCC CGC TGT TGC
MgCl$_2$ (25 mM)
ddH$_2$0
Taq polymerase (5 U/µL)
Mineral oil
Positive control (purified *P. falciparum* and *P. vivax* DNA)

Note: Before preparing the PCR Master Mix, go to the **Black Area** to enter the appropriate program in the thermocycler. If the program has already been entered, review it to ensure no changes have been inadvertently introduced; if so, correct the program and store it for later use. If the PCR will be manually amplified, prepare three water baths at the following temperatures: 55°C, 72°C, and 93°C, and ensure that these temperatures are stably maintained.

1. Calculate the amount of PCR Master Mix that will be necessary for the desired number of reactions, each containing 20 µL of Master Mix. For every 10 reactions, add 1 extra volume of Master Mix to compensate for volume lost during pipetting.
2. Fill out the PCR Worksheet according to the following table.

3.

Ingredient	Description	Stock conc.	Vol/25 µL rxn	Final conc.
Buffer 10X	Buffer B	10X	2.5 µL	1X
dNTPs	20 mM total dNTPs	5 mM A,C,G,T	1.0 µL	0.2 mM A,C,G,T
Primer 1	K114-P1	10 µM	0.5 µL	0.2 µM
Primer 2	K114-P2	10 µM	0.5 µL	0.2 µM
Primer 3	PV1	10 µM	0.5 µL	0.2 µM
Primer 4	PV2	10 µM	0.5 µL	0.2 µM
MgCl$_2$		25 mM	1.5 µL	1.5 mM
H$_2$0	ddH$_2$0		12.875 µL	
Taq	*Taq*	5 U/µL	0.125 µL	0.025 U/µL

Vol. of Master Mix	20 µL
Vol. of sample (to be added in step 13)	5 µL
Total reaction volume	25 µL

4. Label the appropriate tubes (0.5-mL or 0.2-mL tubes for thermocyclers; 1.5-mL screw-cap tubes for manual amplification).
5. Thaw aliquot(s) of each reagent. Vortex each thawed solution well and briefly spin the tubes (pulse spin) in a microcentrifuge to collect all the liquid at the bottom of the tubes.

Keep all the ingredients and tubes on ice at all times.

6. In the **White Area**, using a **white** color-coded pipettor, prepare the PCR Master Mix with all the ingredients except the *Taq* polymerase. Check off each ingredient on the Worksheet after adding it to the Master Mix.
7. Mix well using a vortex or a large pipettor.

8. Add the *Taq* polymerase and mix by pipetting carefully with a pipettor set at half the total volume of the PCR Master Mix. Be careful not to create bubbles.

9. Distribute 20 µL of the PCR Master Mix into each labeled tube.

10. Add 2 drops of mineral oil to each tube using a 1000-µL pipettor.

11. Add 5 µL of ddH$_2$O to prepare a "white area" negative control across the layer of mineral oil.

12. Transfer the tubes from the **white** ice bucket to a **grey** ice bucket.

B. Sample Addition: **Grey Area**

13. In the **Grey Area**, using a **grey** color-coded pipettor, add 5 µL of the sample[16] or control to the appropriate tube, *across* the layer of mineral oil. The controls should be added in the order of the most negative to the most positive. Use a new pipet tip for each sample. Remember to include a negative control consisting of the Grey Area water.

C. Amplification Procedure: **Black Area**

EQUIPMENT
Thermocycler or water baths at 54°C, 72°C, and 95°C
Microcentrifuge

14. Amplification profile:
    93°C   30 sec
    55°C   1 min   40 cycles   Amplification
    72°C   1 min

Product size: A product of 206 base pairs is indicative of the presence of *P. falciparum* DNA, while a product of 183 base pairs is generated from *P. vivax* (Figure 5.7).

III. Product Analysis

Use a 2% agarose gel and the procedure in section 5.1.2.

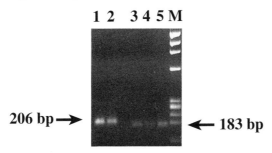

Fig. 5.7. Detection of *P. falciparum* and *P. vivax* by multiplex PCR and gel electrophoresis. Patient blood samples were prepared using the saponin lysis procedure prior to amplification. Lane 1, specimen C; lane 2, J; lane 3, H; lane 4, 49; lane 5, 45; lane M, φX174/HaeIII DNA markers (*see* Appendix B). Expected product sizes: *P. falciparum*, 206 bp; *P. vivax*, 183 bp. Samples in lanes 1 and 2 are positive for *P. falciparum*; samples in lanes 3, 4, and 5 are positive for *P. vivax*.

---

16. When analyzing clinical specimens, 5 µL of each sample should be used as template; however, when amplifying purified DNA or lysates of cultured strains, 1–2.5 µL is sufficient template for each PCR reaction. In the latter case, the volume can be adjusted to 5 µL with ddH$_2$O.

5.1.7   *Vibrio cholerae*

Clinical Manifestations and Epidemiology

Vibrio cholerae is a pathogenic Gram-negative bacillus that can cause epidemic disease in humans exposed to contaminated food or water sources. For centuries, epidemics of cholera have devastated human populations throughout the world. The seventh pandemic began in 1961 in Asia. In 1991, the pandemic was introduced to Latin America and rapidly disseminated across the continent. Toxigenic *V. cholerae* has been associated exclusively with the O1 serotype; however, in 1992, a new serotype, O139, appeared in Bangladesh (Shears, 1994). The *V. cholerae* O1 serotype is divided into two biotypes, the classic biotype and the milder El Tor biotype, each of which is further subdivided into three serotypes: Ogawa, Inaba, and Hikojima (Nalin and Morris, 1991). Cholera manifests itself by the secretion of enormous amounts of watery diarrhea (up to 20 liters a day) and vomiting, rapidly causing dehydration and severe electrolyte imbalance. If the lost fluid and electrolytes are quickly and adequately replaced by oral rehydration therapy or intravenous administration of plasma, over 99% of patients recover; if not, mortality can be up to 50% (Nalin and Morris, 1991; Vaughan, 1982). *V. cholerae* is only toxigenic if it carries the *ctx* operon, which encodes the subunits of cholera toxin. Cholera toxin is composed of one A and five B subunits; the A subunit is post-translationally cleaved into two fragments, A_1 and A_2. The B subunit binds to the GM_1 ganglioside in the membrane of cells lining the intestinal lumen, allowing the A_1 fragment to enter the cell. Once inside, the A_1 fragment catalyzes the adenyl diphosphonucleotide (ADP) ribosylation of adenylate cyclase, causing this enzyme to generate unregulated amounts of cyclic AMP. cAMP then stimulates elevated levels of water and electrolyte secretion by the intestinal endothelial cells (Holmgren, 1981; Vaughan, 1982).

Classical Methods of Diagnosis

Clinical diagnosis of cholera is based on rapid onset of vomiting and the characteristic "rice-water" diarrhea. Identification of the *Vibrio* is classically accomplished by culturing the organism on the appropriate medium (e.g., thiosulfate-citrate-bile salt-sucrose [TCBS] or MacConkey's agar), with or without an enrichment step in alkaline peptone water for 6–18 hours. *V. cholerae* colonies are yellow in color and oxidase-positive. Confirmation of suspected *V. cholerae* is achieved by seroagglutination with group-specific (O1) followed by type-specific antisera. This process takes a minimum of 72 hours. Patient sera can also be tested for vibriocidal and antitoxin antibodies. A sharp rise in antibody titer between acute and convalescent serum samples or the presence of very high titers in convalescent sera indicates infection with *V. cholerae* (Nalin and Morris, 1991). To determine whether *V. cholerae* isolates are toxigenic, cholera toxin can be detected using a GM_1-ELISA, a reverse passive latex agglutination test (RPLA), or a cholera toxin bead-ELISA (Ramamurthy et al., 1992).

PCR-Based Procedures

Several PCR protocols have been developed for detection of the cholera toxin gene, amplifying a region of the *ctx* A gene (Fields et al., 1992; Lee et al., 1993), the *ctx* B gene (Shirai et al., 1991), or both (Shangkuan et al., 1995; Varela et al., 1993). One assay involves a multiplex PCR to simultaneously identify cholera toxin-producing *V. cholerae* and to biotype *V. cholerae* O1 (Shangkuan et al., 1995). PCR assays have been described for detection of *V. cholerae* O139 (Falklind et al., 1996). PCR-based methods have also been used to generate fingerprints for typing O1, O139, and non-O1 strains of *V. cholerae* (Coelho et al., 1995; Rivera et al., 1995). Different sample types can be analyzed by PCR; namely, isolated bacterial colonies (Fields et al., 1992; Shangkuan et al., 1995; Shirai et al., 1991), clinical specimens such as stool (Ramamurthy et al., 1993; Shirai et al., 1991; Varela et al., 1994), and food (DePaola and Hwang, 1995; Karunasagar et al., 1995; Koch et al., 1993) and water sources suspected of contamination. Procedures for concentrating bacteria in water samples (Bej et al., 1991) have been modified and combined with PCR detection of *V. cholerae*.[17]

Points to Consider in Using PCR

While PCR is a rapid, sensitive, and specific method for detecting toxigenic *V. cholerae*, it is important to define situations where it is really advantageous. Since treatment must be administered immediately and symptoms are fairly characteristic, clinical diagnosis of cholera is often sufficient. In addition, if a patient is sick due to infection with *V. cholerae*, it can be assumed that the bacteria are toxigenic. However, PCR tests are particularly useful when rapid confirmation of diagnosis is required.[18] Another important application of PCR is the identification of toxigenic *V. cholerae* in environmental samples and isolates, since not all O1 strains of the bacillus carry the toxin gene.

---

17. E. Harris, unpublished results.
18. For instance, rapid official confirmation of death due to cholera is necessary for expeditious disposal of the corpse in order to prevent further contamination.

PCR Detection of Toxigenic *Vibrio cholerae*

This protocol is used to amplify a 302-bp fragment of the *Vibrio cholerae ctx* B gene, which encodes the B subunit of cholera toxin (Shirai et al., 1991). This approach allows identification of *V. cholerae* as well as detection of the toxin-encoding *ctx* operon, which classifies the pathogen as toxigenic.

I. Sample Preparation: Grey Area

ADDITIONAL EQUIPMENT AND MATERIALS
Boiling water bath (100°C)
Incubator (37°C)
Sterile toothpicks
Collection vials
Floating rack for microcentrifuge tubes (plastic or Styrofoam)

REAGENTS
Sterile ddH$_2$0 (double-distilled water)
Petri plates containing Tryptic Soy Agar (TSA)
Alkaline peptone water
Mineral oil

A. Preparation of Suspected Cholera Stool Specimens

1. Collect stool specimens in the appropriately labeled collection vials.
2. Enrich in alkaline peptone water for 6–12 hours (optional).
3. Boil a 100-µL aliquot of each sample in a screw-cap microcentrifuge tube for 5 minutes.
4. Centrifuge the tubes for 5 minutes in a microcentrifuge at ambient temperature.
5. Transfer the supernatant to a sterile microcentrifuge tube. Proceed directly to the Amplification step or store the tubes at −20°C until further use. If the supernatant is not promptly transferred to a new tube, be sure to repeat the centrifugation in step 4 after thawing the samples and before proceeding to the Amplification.
6. Prior to amplification, prepare 1:10 and 1:100 dilutions of each sample in sterile ddH$_2$0. For the PCR amplification, use 5 µL of undiluted samples, 5 µL of the sample diluted 1:10, and 5 µL of the sample diluted 1:100 (if necessary). Dilution is a simple method for overcoming potential inhibition of the amplification reaction.

B. "Bacterial Lysis" Method for Preparation of V. cholerae Isolates

1. Label sterile 1.5-mL screw-cap microcentrifuge tubes by writing the appropriate number on the tube *and* on the cap with a permanent marker.
2. Transfer 100 µL of sterile ddH$_2$0 to each labeled tube.
3. Label a Petri plate containing TSA with the numbers of the colonies to be examined.
4. With a sterile toothpick, pick a colony of the putative *V. cholerae* isolates and touch the toothpick to the agar in a spot that corresponds to the number of the colony. Immerse the same toothpick in the appropriate tube containing 100 µL of sterile distilled water and agitate the toothpick in the water.
5. Incubate the tubes at 100°C in the water bath for 5 minutes.
6. Store the tubes at −20°C until further use (2–5 µL will be used for the PCR reaction).
7. Incubate the plate overnight at 37°C, then store at 4°C.

C. *"Direct Method" for Preparation of V. cholerae Isolates*

1. Label a Petri plate containing TSA with the numbers of the colonies to be examined.
2. Prepare the PCR Master Mix as described below under Amplification and label the appropriate PCR reaction tubes.
3. Aliquot 25 µL of the PCR mix into each labeled PCR reaction tube.
4. With a sterile toothpick, pick a colony of putative *V. cholerae* isolates and touch the toothpick to the agar in a spot that corresponds to the number of the colony. Immerse the same toothpick in the appropriately labeled tube containing the PCR Mix and agitate the toothpick in the solution.
5. Add 1 drop of mineral oil to each tube using a 1000-µL pipettor. Close the tubes.
6. Carry out the PCR amplification, using a thermocycler or manual amplification with water baths.
7. Incubate the plate overnight at 37°C, then store at 4°C.

II. Amplification

A. *Preparation of PCR Master Mix and Reaction Tubes:* **White Area**

REAGENTS
10X Buffer A (100 m*M* Tris [pH 9.0)], 500 m*M* KCl, 1% Triton® X-100)
dNTPs (5 m*M* each dATP, dCTP, dGTP, dTTP; 20 m*M* total dNTPs)
Primers (10 µ*M*)
  COL1: 5′-CTC AGA CGG GAT TTG TTA GGC ACG
  COL2: 5′-TCT ATC TCT GTA GCC CCT ATT ACG
MgCl$_2$ (25 m*M*)
ddH$_2$0
Taq polymerase (5 U/µL)
Mineral oil
Positive control (toxigenic *V. cholerae* DNA or lysed toxigenic *V. cholerae*)

Note: Before preparing the PCR Master Mix, go to the **Black Area** to enter the appropriate program in the thermocycler. If the program has already been entered, review it to ensure no changes have been inadvertently introduced; if so, correct the program and store it for later use. If the PCR will be manually amplified, prepare three water baths at the following temperatures: 60°C, 72°C, and 94°C, and ensure that these temperatures are stably maintained.

1. Calculate the amount of PCR Master Mix that will be necessary for the desired number of reactions, each with a total reaction volume of 25 µL. For every 10 reactions, add 1 extra volume of Master Mix to compensate for volume lost during pipetting. With the Bacterial Lysis Method and Stool Specimens, each 25-µL reaction will contain 22.5 µL of the PCR Master Mix and 2.5 µL of the sample, whereas with the Direct Method, each reaction contains 25 µL of the PCR Master Mix.
2. Fill out the PCR Worksheet according to the following table.

3.

Ingredient	Description	Stock conc.	Vol/25 µL rxn	Final conc.
Buffer 10X	Buffer A	10X	2.5 µL	1X
dNTPs	20 mM total dNTPs	5 mM A,C,G,T	1 µL	0.2 mM A,C,G,T
Primer 1	COL1	10 µM	0.625 µL	0.25 µM
Primer 2	COL2	10 µM	0.625 µL	0.25 µM
MgCl$_2$		25 mM	1.5 µL	1.5 mM
H$_2$O	ddH$_2$O		16.05 µL (Lysis)	
			18.55 µL (Direct)	
Taq	*Taq*	5 U/µL	0.2 µL	0.05 U/µL
Vol. of Master Mix			25 µL (Direct Method)	
			22.5 µL (Lysis Method/Stool Specimens)	
Vol. of sample (to be added in step 13)			2.5 µL (Lysis Method/Stool Specimens)	
Total reaction volume			25 µL	

4. Label the appropriate tubes (0.5-mL or 0.2-mL tubes for thermocyclers; 1.5-mL screw-cap tubes for manual amplification).
5. Thaw aliquot(s) of each reagent. Vortex each thawed solution well and briefly spin the tubes (pulse spin) in a microcentrifuge to collect all the liquid at the bottom of the tubes.

Keep all the ingredients and tubes on ice at all times.

6. In the **White Area**, using a **white** color-coded pipettor, prepare the PCR Master Mix with all the ingredients except the *Taq* polymerase. Check off each ingredient on the Worksheet after adding it to the Master Mix.
7. Mix well using a vortex or a large pipettor.
8. Add the *Taq* polymerase and mix by pipetting carefully with a pipettor set at half the total volume of the PCR Master Mix. Be careful not to create bubbles.
9. Distribute 22.5 µL of the PCR Master Mix (Lysis Method/Stool Specimen) or 25 µL of the Master Mix (Direct Method) into each labeled tube.
10. Add 1 drop of mineral oil to each tube using a 1000-µL pipettor.
11. Add 2.5 µL of ddH$_2$O to prepare a "white area" negative control across the layer of mineral oil (Lysis Method/Stool Specimen).
12. Transfer the tubes from the **white** ice bucket to a **grey** ice bucket.

*B. Sample Addition: **Grey Area***

13. In the **Grey Area**, using a **grey** color-coded pipettor, add 2.5 µL of the sample (Lysis Method/Stool Specimens) or control to the appropriate tube, *across* the layer of mineral oil. The controls should be added in the order of the most negative to the most positive. Use a new pipet tip for each sample. Remember to include a negative control consisting of the Grey Area water. *See* section I.C for sample addition when using the Direct Method.

C. Amplification Procedure: **Black Area**

EQUIPMENT
Thermocycler or water baths at 60°C, 72°C, and 94°C
Microcentrifuge

14. Amplification profile:

94°C	1 min		
60°C	1.5 min	30 cycles	Amplification
72°C	1.5 min		

Product size: This amplification generates a product of 302 base pairs that is indicative of the presence of *Vibrio cholerae* containing the cholera toxin operon, *ctx* (Figure 5.8).

III. Product Analysis

Use a 1.5% agarose gel and the procedure in section 5.1.2.

1 2 3 4 5 M 6 7 8

302 bp →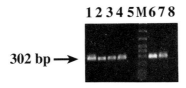

Fig. 5.8. Amplification of the toxin gene from Ecuadorian strains of *Vibrio cholerae*. Colonies were isolated, resuspended in sterile distilled water, and boiled for 5 minutes. PCR products were analyzed by gel electrophoresis. Lane 1, patient 5 (*V. cholerae* O1); lane 2, patient 6 (*V. cholerae* O1); lane 3, patient 7 (*V. cholerae* O1); lane 4, patient 2 plus *V. cholerae* DNA (inhibition control); lane 5, water (negative control); lane M, Amplisize DNA Size Standards (*see* Appendix C; lowest band shown, 50 bp); lane 6, *V. cholerae* O1 Inaba DNA (positive control); lane 7, patient 8 (*V. cholerae* O1); lane 9, *Vibrio parahaemolyticus* (specificity control). Expected product size, 302 bp.

5.1.8 Diarrheagenic *E. coli* and *Shigella*

Clinical Manifestations and Epidemiology

Diarrheagenic *Escherichia coli* (*E. coli*) are Gram-negative bacteria that have been divided into at least six categories with different virulence factors, distinct O (lipopolysaccharide) and H (flagellar) antigens, and differing clinical syndromes and epidemiologic patterns. These include enterotoxigenic *E. coli* (ETEC), enteropathogenic *E. coli* (EPEC), enteroinvasive *E. coli* (EIEC), enterohemorrhagic *E. coli* (EHEC), enteroadherent *E. coli* (EAEC), and enteroaggregative *E. coli* (EAggEC). The three types that are most prevalent in developing countries, ETEC, EPEC, and EIEC, will be described in this section, along with another Gram-negative bacterium, *Shigella* (*S. dysenteriae, S. flexneri, S. boydii*, and *S. sonnei*), which is taxonomically related to EIEC.

Diarrheal illnesses are associated with poverty, overcrowding, poor hygiene, inadequate water supplies, and malnutrition; therefore, they are common in developing countries and in marginalized communities in developed countries. Infected humans are presumably the primary reservoir of diarrheagenic ETEC, EPEC, and EIEC. ETEC is associated with watery diarrhea, nausea, abdominal cramps, and low-grade fever and is a major cause of of travelers' diarrhea and of diarrheal disease in children in developing countries. EPEC causes a watery diarrhea that may become persistent, lasting over 2 weeks. Severe disease associated with EPEC infections is almost entirely limited to infants under 6 months of age, and EPEC has often been incriminated in institutional outbreaks in hospitals and nurseries (Eisenstein, 1995). EIEC and *Shigella* cause invasive inflammatory diarrhea (dysentery) with characteristic blood- and mucus-containing stools, rectal tenesmus, abdominal cramping pain, and fever, and are responsible for endemic and epidemic diarrheal illnesses in all age groups in both developed and developing countries. A small inoculum of *Shigella* (10–1000 organisms) can cause disease, whereas the infective dose for EIEC is roughly 1000 times higher (Acheson and Keusch, 1995). ETEC and EPEC cause noninvasive diarrhea, which is best treated with oral rehydration therapy rather than with antibiotics. On the other hand, antibiotic treatment is indicated for inflammatory diarrhea caused by EIEC and *Shigella*.

ETEC colonize the proximal small intestine by means of fimbrial attachments and colonization factors and cause disease by producing either a heat-labile (LT) or a heat-stable (ST) toxin, or both. LT is a small polypeptide closely related to the cholera toxin (*see* section 5.1.7) and results in intracellular accumulation of cAMP, whereas ST, also a small polypeptide, activates guanylate cyclase, leading to an accumulation of cGMP. The end result of these biochemical imbalances is unregulated secretion of electrolytes and massive fluid loss. EPEC attach to epithelial cells, and this attachment is mediated by fimbrial structures known as bundle-forming pili (BFP), which are encoded by a gene on the enteroadherence factor (EAF) plasmid. Another virulence property exhibited by EPEC, the attachment and effacement of microvilli, requires chromosomal genes. The ability of EIEC and *Shigella* to invade, replicate within, and destroy epithelial cells lining the colon is conferred by multiple genes located on the virulence plasmid and in the chromosome (Levine, 1991).

Classical Methods of Diagnosis

Classical microbiological techniques are used to identify *E. coli*, first by plating on media such as MacConkey agar, which is selective for *Enterobacteriae*. The different diarrheagenic *E. coli* are indistinguishable from each other by biochemical tests. They can be grouped according to agglutination with antibodies specific to either the O or H antigen. To identify ETEC, toxin production must be demonstrated using immunoassays or bioassays. EPEC can be identified by agglutination with antisera against O serogroups or localized adherence to Hep-2 cells in culture (Levine, 1991). EIEC can be identified using an immunoassay that detects specific outer membrane proteins associated with invasiveness or by a laborious bioassay (the guinea pig keratoconjunctivitis test). EIEC can be distinguished from *Shigella* by biochemical methods; for example, EIEC is capable of lactose fermentation, whereas *Shigella* is not (Acheson and Keusch, 1995).

PCR-Based Procedures

Most PCR protocols for identification of diarrheagenic *E. coli* target genes that encode virulence factors associated with the different *E. coli* pathogens. As in the PCR amplification of cholera toxin (section 5.1.7), this strategy allows the simultaneous identification of the organism as *E. coli* and classification of the bacteria based on a particular virulence factor. For identification of ETEC, assays have been described for amplifying only the gene encoding the LT toxin (Deng et al., 1996; Lang et al., 1994; Olive, 1989; Oyofo et al., 1996; Tamanai-Shacoori et al., 1994; Victor et al., 1991) or the genes coding for both LT and ST (Abe et al., 1992; Candrian et al., 1991; Frankel et al., 1989; Schultsz et al., 1994; Stacy-Phipps et al., 1995; Tornieporth et al., 1995). EPEC can be identified by amplification of the adherence-associated BFP gene (Gunzburg et al., 1995; Tornieporth et al., 1995) or the EAF plasmid (Franke et al., 1994). For detection of EIEC and *Shigella*, the *ial* and *virF* loci on the virulence plasmid (Frankel et al., 1990; Islam and Lindberg, 1992; Sethabutr et al., 1993; Yavzori et al., 1994; Ye et al., 1993), the *ipaH* repetitive element found on both the plasmid and the chromosome (Oyofo et al., 1996; Sethabutr et al., 1993; Tornieporth et al., 1995), or the IS*630* sequence (Houng et al., 1997) can all be amplified. These sequences can be detected either separately or in multiplex reactions (Frankel et al., 1989; Lang et al., 1994; Oyofo et al., 1996; Stacy-Phipps et al., 1995). Most protocols referred to above describe identification of the bacteria directly from stool samples; however, since substances in feces can inhibit amplification, certain techniques must be used to further purify the extracted DNA prior to PCR (Lou et al., 1997; Stacy-Phipps et al., 1995). Food sources can also be evaluated for the presence of these diarrheagenic bacteria (Candrian et al., 1991; Deng et al., 1996), as can environmental water samples (Lang et al., 1994; Tamanai-Shacoori et al., 1994).

Genetic typing of various strains of diarrheagenic *E. coli* has been reported using RAPD analysis (Wang et al., 1993), while *Shigella* serotypes can be distinguished using primers directed to the *rfc* locus (Houng et al., 1997). However, many of the DNA-based methods that have been described for typing a wide variety of bacteria (including *E. coli*) do not differentiate the different categories of diarrheagenic *E. coli* because they do not identify the virulence genes responsible for the distinct pathologies.

Points to Consider in Using PCR

PCR is a useful diagnostic tool for EIEC or *Shigella*, because these invasive infections require treatment with antibiotics. Diarrheal illnesses caused by the non-invasive ETEC and EPEC can be treated with standard oral rehydration therapy; thus, PCR identification of the bacteria is not necessary for diagnosis and treatment. In these cases, PCR is useful for epidemiological investigations to understand the source of the outbreaks, identify risk factors, and design control measures. For example, using these techniques, it was found that EPEC in Salvador, Brazil, was entirely hospital-associated (Seigel et al., 1996), whereas ETEC tends to be community-associated. PCR is also helpful for identification of the various diarreagenic *E. coli* bacteria in food and water sources for confirmation of epidemiological findings.

When using PCR to analyze human samples, it is important to recognize the advantage offered by combining microbiological and DNA-based techniques. By first culturing the sample on selective plates and then using PCR to identify the resulting colonies, rather than amplifying directly from stool samples, the bacterial load can be determined. This is important since the *number* of a particular diarrheagenic bacteria in the stool correlates with clinical manifestation of disease and distinguishes a nonsymptomatic carrier from a symptomatic case. In other words, a stool sample may be positive for several diarrheagenic bacteria, but the elevated numbers of one particular pathogen would indicate that it is the predominant cause of diarrheal disease, whereas the individual would be considered a carrier of the other detected microorganisms. This valuable information is not available when PCR is used directly from stool because it is not a quantitative method.

PCR Differentiation of Diarrheagenic *Escherichia coli* and *Shigella*

The following protocols can be used to amplify three distinctly sized products from different diarrheagenic *Escherichia coli* and *Shigella*. Diagnostic fragments are generated from the heat-labile (LT) and heat-stable (ST) toxin genes of enterotoxigenic *E. coli* (ETEC) and from the *ial* invasion-associated locus of *Shigella* (Frankel et al., 1989). Another more recent publication describes a protocol for amplifying four different-sized products from the LT and STa genes of ETEC, the *ipaH* invasion-associated gene of enteroinvasive *E. coli* (EIEC) and *Shigella*, and the bundle-forming pilus (BFP) gene of enteropathogenic *E. coli* (EPEC).[19]

I. Sample Preparation: Grey Area

ADDITIONAL EQUIPMENT AND MATERIALS
Boiling water bath (100°C)
Incubator (37°C)
Bunsen burner
Collection vials
Floating rack for microcentrifuge tubes (plastic or Styrofoam)
Sterile 1.5-mL screw-cap microcentrifuge tubes
Sterile wooden toothpicks or inoculating loop

REAGENTS
Sterile ddH$_2$0 (double-distilled water)
Sterile phosphate buffered saline (PBS)
Cary-Blair transport medium (*see* Appendix B)
Petri plates with MacConkey agar[20]

1. Place rectal swabs from patients in Cary-Blair transport medium. Plate onto Petri plates containing MacConkey agar and incubate overnight at 37°C.
2. Label sterile 1.5-mL screw-cap microcentrifuge tubes by writing the appropriate number on the tube *and* on the cap with a permanent marker.

---

19. Each amplification is conducted separately, with a single primer pair directed to one of the four targets. Reaction conditions for these amplifications are similar to those described above, except that the magnesium chloride concentration in each amplification is 1 mM, and each primer concentration is 1 μM. The amplification profile consists of 30 cycles of 94°C for 1 min, 56°C for 2 min, and 72°C for 1 min, yielding a 708-bp fragment from the LT gene of ETEC, a 182-bp product from the STa gene of ETEC, a 324-bp fragment from the BFP gene of EPEC, and a 424-bp product from the *ipaH* locus of EIEC and *Shigella*. The primer sequences are as follows: ET-LT1: 5'-GCG ACA AAT TAT ACC GTG CT; ET-LT2: 5'-CCG AAT TCT GTT ATA TAT GT; ET-ST1: 5'-CTG TAT TGT CTT TTT CAC CT; ET-ST2: 5'-GCA CCC GGT ACA AGC AGG AT; EP1: 5'-CAA TGG TGC TTG CGC TTG CT; EP2: 5'-GCC GCT TTA TCC AAC CTG GT; EI-1: 5'-GCT GGA AAA ACT CAG TGC CT; EI-2:5'-CCA GTC CGT AAA TTC ATT CT (Tornieporth et al., 1995).
20. MacConkey medium contains deoxycholate, which can interfere with amplification. Therefore, colonies grown on MacConkey agar should be washed in PBS two or three times before lysing the bacteria.

3. Transfer 300 µL of sterile PBS to each labeled tube.

4. Using a sterile toothpick or inoculating loop, transfer the bacterial colonies from each plate into the 300 µL of sterile PBS in the appropriately labeled microcentrifuge tube and mix.

5. Centrifuge the tubes for 2 minutes in a microcentrifuge, remove the supernatant, and resuspend the bacteria in 300 µL of sterile PBS.

6. Repeat step 5 but resuspend the bacteria in 300 µL of sterile ddH$_2$0.

7. Incubate the tubes at 100°C in the boiling water bath for 10 minutes, using a floating rack.

8. Mix the lysate by pipetting and centrifuge the tubes for 2 minutes at ambient temperature.

9. Transfer the supernatant to a sterile microcentrifuge tube. Proceed directly to the Amplification step or store the tubes at −20°C until further use. If the supernatant is not promptly transferred to a new tube, be sure to repeat the centrifugation in step 8 after thawing the samples and before proceeding to the Amplification.

II. Amplification

A. Preparation of PCR Master Mix and Reaction Tubes: **White Area**

REAGENTS

10X Buffer B (100 m*M* Tris [pH 8.3], 500 m*M* KCl)

dNTPs (5 m*M* each dATP, dCTP, dGTP, dTTP; 20 m*M* total dNTPs)

Primers (10 µ*M*)

   LT-1: 5′-GGC GAC AGA TTA TAC CGT GC

   LT-2: 5′-CCG AAT TCT GTT ATA TAT GTC

   ST-1: 5′-TCT GTA TTG TCT TTT TCA CC

   ST-2: 5′-TTA ATA GCA CCC GGT ACA AGC

   Sh-1: 5′-CTG GAT GGT ATG GTG AGG

   Sh-2: 5′-GGA GGC CAA CAA TTA TTT CC

MgCl$_2$ (25 m*M*)

ddH$_2$0

Taq polymerase (5 U/µL)

Mineral oil

Positive control (purified DNA or boiled lysates of reference strains of the different diarrheagenic *E. coli* and *Shigella*)

Note: Before preparing the PCR Master Mix, go to the **Black Area** to enter the appropriate program in the thermocycler. If the program has already been entered, review it to ensure no changes have been inadvertently introduced; if so, correct the program and store it for later use. If the PCR will be manually amplified, prepare three water baths at the following temperatures: 45°C, 53°C, 72°C, and 94°C, and ensure that these temperatures are stably maintained.

1. Calculate the amount of PCR Master Mix that will be necessary for the desired number of reactions, each containing 22.5 µL of Master Mix. For every 10 reaction volumes, add 1 extra volume of Master Mix to compensate for volume lost during pipetting.

2. Fill out the PCR Worksheet according to the following table.

3. a. For the ETEC LT gene:

Ingredient	Description	Stock conc.	Vol/25 µL rxn	Final conc.
Buffer 10X	Buffer B	10X	2.5 µL	1X
dNTPs	20 mM total dNTPs	5 mM A,C,G,T	1.0 µL	0.2 mM A,C,G,T
Primer 1	LT-1	10 µM	1.0 µL	0.4 µM
Primer 2	LT-2	10 µM	1.0 µL	0.4 µM
MgCl$_2$		25 mM	2.5 µL	2.5 mM
H$_2$0	ddH$_2$0		14.375 µL	
Taq	*Taq*	5 U/µL	0.125 µL	0.025 U/µL

Vol. of Master Mix   22.5 µL
Vol. of sample (to be added in step 13)   2.5 µL
Total reaction volume   25 µL

b. For the ETEC ST gene:

Ingredient	Description	Stock conc.	Vol/25 µL rxn	Final conc.
Buffer 10X	Buffer B	10X	2.5 µL	1X
dNTPs	20 mM total dNTPs	5 mM A,C,G,T	1.0 µL	0.2 mM A,C,G,T
Primer 1	ST-1	10 µM	1.0 µL	0.4 µM
Primer 2	ST-2	10 µM	1.0 µL	0.4 µM
MgCl$_2$		25 mM	2.5 µL	2.5 mM
H$_2$0	ddH$_2$0		14.375 µL	
Taq	*Taq*	5 U/µL	0.125 µL	0.025 U/µL

Vol. of Master Mix   22.5 µL
Vol. of sample (to be added in step 13)   2.5 µL
Total reaction volume   25 µL

c. For the *Shigella ial* locus:

Ingredient	Description	Stock conc.	Vol/25 µL rxn	Final conc.
Buffer 10X	Buffer B	10X	2.5 µL	1X
dNTPs	20 mM total dNTPs	5 mM A,C,G,T	1.0 µL	0.2 mM A,C,G,T
Primer 1	Sh-1	10 µM	1.0 µL	0.4 µM
Primer 2	Sh-2	10 µM	1.0 µL	0.4 µM
MgCl$_2$		25 mM	2.5 µL	2.5 mM
H$_2$0	ddH$_2$0		14.375 µL	
Taq	*Taq*	5 U/µL	0.125 µL	0.025 U/µL

Vol. of Master Mix   22.5 µL
Vol. of sample (to be added in step 13)   2.5 µL
Total reaction volume   25 µL

4. Label the appropriate tubes (0.5-mL or 0.2-mL tubes for thermocyclers; 1.5-mL screw-cap tubes for manual amplification).

5. Thaw aliquot(s) of each reagent. Vortex each thawed solution well and briefly spin the tubes (pulse spin) in a microcentrifuge to collect all the liquid at the bottom of the tubes.

Keep all the ingredients and tubes on ice at all times.

6. In the **White Area**, using a **white** color-coded pipettor, prepare the PCR Master Mix with all the ingredients except the *Taq* polymerase. Check off each ingredient on the Worksheet after adding it to the Master Mix.

7. Mix well using a vortex or a large pipettor.

8. Add the *Taq* polymerase and mix by pipetting carefully with a pipettor set at half the total volume of the PCR Master Mix. Be careful not to create bubbles.

9. Distribute 22.5 µL of the PCR Master Mix into each labeled tube.

10. Add 1 drop of mineral oil to each tube using a 1000-µL pipettor.

11. Add 2.5 µL of ddH$_2$O to prepare a "white area" negative control across the layer of mineral oil.

12. Transfer the tubes from the **white** ice bucket to a **grey** ice bucket.

B. *Sample Addition: **Grey Area***

13. In the **Grey Area**, using a **grey** color-coded pipettor, add 2.5 µL of the sample or control to the appropriate tube, *across* the layer of mineral oil. The controls should be added in the order of the most negative to the most positive. Use a new pipet tip for each sample. Remember to include a negative control consisting of the Grey Area water.

C. *Amplification Procedure: **Black Area***

EQUIPMENT
Thermocycler or water baths at 45°C, 53°C, 72°C, and 94°C
Microcentrifuge

14. Amplification profile:

94°C	1 min		
45°C	1 min	5 cycles	Amplification
72°C	1 min		
94°C	1 min		
53°C	1 min	25 cycles	Amplification
72°C	1 min		
72°C	3 min	1 cycle	Final extension

Product size: The following products are obtained from these amplifications: a 750-bp fragment from the LT gene of ETEC, a 186-bp product from the ST gene of ETEC, and a 320-bp product from the *ial* locus of *Shigella*.

III. Product Analysis

Use a 1.5% agarose gel and the procedure in section 5.1.2.

5.1.9   *Chlamydia trachomatis* and *Neisseria gonorrhoeae*

Chlamydia trachomatis and *Neisseria gonorrhoeae* are both important causes of sexually transmitted diseases; these bacteria are associated with similar symptoms but require different treatment regimens. The protocols provided below describe PCR amplifications that detect each pathogen separately as well as a multiplex amplification that detects both pathogens simultaneously, but with slightly lower sensitivity.

Chlamydia trachomatis: Clinical Manisfestations and Epidemiology

C. trachomatis,[21] which is divided into 18 serovars, is one of the most common sexually transmitted bacterial diseases, causing more than 50 million new cases annually (Black, 1997). It causes urogenital tract disease, trachoma and inclusion conjunctivitis (ocular disease), and lymphogranuloma venereum (LGV); different serovars tend to be associated with each type of disease (Taylor and Bell, 1991). Although nearly 70–80% of infected women are asymptomatic, when symptoms do occur they include cervicitis, urethritis, and endometritis. Untreated *C. trachomatis* infections can cause pelvic inflammatory disease (PID), infertility, scarring, and ectopic pregnancies; the risk of developing these sequelae may increase with each successive infection. Since immunity is only partially protective, recurrent infections are common. In men, clinical manifestations are similar to gonorrhea, and sequelae include epididymitis and arthritis; up to 50% of men experience asymptomatic infections. Risk factors include youth, multiple sexual partners, failure to use contraception barriers, and concurrent gonococcal infection. The high percentage of asymptomatic infections result in a large reservoir of carriers who can unknowingly transmit the pathogen to sexual partners. In addition, 65% of newborns born to infected untreated mothers become infected during vaginal delivery, and *C. trachomatis* is one of the most common causes of neonatal conjunctivitis and pneumonia.

 Chlamydia are nonmotile, Gram-negative bacteria, which are obligate intracellular pathogens because they require an exogenous source of the high-energy compound, adenosine triphosphate (ATP) (Black, 1997). The infectious form of *Chlamydia*, the elementary body, induces phagocytosis and develops within the host cell phagosome to a metabolically active and dividing reticulate body. This reticulate body then reforms elementary bodies that are released to infect other cells (Taylor and Bell, 1991).

C. trachomatis: Classical Methods of Diagnosis

Culture was considered the reference method for diagnosis of chlamydial infections until recently. It is now recognized that nucleic acid amplification techniques are more sensitive than culture. Specimens must be inoculated onto cell culture monolayers and then visualized 2–3 days later by staining with fluorescently labeled antibodies specific to the *C. trachomatis* major outer membrane protein (MOMP) or to the genus-specific lipopolysaccharide (LPS). Limitations of culture include the high

---

21. The genus *Chlamydia* consists of four species: *C. trachomatis*, *C. psittaci*, *C. pneumoniae*, and *C. pecorum*.

cost, technical expertise, and length of time required to obtain results. Direct cyto-logic examination using Giemsa stain can be useful for diagnosis of neonatal inclusion conjuntivitis, but requires substantial expertise. The direct fluorescent-antibody (DFA) also requires microscopic examination by experienced personnel, but the sensitivity and specificity are much higher, especially using anti-MOMP monoclonal antibodies (80–90% sensitivity and 98–99% specificity relative to culture) (Black, 1997). Many commercial tests are based on detection of chlamydial LPS by enzyme immunoassay (EIA) (e.g., Chlamydiazyme, Abbott Diagnostics, North Chicago, IL). The overall sensitivity ranges from 73–86%, and specificity from 98–99%, depending on the manufacturer and the specimen type (urine, endocervical swabs, or male urethral samples). Serological tests are only useful for diagnosis of chlamydial pneumonitis in infants and LGV, but not for genital tract infections. DNA probes that hybridize to species-specific sequences of the 16S rRNA (PACE 2, Gen-Probe Inc., San Diego, CA) have an overall sensitivity of 85% and specificity of 98–99% relative to culture. For comparison, the limit of detection of each diagnostic technique is: 1–10 organisms for nucleic acid amplification techniques, 5–100 organisms for culture, 10–500 organisms for DFA, 500–10,000 organisms for DNA probes, and 5000–100,000 organisms for EIA (Black, 1997).

C. trachomatis: PCR-Based Detection Procedures

PCR assays for detection of *C. trachomatis* target either the cryptic plasmid (Claas et al., 1990; Griffais and Thibon, 1989; Loeffelholz et al., 1992; Lucotte et al., 1992; Mahony et al., 1992; Naher et al., 1991; Ossewaarde et al., 1992; Ostergaard et al., 1990; Ratti et al., 1991; Welch et al., 1990), which is present at 7–10 copies per cell, or chromosomal sequences, including the MOMP gene (Bobo et al., 1990; Dean et al., 1992; Dutilh et al., 1989; Holland et al., 1990; Ossewaarde et al., 1992; Palmer et al., 1991; Taylor-Robinson et al., 1992), the 16S rRNA (Claas et al., 1990, 1991), or the cysteine-rich outer membrane protein gene (Watson et al., 1991). Plasmid-based PCR assays appear to be more sensitive than amplifications that target chromosomal elements (Mahony et al., 1993; Roosendaal et al., 1993). Some strains of *C. trachomatis* lack the cryptic plasmid (An et al., 1992; Peterson et al., 1990), but these cases are rare (Black, 1997; Roosendaal et al., 1993). Multiplex assays for simultaneous detection of *C. trachomatis* and *N. gonorrhoeae* have also been described (Mahoney et al., 1995; Wong et al., 1995). A competitive PCR based on the MOMP gene has been developed to quantitate *C. trachomatis* (Frost et al., 1995). Overall, PCR appears to be more sensitive than culture for detection of *C. tra-chomatis* (Black, 1997).

Several commercial PCR-based detection systems are available that target the cryptic plasmid (e.g., Amplicor, Roche Diagnostic Systems, Branchburg, NJ) or the MOMP gene (Genemed Biotechnologies, San Francisco, CA). The Amplicor test has been widely used in developed countries, and many reports have been published evaluating its performance in clinical laboratory settings (Black, 1997). Roche Diagnostic Systems also manufactures a PCR assay for detection of both *C. tra-*

chomatis and *N. gonorrhoeae* (Amplicor CT/NG). Another commercially available amplification technique for diagnosis of chlamydial infections is the Ligase Chain Reaction (Abbott Laboratories, Abbott Park, IL), which uses primers directed to the cryptic plasmid. The Q-β replicase system is another, more complex amplification system that has been applied to detection of *Chlamydia* by targeting the 16S rRNA genes (An et al., 1995)

Clinical samples used for PCR diagnosis of urogenital infections include urine, urethral specimens, endocervical swabs, and tampon-collected genital cells (Black, 1997; Tabrizi et al., 1996, 1997). Peripheral blood, peripheral blood leukocytes, synovial fluid, and synovial-membrane biopsies are used for diagnosis of *Chlamydia*-induced reactive arthritis (Taylor-Robinson et al., 1992), and conjunctival samples can be processed for detection of ocular chlamydial infections (Dean et al., 1989).

C. trachomatis serovars can be typed by PCR amplification of the MOMP gene (*omp1*) followed by restriction enzyme digestion (Frost et al., 1991; Gaydos et al., 1992; Lan et al., 1993; Rodriguez et al., 1991; Sayada et al., 1991). Higher sensitivity has been reported using a nested PCR of *omp1* for subsequent RFLP analysis (Lan et al., 1994). Fluorescently labeled genotype-specific MOMP gene primers have been used to differentiate serovars by nested amplification of conjunctivitis samples followed by polyacrylamide gel electrophoresis (Pecharatana et al., 1993). Genotyping of individual chlamydial strains has been accomplished by amplification and sequencing of *omp1* (Dean et al., 1992, 1995; Dean and Stephens., 1994). Differentiation of *Chlamydia* species has also been conducted by RAPD analysis (Scieux et al., 1993).

Neisseria gonorrhoeae: Clinical Manisfestations and Epidemiology

Gonorrhea is one of the oldest known human diseases and is still a major sexually transmitted disease today. *N. gonorrhoeae*, a Gram-negative diplococcus, is estimated to cause 78 million new infections per year (WHO, 1995). After reaching a peak in 1978, incidence of gonorrhea has declined steadily in the United States and in other industrialized countries. However, gonorrhea and its complications remain a major problem in developing countries. Transmission is almost exclusively via sexual contact or perinatally. The most common symptom of gonorrhea in men is purulent urethritis; clinical manifestations in women are endocervicitis and vaginitis. Complications include pelvic inflammatory disease, acute salpingitis, infertility, and ectopic pregnancy in women and acute epididymitis in men (Handsfield and Sparling, 1995). Asymptomatic infections can occur in both sexes; these carriers are epidemiologically important since they are not treated and serve as reservoirs of transmission. Repeated infections do not produce immunity to reinfection. Perinatal transmission of *N. gonorrhoeae* results in severe conjunctivitis, arthritis, and septicemia (Bell and Perine, 1991). Resistance to antibiotics such as penicillin and tetracyclines is widespread, and can be caused by either chromosomal or plasmid-encoded genes.[22]

N. gonorrhoeae: Classical Methods of Diagnosis

Direct Gram stain of *N. gonorrhoeae* is useful for diagnosis of symptomatic urethritis in men but is much less sensitive for asymptomatic infections and diagnosis
of gonorrhea in women. The standard diagnostic technique involves culture of specimens on nonselective medium (e.g., chocolate agar) or selective medium; the small
mucoid colonies that result are Gram-stained and tested for oxidase. Specimens for
N. gonorrhoeae can be differentiated from other species of *Neisseria* by the ability
of *N. gonorrhoeae* to ferment glucose but not lactose, maltose, or sucrose. Co-agglu-
tination using monoclonal antibodies, determination of nutritional requirements, and
biochemical analysis of enzymes are examples of confirmatory tests (Bell and
Perine, 1991). A major advantage of culture is that the isolated strains can be tested
for antibiotic resistance. Enzyme immunoassays, fluorescein-conjuguated monoclonal antibodies, and DNA probes are all less sensitive than culture (Handsfield and
Sparling, 1995). Serological tests are not useful for diagnosis since they do not distinguish past from current infections (Bell and Perine, 1991).

N. gonorrhoeae: PCR-Based Detection Procedures

Assays reported for the detection of *N. gonorrhoeae* by PCR amplify the *cppB* gene
on the cryptic plasmid and follow either standard PCR protocols (Ho et al., 1992) or
a single-tube nested PCR format (Herrmann et al., 1996). Duplex PCR protocols
have been described to amplify both *N. gonorrhoeae* and *C. trachomatis* (mentioned
above). Another set of primers directed to the 16S rDNA sequences amplify fragments from all the pathogenic *Neisseria*, but are not specific to *N. gonorrhoeae*
(Murallidhar and Steinman, 1994). Specimens tested by these techniques include
first-void urine samples, cervical and urethral swabs, and cervical swabs smeared on
glass slides, air-dried, and kept at room temperature for 18 months (Herrmann et al.,
1996). As with *C. trachomatis*, self-administered tampon-collected specimens have
been shown to be adequate samples for PCR detection of *N. gonorrhoeae*. This
method is thus useful for diagnosis of sexually transmitted diseases of women living
in remote communities since the samples can be collected by the patients themselves
and shipped to diagnostic facilities for testing (Tabrizi et al., 1997). RAPD-based
typing can distinguish *N. gonorrhoeae* from other *Neisseria* species and differentiate
certain groups within *N. gonorrhoeae* (Zhu et al., 1995).

C. trachomatis and N. gonorrhoeae: Points to Consider in Using PCR

The high sensitivity of PCR-based techniques allows detection of *C. trachomatis* and
N. gonorrhoeae in samples (e.g., urine) collected by noninvasive procedures. This is a
significant advantage since many chlamydial and gonorrheal infections are asymptomatic. The use of easily-collected samples enables more effective screening programs
to be conducted. Multiplex assays for the simultaneous detection of both pathogens are

---

22. For example, some plasmids carry the enzyme beta-lactamase that destroys the beta-lactam ring of
    the penicillin molecule, thereby conferring penicillin resistance to the organism.

particulary useful, since these two organisms cause similar clinical manifestations and are frequently present in simultaneous infections, particularly in women (Handsfield and Sparling, 1995). PCR-based techniques are especially useful for diagnosis of *C. trachomatis* infections because the other diagnostic techniques are difficult and expensive. Since nucleic acid amplification techniques, which are more sensitive than culture, have been employed for detection of this pathogen, it has been shown that the prevalence of *C. trachomatis* infection is higher than was previously believed. The main disadvantage cited for nucleic acid amplification techniques is the high cost associated with performing the tests (Schachter, 1997). In-house PCR assays are more cost-effective, but require rigorous quality control to ensure reproducibility. Lastly, important epidemiological information about *C. trachomatis* can be obtained from studies using PCR-based methods for identifying serovars or genotyping individual strains.

PCR Detection of *Chlamydia trachomatis* and *Neisseria gonorrhoeae*

In these PCR protocols, a 241-bp fragment from the cryptic plasmid of *C. tra-chomatis* and a 390-bp fragment from the *cppB* gene on the cryptic plasmid of *N. gonorrhoeae* are amplified (Mahoney et al., 1995). Since there are multiple copies of these plasmids in each bacterium, these assays are more sensitive than other PCR assays that target only single-copy chromosomal genes. The two PCR protocols described below can be combined into one multiplex amplification that allows simultaneous detection of *C. trachomatis* and *N. gonorrhoeae* (Version 1); however, the sensitivity is slightly lower than if sequences from each pathogen are amplified in separate reactions (Versions 2 and 3).

I. Sample Preparation: Grey Area

ADDITIONAL EQUIPMENT AND MATERIALS
Boiling water bath (100°C)
Collection vials (1-mL cryovials)
Floating rack for microcentrifuge tubes (plastic or styrofoam)
Sterile Dacron®-tipped applicators (Fisherbrand #14–959–90)

REAGENTS
Sterile ddH$_2$0 (double-distilled water)
5% Chelex® 100 (Bio-Rad Laboratories, #143–2832) in ddH$_2$0

A. Preparation of Endocervical Swab Specimens[23]

1. Aliquot 500 µL of 5% Chelex® 100 into 1-mL cryovials.
2. Label the cryovials appropriately before collecting specimens.
3. Take an endocervical swab using a Dacron®-tipped applicator.[24] This is usually done during a pelvic examination.
4. Place the Dacron tip of the swab in the 5% Chelex 100 solution so that it is completely submerged and break off the plastic shaft at the top of the cryovial.
5. Close the cryovial tightly.
6. Agitate thoroughly using a vortex mixer for 30 seconds to 1 minute.
7. Remove the Dacron swab, squeezing out excess liquid by pressing the swab against the side of the vial.
8. Boil the cryovial for 10 minutes in a boiling water bath.
9. Centrifuge the vials for 5 minutes in a microcentrifuge.

---

23. While the preparation of material from endocervical swabs is described here, these PCR amplifications can be conducted with other clinical samples as well, including first-void urine (Mahony et al., 1992), urethral specimens (Mahony et al., 1992), and tampon-collected genital cells (Tabrizi et al., 1996, 1997). Ocular chlamydial infections can be detected by analyzing conjunctival specimens (Dean et al., 1992, 1993).
24. In choosing materials for sample collection, it must be kept in mind that some applicators contain materials that can inhibit *Taq* polymerase. The Dacron®-tipped applicators described in this protocol have been extensively tested and do not inhibit PCR.

10. Prepare 150-μL aliquots of the supernatants. Sample aliquots can be frozen at $-20°C$ until later use or amplified immediately. If the aliquots are frozen, always repeat the centrifugation in step 9 after thawing completely and before proceeding to the amplification.
11. Use 5 μL of the supernatant for each PCR amplification.

II. Amplification

A. Preparation of PCR Master Mix and Reaction Tubes: **White Area**

REAGENTS
10X Buffer B (100 m*M* Tris [pH 8.3)], 500 m*M* KCl)
dNTPs (5 m*M* each dATP, dCTP, dGTP, dTTP; 20 m*M* total dNTPs)
Primers (10 μ*M*)
   KL1: 5′-TCC GGA GCG AGT TACG AAG A
   KL2: 5′-AAT CAA TGC CCG GGA TTG GT
   HO1: 5′-GCT ACG CAT ACC CGC GTT GC
   HO3: 5′-CGA AGA CCT TCG AGC AGA CA
MgCl$_2$ (25 m*M*)
ddH$_2$0
Taq polymerase (5 U/μL)
Mineral oil
Positive control (purified *C. trachomatis* and *N. gonorrhoeae* DNA)

Note: Before preparing the PCR Master Mix, go to the **Black Area** to enter the appropriate program in the thermocycler. If the program has already been entered, review it to ensure no changes have been inadvertently introduced; if so, correct the program and store it for later use. If the PCR will be manually amplified, prepare three water baths at the following temperatures: 55°C, 72°C, and 94°C, and ensure that these temperatures are stably maintained.

1. Calculate the amount of PCR Master Mix that will be necessary for the desired number of reactions, each containing 20 μL of Master Mix. For every 10 reactions, add 1 extra volume of Master Mix to compensate for volume lost during pipetting.
2. Fill out the PCR Worksheet according to the following table.

   Version 1: Multiplex PCR of *C. trachomatis* and *N. gonorrhoeae*

Ingredient	Description	Stock conc.	Vol/25 μL rxn	Final conc.
Buffer 10X	Buffer B	10X	2.5 μL	1X
dNTPs	20 m*M* total dNTPs	5 m*M* A,C,G,T	1.0 μL	0.2 m*M* A,C,G,T
Primer 1	KL1	10 μ*M*	2.5 μL	1 μ*M*
Primer 2	KL2	10 μ*M*	2.5 μL	1 μ*M*
Primer 3	HO1	10 μ*M*	2.5 μL	1 μ*M*
Primer 4	HO3	10 μ*M*	2.5 μL	1 μ*M*
MgCl$_2$		25 m*M*	2.0 μL	2.0 m*M*
H$_2$O	ddH$_2$O		4.25 μL	
Taq	*Taq*	5 U/ul	0.25 μL	0.05 U/μL
Vol. of Master Mix			20 μL	
Vol. of sample (to be added in step 13)			5 μL	
Total reaction volume			25 μL	

Version 2: Amplification of only *C. trachomatis*

Ingredient	Description	Stock conc.	Vol/25 µL rxn	Final conc.
Buffer 10X	Buffer B	10X	2.5 µL	1X
dNTPs	20 m*M* total dNTPs	5 m*M* A,C,G,T	1.0 µL	0.2 m*M* A,C,G,T
Primer 1	KL1	10 µ*M*	2.5 µL	1 µ*M*
Primer 2	KL2	10 µ*M*	2.5 µL	1 µ*M*
MgCl₂		25 m*M*	2.0 µL	2.0 m*M*
H₂O	ddH₂O		9.25 µL	
Taq	*Taq*	5 U/ul	0.25 µL	0.05 U/µL

Vol. of Master Mix		20 µL
Vol. of sample (to be added in step 13)		5 µL
Total reaction volume		25 µL

Version 3: Amplification of only *N. gonorrhoeae*

Ingredient	Description	Stock conc.	Vol/25 µL rxn	Final conc.
Buffer 10X	Buffer B	10X	2.5 µL	1X
dNTPs	20 m*M* total dNTPs	5 m*M* A,C,G,T	1.0 µL	0.2 m*M* A,C,G,T
Primer 1	HO1	10 µ*M*	2.5 µL	1 µ*M*
Primer 2	HO3	10 µ*M*	2.5 µL	1 µ*M*
MgCl₂		25 m*M*	2.0 µL	2.0 m*M*
H₂O	ddH₂O		9.25 µL	
Taq	*Taq*	5 U/ul	0.25 µL	0.05 U/µL

Vol. of Master Mix		20 µL
Vol. of sample (to be added in step 13)		5 µL
Total reaction volume		25 µL

4. Label the appropriate tubes (0.5-mL or 0.2-mL tubes for thermocyclers; 1.5-mL screw-cap tubes for manual amplification).

5. Thaw aliquot(s) of each reagent. Vortex each thawed solution well and briefly spin the tubes (pulse spin) in a microcentrifuge to collect all the liquid at the bottom of the tubes.

Keep all the ingredients and tubes on ice at all times.

6. In the **White Area**, using a **white** color-coded pipettor, prepare the PCR Master Mix with all the ingredients except the *Taq* polymerase. Check off each ingredient on the Worksheet after adding it to the Master Mix.

7. Mix well using a vortex or a large pipettor.

8. Add the *Taq* polymerase and mix by pipetting carefully with a pipettor set at half the total volume of the PCR Master Mix. Be careful not to create bubbles.

9. Distribute 20 µL of the PCR Master Mix into each labeled tube.

10. Add 1 drop of mineral oil to each tube using a 1000-µL pipettor.

11. Add 5 µL of ddH₂O to prepare a "white area" negative control across the layer of mineral oil.

12. Transfer the tubes from the **white** ice bucket to a **grey** ice bucket.

B. Sample Addition: **Grey Area**

13. In the **Grey Area**, using a **grey** color-coded pipettor, add 5 µL of the sample[25] or control to the appropriate tube, *across* the layer of mineral oil. The controls should be added in the order of the most negative to the most positive. Use a new pipet tip for each sample. Remember to include a negative control consisting of the Grey Area water.

C. Amplification Procedure: **Black Area**

EQUIPMENT
Thermocycler or water baths at 55°C, 72°C, and 94°C
Microcentrifuge

14. Amplification profile:

94°C	1 min		
55°C	1 min	35 cycles	Amplification
72°C	2 min		

Product size: A product of 241 base pairs is generated from *C. trachomatis* and a product of 390 base pairs is amplified from *N. gonorrhoeae* (Figure 5.9).

III. Product Analysis

Use a 1.5% agarose gel and the procedure in section 5.1.2.

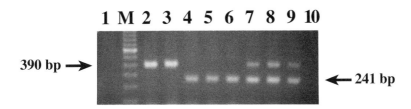

Fig. 5.9. Multiplex PCR amplification of *Chlamydia trachomatis* and *Neisseria gonorrhoeae*. Endocervical swabs were collected from sex workers in Managua, Nicaragua, placed in Chelex® 100, and boiled to liberate bacterial DNA. The samples were amplified using a multiplex PCR assay; products were analyzed by gel electrophoresis. Lane M, 100-bp ladder (*see* Appendix C; lowest band shown, 100 bp); lane 1, negative control (water); lanes 2 and 3, patients positive for *N. gonorrhoeae* only; lanes 4–6, patients positive for *C. trachomatis* only; lanes 7 and 8, patients positive for both *C. trachomatis* and *N. gonorrhoeae*; lane 9, positive control for *C. trachomatis* and *N. gonorrhoeae*; lane 10, final negative control (water). Expected product sizes: *C. trachomatis*, 241 bp; *N. gonorrhoeae*; 390 bp.

---

25. When analyzing clinical specimens, 5 µL of each sample should be used as template; however, when amplifying purified DNA, 1–2.5 µL is sufficient template for each PCR reaction. In the latter case, the volume can be adjusted to 5 µL with ddH₂O.

5.1.10   *Leptospira*

Clinical Manifestations and Epidemiology

Leptospirosis is an acute systemic disease caused by spirochetes belonging to the genus *Leptospira*. The seven pathogenic species (*L. interrogans*, *L. borgpetersenii*, *L. weilii*, *L. noguchii*, *L. santarosai*, *L. inadai*, and *L. kirschneri*) are further divided into multiple serogroups and serovars[26] (Yasuda et al., 1987). *Leptospira* are shed in the urine of infected mammalian hosts, with rodents being the most important animal reservoir. Humans become infected by contact with contaminated water or moist soil. While leptospirosis is a zoonosis that has been traditionally associated with rural wild and domesticated animals and humans working with these animals, it is now emerging as a major infectious cause of renal failure and hepatitis in human populations in urban centers of developing countries. It is of greatest public health importance in Southeast Asia and Latin America, where serological prevalence was reported as 27% in Thailand, 23% in Vietnam, and 37% in rural Belize (Watt, 1991). Leptospirosis is characterized by an abrupt-onset "flu-like" illness with fever, myalgia, headache, and nausea. In 5–10% of infected individuals, it is complicated by jaundice, renal failure, hemorrhage, and vascular collapse (Weil's syndrome). Differential diagnoses include illnesses such as dengue fever, malaria, typhoid fever, and scrub typhus (Watt, 1991). Rapid diagnosis is critical for early treatment with antibiotics and hemodialysis, as these can substantially decrease mortality.

Classical Methods of Diagnosis

The microscopic agglutination assay is considered the reference method for serological diagnosis of leptospirosis. This technique is labor-intensive, expensive, and requires testing acute and convalescent sera against a large panel of standard *Leptospira* strains. In addition, serological tests cannot contribute to early diagnosis, because antibodies only become detectable approximately 7 days after onset of the disease (Watt, 1991). Culturing *Leptospira* can take up to 8 weeks and is therefore too lengthy for rapid diagnosis. Microscopy is unreliable and insensitive, while immunochemical staining (White and Ristic, 1959) and DNA hybridization techniques (Terpstra et al., 1986) are useful but have fairly low sensitivity.

PCR-Based Procedures

Several PCR-based tests for *Leptospira* have been developed and can be applied directly to clinical specimens (e.g., serum, urine). The primers are directed to the 16S rRNA gene (Merien et al., 1992; Wagenaar et al., 1994), the 23S rRNA gene (Woo et al., 1997) or other genomic sequences (Gravecamp et al., 1993; Kee et al., 1994; Masri

---

26. Each *Leptospira* species is composed of serogroups, each of which is further subdivided into several serological variants or serovars.

et al., 1997; Savio et al., 1994; van Eys et al., 1989). The sensitivities of these assays range from 50–100%, with 100% specificity (Bal et al., 1994; Brown et al., 1995; Gravecamp, et al., 1993; Merien et al., 1995). PCR-based typing methods with primers directed to repetitive sequences (IS*1533*) can differentiate *Leptospira* serovars directly from infected urine (Zuerner et al., 1995). Restriction digestion of amplified fragments can also be used for serovar identification (Savio et al., 1994; Woodward and Redstone, 1993), as can arbitrarily primed PCR (AP-PCR) (Brown and Levett, 1997; Ralph et al., 1993) and random amplified polymorphic DNA (RAPD) (Corney et al., 1993; Gerritsen et al., 1995). Alternatively, low-stringency amplification with diagnostic primers can generate serovar-specific fingerprints (de Caballero et al., 1994).

Points to Consider in Using PCR

As mentioned above, early diagnosis and treatment of leptospirosis is essential for decreasing mortality. In addition, a number of other etiologic agents can cause similar clinical manifestations, making definitive diagnosis of leptospirosis critical. Compared with other diagnostic methods, PCR offers an advantage in its rapidity and specificity. The challenge is to make PCR accessible in health posts, private clinics, and the like, such that specimens can be processed and patients treated in a timely manner. Another important use of PCR is as a tool to facilitate epidemiological studies aimed at identifying risk factors associated with development of severe disease. With this information, preventive measures can be recommended for the community as a whole to decrease *Leptospira* infection and the serious complications of leptospirosis.

PCR Detection of *Leptospira*

This protocol is used to amplify genomic sequences from pathogenic species of *Leptospira* (Gravecamp et al., 1993). It also amplifies sequences from certain non-pathogenic *Leptospira*, such as *L. biflexi* serovar Patoc I.[27] One procedure for preparing isolated *Leptospira* colonies for PCR is provided along with two methods for preparing clinical specimens: a simple extraction procedure and a more extensive purification using guanidine isothiocyanate and silica particles.

I. Sample Preparation: Grey Area

A. "Bacterial Lysis" Method for Preparation of Leptospira Isolates

ADDITIONAL EQUIPMENT AND MATERIALS
Boiling water bath (100°C)
Incubator (37°C)
Sterile toothpicks
Floating rack for microcentrifuge tubes (plastic or Styrofoam)

REAGENTS
Sterile ddH$_2$0 (double-distilled water)
Petri plates containing Cox medium (*see* Appendix B)

1. Label sterile 1.5-mL screw-cap microcentrifuge tubes by writing the appropriate number on the tube *and* on the cap with a permanent marker.
2. Transfer 100 µL of sterile ddH$_2$0 to each labeled tube.
3. Label a Petri plate containing Cox medium with the numbers of the colonies to be examined.
4. With a sterile toothpick, pick a colony of the putative *Leptospira* isolates and touch the toothpick to the agar in a spot that corresponds to the number of the colony. Submerge the same toothpick in the appropriate tube containing 100 ul of sterile distilled water and agitate the toothpick in the solution.
5. Incubate the tubes at 100°C in the water bath for 5 minutes.
6. Store the tubes at $-20°C$ until further use (2–5 µL will be used for the PCR reaction).
7. Incubate the plate overnight at 37°C, then store at 4°C.

Note: The following two protocols for preparation of clinical specimens[28] were contributed by Albert Ko and Lee W. Riley.[29]

---

27. Albert Ko, personal communication; Roman Vallecillo and Eva Harris, unpublished results.
28. The centrifugation method, when coupled with PCR amplification, can detect 20 leptospires per milliliter of specimen. The advantage of the centrifugation method is that it is rapid and inexpensive; the major limitation is that it requires immediate processing of specimens after collection. In contrast, using the second purification procedure, samples can be frozen after collection and subsequently processed. The limit of detection using the purified samples is 200–2000 leptospires per milliliter of specimen. This sensitivity can be increased by using larger quantities of specimens or by combining the amplification with a hybridization step.
29. Albert Ko (Gonçalo Moniz Research Center, Oswaldo Cruz Foundation/Brazilian Ministry of Health, Salvador, Brazil) and Lee W. Riley (School of Public Health, University of California, Berkeley, CA), personal communication.

B. Centrifugation Method for Preparation of Clinical Specimens[30]

ADDITIONAL EQUIPMENT AND MATERIALS
Boiling water bath (100°C)
Vacutainer® tubes with EDTA anticoagulant for blood collection
50-mL polypropylene tubes
Floating rack for microcentrifuge tubes (plastic or Styrofoam)

REAGENTS
Sterile ddH$_2$0 (double-distilled water)
Sterile 1X phosphate buffered saline (PBS), pH 7.4

1. Obtain blood samples by venopuncture using the EDTA-containing Vacutainer® tubes with EDTA. It is recommended to avoid using heparin as an anticoagulant since it may inhibit the PCR reaction. Centrifuge the tubes at 800 rpm for 10 minutes. Separate the plasma without pipetting either red blood cells or the buffy coat and process immediately.
2. Collect urine samples and transfer to polypropylene centrifuge tubes. Centrifuge the tubes at 800 rpm for 10 minutes. Separate the supernatant for immediate use. This step is important because it removes the cellular debris that is common in patients with leptospirosis-induced renal involvement and that may inhibit the PCR reaction.
3. Label sterile 1.5-mL microcentrifuge tubes with a permanent marker. Transfer 1 mL of each clinical specimen or control to the appropriately labeled tubes.
4. Centrifuge the tubes in a microcentrifuge at 12,000g for 10 minutes.
5. Remove the supernatant with a pipet and resuspend the pellet in 0.5–1 mL of 1X PBS (pH 7.4).
6. Centrifuge the tubes at 12,000g for 10 minutes.
7. Repeat steps 5 and 6.
8. Resuspend the pellet in 20 μL of sterile ddH$_2$0.
9. Boil the samples in a water bath at 100°C for 10 minutes.
10. The samples may now be stored at −20°C until the PCR reaction is performed.
11. When ready to use, thaw the samples and centrifuge the tubes at 12,000g for 15 minutes. Use 10 μL of the extract in a 50 μL PCR reaction.

C. Guanidine Isothiocyanate Extraction Procedure[31]

ADDITIONAL EQUIPMENT AND MATERIALS
Water bath at 56°C
Vacutainer tubes for blood collection
Sterile Pasteur pipets and bulbs
Suction apparatus (optional)
Sterile toothpicks
Silica particles (*see* Appendix B)

REAGENTS
Sterile ddH$_2$0 (double-distilled water)
L6 lysis buffer (*see* Appendix B)
L2 washing buffer (*see* Appendix B)

---

30. Adapted from Merien et al. (1992).
31. Adapted from Bal et al. (1994), Boom et al. (1990), and Boom et al. (1991).

Acetone
1X phosphate buffered saline (PBS), pH 7.4
10 m*M* Tris-HCl, pH 8.0

1. Collect blood from patients by venopuncture and allow it to clot in sterile glass tubes. After coagulation (15 minutes), rim the clot with a toothpick and allow the clot to retract (approximately 1 hour at ambient temperature). Centrifuge the tube at 800 rpm for 10 minutes. Separate the serum and store it at −20°C until use.
2. Collect urine samples and transfer to polypropylene centrifuge tubes. Centrifuge the tubes at 800 rpm for 10 minutes. Separate the supernatant and store at −20°C until use.

Note: Centrifugation at 800 rpm does not efficiently pellet leptospires. These steps are not as critical as in the centrifugation method for leptospiral DNA extraction and can be skipped. The advantage is that centrifugation facilitates separation of sera and removal of cellular debris from urine, which can be abundant in patients with renal involvement.

3. Prepare appropriately labeled sterile 1.5-mL microcentrifuge tubes containing 900 μL of L6 lysis buffer.
4. After thawing the samples, distribute 100 μL of the serum or urine into appropriately labeled 1.5-mL microcentrifuge tubes containing 900 μL of lysis buffer.
5. Vortex the slurry of silica particles thoroughly to ensure that the particles are completely resuspended in a homogeneous mixture.
6. Add 10 μL of the silica particle slurry to each tube, including the positive and negative controls, and vortex.
7. Allow the suspension to settle for 10 minutes and then vortex again.
8. Centrifuge the tubes at 12,000g for 1 minute in a microcentrifuge and remove and discard the supernatant. A suction apparatus with autoclaved Pasteur pipets works well for this step.
9. Add 1 mL of L2 washing buffer to each sample and vortex thoroughly.
10. Centrifuge the tubes at 12,000g for 1 minute. Remove and discard the supernatant.
11. Repeat steps 9 and 10.
12. Add 1 mL of 70% ethanol to each sample and vortex thoroughly.
13. Centrifuge the tubes at 12,000g for 1 minute. Remove and discard the supernatant.
14. Repeat steps 12 and 13.
15. Add 1 mL of acetone to each sample and vortex thoroughly.
16. Centrifuge the tubes at 12,000g for 1 minute. Remove and discard the supernatant.
17. Centrifuge the tubes again for 10 seconds. Remove and discard the remainder of the supernatant.
18. Allow the samples to air dry in a horizontal position for 10–15 minutes.
19. Add 20 μL of 10 m*M* Tris-HCl (pH 8.0) and vortex thoroughly.
20. Incubate the tubes in a 56°C water bath for 15 minutes.
21. Vortex again and centrifuge the tubes at 12,000g for 1–2 minutes.
22. Remove the supernatant carefully so as not to take up the silica particles and transfer it to a sterile microcentrifuge tube.
23. Use 10 μL for a 50 μL PCR reaction. The remainder of the sample can be stored at −20°C.

II. Amplification

A. Preparation of PCR Master Mix and Reaction Tubes: **White Area**

REAGENTS
10X Buffer B (100 m*M* Tris [pH 8.3)], 500 m*M* KCl)
dNTPs (5 m*M* each dATP, dCTP, dGTP, dTTP; 20 m*M* total dNTPs)
Primers (10 μ*M*)
  G1: 5'-CTG AAT CGC TGT ATA AAA GT
  G2: 5'-GGA AAA CAA ATG GTC GGA AG
MgCl₂ (25 m*M*)
ddH₂0
Taq polymerase (5 U/μL)
Mineral oil
Positive control (purified *Leptospira* DNA or boiled cultures representing the different pathogenic species)

Note: Before preparing the PCR Master Mix, go to the **Black Area** to enter the appropriate program in the thermocycler. If the program has already been entered, review it to ensure no changes have been inadvertently introduced; if so, correct the program and store it for later use. If the PCR will be manually amplified, prepare three water baths at the following temperatures: 50°C, 72°C, and 94°C, and ensure that these temperatures are stably maintained.

1. Calculate the amount of PCR Master Mix that will be necessary for the desired number of reactions, each containing 40 μL of Master Mix. For every 20 reactions, add 1 extra volume of Master Mix to compensate for volume lost during pipetting.
2. Fill out the PCR Worksheet according to the following table.

3.

Ingredient	Description	Stock conc.	Vol/50 μL rxn	Final conc.
Buffer 10X	Buffer B	10X	5.0 μL	1X
dNTPs	20 m*M* total dNTPs	5 m*M* A,C,G,T	2.0 μL	0.2 m*M* A,C,G,T
Primer 1	G1	10 μ*M*	5.0 μL	1 μ*M*
Primer 2	G2	10 μ*M*	5.0 μL	1 μ*M*
MgCl₂		25 m*M*	2.0 μL	1 m*M*
H₂O	ddH₂O		20.7 μL	
Taq	*Taq*	5 U/μL	0.3 μL	0.03 U/μL
Vol. of Master Mix			40 μL	
Vol. of sample (to be added in step 13)			10 μL	
Total reaction volume			50 μL	

4. Label the appropriate tubes (0.5-mL or 0.2-mL tubes for thermocyclers; 1.5-mL screw-cap tubes for manual amplification).
5. Thaw aliquot(s) of each reagent. Vortex each thawed solution well and briefly spin the tubes (pulse spin) in a microcentrifuge to collect all the liquid at the bottom of the tubes.

Keep all the ingredients and tubes on ice at all times.

6. In the **White Area,** using a **white** color-coded pipettor, prepare the PCR Master Mix with all the ingredients except the *Taq* polymerase. Check off each ingredient on the Worksheet after adding it to the Master Mix.
7. Mix well using a vortex or a large pipettor.
8. Add the *Taq* polymerase and mix by pipetting carefully with a pipettor set at half the total volume of the PCR Master Mix. Be careful not to create bubbles.

9. Distribute 40 μL of the PCR Master Mix into each labeled tube.

10. Add 2 drops of mineral oil to each tube using a 1000-μL pipettor.

11. Add 10 μL of ddH$_2$O to prepare a "white area" negative control across the layer of mineral oil.

12. Transfer the tubes from the **white** ice bucket to a **grey** ice bucket.

B. Sample Addition: **Grey Area**

13. In the **Grey Area**, using a **grey** color-coded pipettor, add 10 μL of the sample or control to the appropriate tube, *across* the layer of mineral oil. The controls should be added in the order of the most negative to the most positive. Use a new pipet tip for each sample. Remember to include a negative control consisting of the Grey Area water.

C. Amplification Procedure: **Black Area**

EQUIPMENT
Thermocycler or water baths at 50°C, 72°C, and 94°C
Microcentrifuge

14. Amplification profile:

94°C	3 min	1 cycle	Initial denaturation
94°C	1.5 min		
50°C	1 min	35 cycles	Amplification
72°C	2 min		
72°C	10 min	1 cycle	Final extension

Product size: Primer pair G1/G2 generates a 285-bp product from the six pathogenic species *L. interrogans, L. borgpetersenii, L. weilii, L. noguchii, L. santarosai.,* and *L. inadai.*

III. Product Analysis

Use a 1.5% agarose gel and the procedure in section 5.1.2.

5.1.11   *Trypanosoma cruzi*

Clinical Manifestations and Epidemiology

Chagas disease, or American trypanosomiasis, is still a serious public health problem in many Latin American countries. The World Health Organization estimates that 16 to 18 million people are infected with the kinetoplastid parasite *Trypanosoma cruzi*, and 50,000 people die each year from Chagas disease (WHO, 1991). *T. cruzi* is transmitted by triatomine insects or by transfusion with infected blood. The acute phase of the disease, with elevated parasitemia, is associated with mild and nonspecific symptoms that resolve over a period of weeks to months. The chronic form of the disease becomes apparent only years or decades after the initial infection, when very few parasites are circulating. The parasites reside in muscle tissue, causing heart failure or hypertrophy of the esophagus or colon (megasyndrome) (Kirchhoff, 1995). Distinct disease manifestations, which may be related to genetic differences in the parasite, are associated with different geographical regions. For instance, there are more cases of megasyndrome in South America than in Central America.

Classical Methods of Diagnosis

Classical methods of diagnosis include serologic tests (IgG detection in chronic disease) and parasite detection via microscopy, hemoculture, and xenodiagnosis. Microscopy can be useful for detection of *T. cruzi* parasites in blood smears during the symptomatic acute phase of the disease. Both hemoculture and xenodiagnosis require over 1 month to complete and are often less than 50% sensitive compared with serologic results. In addition, hemoculture is prone to microbiological contamination, and xenodiagnosis is an unpleasant and difficult procedure. The main problem with serologic tests conducted with crude parasite antigen is the cross-reactivity with host antibodies against a range of other pathogens, *Leishmania* in particular (Kirchhoff, 1995). However, recent reports of specific *T. cruzi* antigens for new-generation serologic tests are promising and will most likely constitute the best option for large-scale screening, as long as the geographical variation in immunogenicity of parasite antigens is taken into consideration.

PCR-Based Procedures

Various approaches to PCR detection of *T. cruzi* have been described, targeting different repetitive sequences, such as the kinetoplast minicircle DNA, which is present at 120,000 copies per parasite (Sturm et al., 1989); the satellite DNA, repeated 100,000 times per genome (Diaz et al., 1992; Moser et al., 1989); ribosomal RNA, with 60,000 copies per parasite (Souto and Zingales, 1993); interspersed repetitive DNA, repeated 10,000 times per genome (Requena et al., 1992); the ribosomal intergenic DNA, with 400 repeats per genome (Novak et al., 1993); the mini-exon repeat, present 200–400 times (Souto et al., 1996); and a nuclear sequence coding for a flagellar protein, with 20 copies per parasite (Silber et al., 1997). A number of studies in patients with both acute and chronic disease have demonstrated PCR to have a significantly higher sensitivity (90–100%) than the other parasitological methods (which range in sensitivity from 17–70%), as compared with serology (Avila et al., 1993; Britto et al., 1995; Wincker et al., 1994a, 1994b). PCR has also been applied to detection of *T. cruzi* in its triatomine vectors (Breniere et al., 1995; Russomando et al., 1996; Shikanai-Yasuda et al., 1996).

Various PCR-based techniques have been used to characterize the distinct phylogenetic lineages of *T. cruzi*, and these results have been shown to concur with phylogenetic classifications obtained using the classical multilocus enzyme electrophoresis method (Souto et al., 1996; Tibayrenc et al., 1993). One such technique is random amplified polymorphic DNA (RAPD) analysis (Souto et al., 1996; Steindel et al., 1993; Tibayrenc et al., 1993); another is amplification of polymorphic loci such as the ribosomal intergenic spacer (Gonzalez et al., 1994), the mini-exon repeat, or ribosomal DNA (Souto et al., 1996). This genetic fingerprinting is useful for identifying the strains circulating in specific regions, for distinguishing *T. cruzi* parasites associated with sylvatic and domestic cycles of transmission, and for investigating the biological characteristics of particular strains associated with different clinical manifestations (Revollo et al., 1998).

Points to Consider in Using PCR

It has clearly been shown in the reports cited above that PCR is the most sensitive parasitological method for detection of *T. cruzi*. The important question to consider is whether PCR diagnosis is necessary and whether it is the wisest use of scarce resources. For instance, it may be more useful to concentrate efforts on effective control of the vector of transmission rather than to increase the sensitivity of diagnosis. The new, more specific serological assays are more amenable to large-scale screening than are molecular biology techniques. However, there are clearly situations where PCR is avantageous, and each application must be carefully evaluated to determine the utility of PCR. Examples of appropriate use of PCR include diagnosis of Chagas disease in infants or chronic patients or rapid typing of *T. cruzi* strains in humans, insect vectors, or animal reservoirs. Such information may lead to the development of more effective therapeutic and control strategies.

PCR Detection of *Trypanosoma cruzi*

This protocol is used to amplify a 330-bp product from the minicircle DNA of *Trypanosoma cruzi* (Avila et al., 1991, 1993). Since there are 120,000 copies of the minicircle in each parasite, this is a very sensitive assay and can detect as little as one parasite in 20 mL of blood (Avila et al., 1991). The guanidine lysis buffer provides a useful method for stable storage of blood samples stably at either ambient temperature or at 4°C. Boiling these lysates breaks up the network of the kinetoplast minicircles, making them accessible as targets for amplification (Britto et al., 1993).

I. Sample Preparation: Grey Area

ADDITIONAL EQUIPMENT AND MATERIALS
Boiling water bath (100°C)
Vials for blood collection
Polypropylene tubes (15 mL or 50 mL)
Floating rack for microcentrifuge tubes (plastic or Styrofoam)

REAGENTS
Sterile ddH$_2$0 (double-distilled water)
Guanidine lysis buffer (6 *M* guanidine HCl, 0.2 *M* EDTA [pH 8.0])
Phenol saturated with Tris-HCl, pH 8.0[32]
Chloroform[32]
Phenol/chloroform (1:1)[32]
3 *M* sodium acetate, pH 5.2
100% ethanol
70% ethanol
Glycogen (100 µg/mL)

1. Prepare polypropylene tubes containing 1 volume of guanidine lysis buffer. Add 1 volume of freshly-drawn whole blood and mix immediately.
2. Boil for 15 minutes in a boiling water bath.
3. Transfer 100 µL of the blood lysate to a sterile microcentrifuge tube and add 100 µL of a 1:1 mixture of phenol/chloroform. Mix well using a vortex. Store the remainder of the blood lysate at 4°C.
4. Centrifuge the tubes for 10 minutes in a microcentrifuge.
5. Remove the aqueous upper layer and transfer it to a new microcentrifuge tube.
6. Add 100 µL of chloroform and mix well using a vortex.
7. Repeat steps 4 and 5.
8. Add 1/10 volume 3 *M* sodium acetate (pH 5.2) and 2 volumes of ice-cold absolute ethanol. (1 µg/mL glycogen may be used as carrier, if desired.)
9. Centrifuge the tubes for 20 minutes in a microcentrifuge at 4°C.
10. Remove the supernatant carefully and discard it. Add 100 µL of 70% ethanol to the pellet.

---

32. Phenol and chloroform waste should be collected in a separate container and transferred to the organic waste container stored in the chemical fume hood.

11. Centrifuge the tubes for 10 minutes.
12. Remove the supernatant carefully and discard it. Air dry the pellet in a horizontal position for 15 minutes or until dry.
13. Resuspend the pellet in 50 μL of sterile ddH$_2$O.

II. Amplification

A. *Preparation of PCR Master Mix and Reaction Tubes:* **White Area**

REAGENTS
10X Buffer B (100 mM Tris [pH 8.3)], 500 mM KCl)
dNTPs (5 mM each dATP, dCTP, dGTP, dTTP; 20 mM total dNTPs)
Primers (10 μM)
  S35: 5′-AAA TAA TGT ACG GGK GAG ATG CAT GA (where K = G/T)
  S36: 5′-GGG TTC GAT TGG GGT TGG TGT
MgCl$_2$ (25 mM)
Bovine serum albumin (BSA; 10 mg/mL)
ddH$_2$0
Taq polymerase (5 U/μL)
Mineral oil
Positive control (purified *T. cruzi* DNA)

Note: Before preparing the PCR Master Mix, go to the **Black Area** to enter the appropriate program in the thermocycler. If the program has already been entered, review it to ensure no changes have been inadvertently introduced; if so, correct the program and store it for later use. If the PCR will be manually amplified, prepare three water baths at the following temperatures: 60°C, 72°C, and 94°C, and ensure that these temperatures are stably maintained.

1. Calculate the amount of PCR Master Mix that will be necessary for the desired number of reactions, each containing 22.5 μL of Master Mix. For every 10 reactions, add 1 extra volume of Master Mix to compensate for volume lost during pipetting.
2. Fill out the PCR Worksheet according to the following table.

3.

Ingredient	Description	Stock conc.	Vol/25 μL rxn	Final conc.
Buffer 10X	Buffer B	10X	2.5 μL	1X
dNTPs	20 mM total dNTPs	5 mM A,C,G,T	1.0 μL	0.2 mM A,C,G,T
Primer 1	S35	10 μM	2.5 μL	1 μM
Primer 2	S36	10 μM	2.5 μL	1 μM
MgCl$_2$		25 mM	5.0 μL	5 mM
BSA		10 mg/mL	0.25 μL	0.1 mg/mL
H$_2$O	ddH$_2$O		8.6 μL	
Taq	*Taq*	5 U/μL	0.15 μL	0.03 U/μL

Vol. of Master Mix		22.5 μL
Vol. of sample (to be added in step 13)		2.5 μL
Total reaction volume		25 μL

4. Label the appropriate tubes (0.5-mL or 0.2-mL tubes for thermocyclers; 1.5-mL screw-cap tubes for manual amplification).
5. Thaw aliquot(s) of each reagent. Vortex each thawed solution well and briefly spin the tubes (pulse spin) in a microcentrifuge to collect all the liquid at the bottom of the tubes.

Keep all the ingredients and tubes on ice at all times.

6. In the **White Area**, using a **white** color-coded pipettor, prepare the PCR Master Mix with all the ingredients except the *Taq* polymerase. Check off each ingredient on the Worksheet after adding it to the Master Mix.
7. Mix well using a vortex or a large pipettor.
8. Add the *Taq* polymerase and mix by pipetting carefully with a pipettor set at half the total volume of the PCR Master Mix. Be careful not to create bubbles.
9. Distribute 22.5 µL of the PCR Master Mix into each labeled tube.
10. Add 1 drop of mineral oil to each tube using a 1000-µL pipettor.
11. Add 2.5 µL of ddH$_2$O to prepare a "white area" negative control across the layer of mineral oil.
12. Transfer the tubes from the **white** ice bucket to a **grey** ice bucket.

B. Sample Addition: **Grey Area**

13. In the **Grey Area**, using a **grey** color-coded pipettor, add 2.5 µL of the sample or control to the appropriate tube, *across* the layer of mineral oil. The controls should be added in the order of the most negative to the most positive. Use a new pipet tip for each sample. Remember to include a negative control consisting of the Grey Area water.

C. Amplification Procedure: **Black Area**

EQUIPMENT
Thermocycler or water baths at 60°C, 72°C, and 94°C
Microcentrifuge

14. Amplification profile:

94°C	1 min		
60°C	1 min	30 cycles	Amplification
72°C	1 min		

Product size: This amplification generates a product of 330 base pairs, which is indicative of the presence of *T. cruzi* minicircle kDNA.

III. Product Analysis

Use a 1.5% agarose gel and the procedure in section 5.1.2.

Characterization of *Trypanosoma cruzi* by RAPD

Random amplified polymorphic DNA (RAPD) is a PCR-based procedure that uses a single arbitrary primer to generate distinctive patterns (fingerprints) from different DNA templates. This protocol describes two arbitrary primers that have been used to characterize strains of *Trypanosoma cruzi* (Tibayrenc et al., 1993). Purified *T. cruzi* DNA must be used as a template in this reaction, since the arbitrary primers also amplify products from the human DNA present in clinical samples or the insect DNA in vector specimens. When performing RAPD analysis, care must be taken not to contaminate the PCR reactions with extraneous DNA, because any DNA can generate a product. Several nanograms of DNA are required to generate RAPD fingerprints, as opposed to several femtograms for standard diagnostic PCR. To generate a reproducible pattern, it is imperative to utilize absolutely identical conditions for each amplification, including the same lots of the reagents, the same pipettors, and the same thermocycler. RAPD is a powerful but finicky technique, and extreme care is necessary to obtain reproducible, informative results (Black, 1993).

I. Sample Preparation: Grey Area

ADDITIONAL EQUIPMENT AND MATERIALS
Water bath at 55°C
50-mL polypropylene centrifuge tube
Pasteur pipets
Razor blade

REAGENTS
Sterile ddH$_2$0 (double-distilled water)
Sterile 1X phosphate buffered saline, pH 7.4
20% sodium dodecyl sulfate (SDS)
NET lysis buffer (*see* Appendix B)
Proteinase K (20 mg/mL)
Phenol saturated with Tris-HCl, pH 8.0[33]
Chloroform:isoamyl alcohol (24:1)[33]
3 *M* sodium acetate, pH 4.0
100% ethanol
70% ethanol

A. Proteolysis

Steps 1, 3, and 5 must be performed in a laminar flow hood, taking the appropriate biosafety precautions.

1. Transfer 35 mL of a culture of *T. cruzi* into a 50-mL polyproylene centrifuge tube and close the tube tightly.
2. Centrifuge the tube with the *T. cruzi* culture at 3500 rpm for 10 minutes.
3. Discard the supernatant and resuspend the pellet in 10 mL of PBS (pH 7.4).
4. Centrifuge the tube at 3500 rpm for 10 minutes.

---

33. Phenol and chloroform waste should be collected in a separate container and transferred to the organic waste container stored in the chemical fume hood.

5. Discard the supernatant, leaving a few drops of PBS in which to resuspend the parasites.

Always keep the samples on ice.

6. Label five 1.5-mL microcentrifuge tubes for each sample. (Label them 1–5 with a permanent marker.)
7. Transfer 100 µL of the resuspended parasites to tube 1 and add 2 volumes (200 µL) of NET lysis buffer.
8. Add 15 µL of 20% SDS, for a final concentration of 1%.
9. Mix gently by inversion.
10. Incubate overnight in a water bath at 55°C.

B. Extraction with Organic Solvents

11. For each SDS-treated sample, prepare five yellow pipet tips with the tip cut off with a razor blade; these will be used to recover the aqueous phase after the extractions with organic solvents.
12. To each sample, add an equal volume of phenol (pH 8.0) (approximately 300 µL). Mix gently by inversion.
13. Centrifuge the tubes at 12,000g in a microcentrifuge for 10 minutes at ambient temperature.
14. Carefully pipette off the aqueous upper phase with a yellow cut-off pipet tip and transfer the supernatant to tube 2.
15. Repeat steps 12–14 and transfer the aqueous phase to tube 3.
16. Add an equal volume of chloroform:isoamyl alcohol (24:1) (approximately 300 µL). Mix gently by inversion.
17. Centrifuge the tubes at 12,000g for 5 minutes at ambient temperature.
18. Carefully pipet off the aqueous upper phase with a yellow cut-off pipet tip and transfer the supernatant to tube 4.
19. Repeat steps 16–18 and transfer the aqueous phase to tube 5.

C. Ethanol precipitation

20. Measure the volume of each recovered supernatant.
21. Add 1/10 volume 3 M sodium acetate (pH 4.0) and 2.5 volumes of ice-cold absolute ethanol.
22. Incubate overnight at $-20°C$ or 1 hour at $-70°C$.
23. Centrifuge the tubes for 30 minutes at 12,000g at 4°C if possible; if not, at ambient temperature.
24. Remove the supernatant carefully so as not to lose the DNA pellet. Add 200 µL of 70% ethanol.
25. Centrifuge the tubes at 12,000g for 10 minutes at ambient temperature.
26. Remove the supernatant carefully and discard it.
27. Repeat steps 24–26.
28. Let the DNA pellet air dry in a horizontal position in an oven at 37°C or at ambient temperature.
29. Resuspend the DNA pellet in 50 µL of sterile ddH$_2$O.
30. Measure the concentration of DNA using a UV spectrophotometer or estimate the DNA concentration using a UV transilluminator according to the procedure described in section 3.3.1.
31. Prepare a 2.5 ng/µL stock of DNA and use 4 µL (10 ng) for each 50-µL RAPD reaction (20 ng for each 100-µL RAPD reaction).

II. Amplification

A. Preparation of PCR Master Mix and Reaction Tubes: **White Area**

REAGENTS
10X Buffer B (100 m*M* Tris [pH 8.3)], 500 m*M* KCl)
dNTPs (5 m*M* each dATP, dCTP, dGTP, dTTP; 20 m*M* total dNTPs)
Primers (10 µ*M*)
  A10: 5'-GTG ATG GCA G
  R16: 5'-CTC TGC GCG T
MgCl$_2$ (25 m*M*)
ddH$_2$0
Taq polymerase (5 U/µL)
Mineral oil
Positive control (purified DNA from *T. cruzi* reference strains that generate known fingerprint patterns)

Note: Before preparing the PCR Master Mix, go to the **Black Area** to enter the appropriate program in the thermocycler. If the program has already been entered, review it to ensure no changes have been inadvertently introduced; if so, correct the program and store it for later use.

Note: the same thermocycler and identical reaction conditions should be used for the analysis of all strains in a particular study.

1. Calculate the amount of PCR Master Mix that will be necessary for the desired number of reactions, each containing 46 µL of Master Mix. For every 20 reactions, add 1 extra volume of Master Mix to compensate for volume lost during pipetting.
2. Fill out the PCR Worksheet according to the following table.

3.

Ingredient	Description	Stock conc.	Vol/50 µL rxn	Final conc.
Buffer 10X	Buffer B	10X	5.0 µL	1X
dNTPs	20 m*M* total dNTPs	5 m*M* A,C,G,T	1.0 µL	0.1 m*M* A,C,G,T
Primer 1	A10 *or* R16	10 µ*M*	2.0 µL	0.4 µ*M*
MgCl$_2$		25 m*M*	3.0 µL	1.5 m*M*
BSA		10 mg/mL	0.5 µL	0.1 mg/mL
H$_2$O	ddH$_2$O		34.25 µL	
Taq	*Taq*	5 U/µL	0.25 µL	0.025 U/µL

Vol. of Master Mix	46 µL
Vol. of sample (to be added in step 13)	4 µL
Total reaction volume	50 µL

4. Label the appropriate tubes (0.5-mL or 0.2-mL tubes).
5. Thaw aliquot(s) of each reagent. Vortex each thawed solution well and briefly spin the tubes (pulse spin) in a microcentrifuge to collect all the liquid at the bottom of the tubes.

Keep all the ingredients and tubes on ice at all times.

6. In the **White Area**, using a **white** color-coded pipettor, prepare the PCR Master Mix with all the ingredients except the *Taq* polymerase. Check off each ingredient on the Worksheet after adding it to the Master Mix.
7. Mix well using a vortex or a large pipettor.
8. Add the *Taq* polymerase and mix by pipetting carefully with a pipettor set at half the total volume of the PCR Master Mix. Be careful not to create bubbles.

9. Distribute 46 μL of the PCR Master Mix into each labeled tube.
10. Add 2 drops of mineral oil to each tube using a 1000-μL pipettor.
11. Add 4 μL of ddH$_2$O to prepare a "white area" negative control across the layer of mineral oil.
12. Transfer the tubes from the **white** ice bucket to a **grey** ice bucket.

B. Sample Addition: **Grey Area**

13. In the **Grey Area**, using a **grey** color-coded pipettor, add 4 μL (10 ng) of the sample or control to the appropriate tube, *across* the layer of mineral oil. The controls should be added in the order of the most negative to the most positive. Use a new pipet tip for each sample. **Remember to include a negative control consisting of the Grey Area water.**

C. Amplification Procedure: **Black Area**

EQUIPMENT
Thermocycler
Microcentrifuge

14. Amplification profile:

94°C	1 min		
36°C	1 min	45 cycles	Amplification
72°C	1 min		
72°C	7 min	1 cycle	Final extension

Interpretation of Results: This protocol generates a pattern of amplified products that is distinct for each strain (Figure 5.10). Since a large number of fragments may be generated, the interpretation of the results can be complex. If the objective is to analyze several unknown strains and compare the resulting patterns with fingerprints of known strains analyzed side by side with the samples, visual interpretation is adequate. As in the case of DRE-PCR characterization of *M. tuberculosis* (section 5.1.5), the patterns can be copied onto graph paper and grouped by number of bands generated. When a similar pattern is detected, the RAPD products of the samples in question should be re-examined side by side by agarose gel electrophoresis. However, if the objective is to construct a phylogenetic tree and to determine the genetic distance between several clones, then more sophisticated analysis is required (Black, 1993). In brief, each fragment is assigned a number and the resulting codes describing the fingerprint of each strain are entered into a computer, which computes the relatedness between the different strains. The similarity between two strains is based on the number of identical fragments they share out of the total number of fragments in each fingerprint pattern.

III. Product Analysis

Use a 1.2% agarose gel and the procedure in section 5.1.2.

Primer: **A10**   **R16**

Strain: 0 1 2 3 M 1 2 3 4 0 M

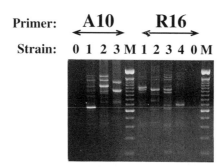

Fig. 5.10. Differentiation of *Trypanosoma cruzi* strains by RAPD analysis. DNA was purified from cultures of *T. cruzi* and amplified using either primer A10 or R16 as indicated. Products were analyzed by gel electrophoresis. 0, water (negative control); 1, strain Tula; 2, strain Esquilo; 3, strain X10; 4, strain MN; M, 100-bp ladder (*see* Appendix C; lowest band shown, 100 bp).

5.2   Nonradioactive DNA Probes: *V. cholerae* Colony Blot

DNA probes can be used to detect specific nucleic acid sequences, although with lower sensitivity than PCR. One advantage of this method is that it is easier to process large numbers of samples at once. The DNA or RNA of interest is usually attached to a solid support, such as a nylon or nitrocellular membrane or a microtiter well. When a nylon or nitrocellular membrane (blot) is used, the nucleic acids can be transferred to the membrane from a gel after electrophoresis or directly from bacterial colonies or phage plaques, or applied directly to the membrane using a dot-blot (or slot-blot) apparatus or a pipettor. The DNA or RNA is then fixed to the membrane using heat or ultraviolet light to crosslink the nucleic acids to the fibers of the membrane. The blot is incubated with a DNA probe, which hybridizes to complementary sequences fixed to the membrane. To detect this hybridization, the probe must be labeled, either with a radioactive isotope or a nonradioactive molecule that can be subsequently visualized. The nonradioactive detection procedure relies on the activity of an enzyme (usually alkaline phosphatase or horseradish peroxidase) conjugated to the probe, which converts specific substrates into a colored product. An alternative detection procedure is the use of substrates that emit light during the enzymatic conversion to the product; this light can be captured on film, much like the classical autoradiogram for visualization of radioactive isotopes. The enzyme can be conjugated directly to the DNA probe, although this tends to be an expensive process. Alternatively, the probe can be labeled with an intermediary molecule, such as biotin or the plant compound digoxigenin, which is recognized by a second molecule that is conjugated to the enzyme. This second molecule is usually streptavidin, which has a high affinity for biotin, or an anti-digoxigenin antibody. For more detailed discussion of DNA probes, see Sambrook et al. (1989).

5.2.1   Labeling DNA Probes Using PCR

This protocol amplifies a 564-bp fragment of the *Vibrio cholerae ctx* A gene, which encodes the A subunit of cholera toxin (Fields et al., 1992; Olsvik et al., 1993). Digoxigenin-labeled nucleotides (dUTP) are included to label the PCR product for subsequent use as a probe in nonradioactive hybridization procedures. DNA fragments can be labeled by incorporation of labeled nucleotides during PCR amplification or by random primed DNA labeling (Boerhinger Mannheim, 1995; Sambrook et al., 1989). Oligonucleotides can be labeled by attaching one labeled nucleotide (or the label itself) directly to the 3′ or 5′ end of the oligonucleotide or by adding multiple labeled nucleotides (10–100) to the 3′ end using the enzyme terminal transferase (3′ tailing) (Boerhinger Mannheim, 1995; Sambrook et al., 1989).

I.ʻ Sample Preparation: Grey Area

ADDITIONAL EQUIPMENT AND MATERIALS
Boiling water bath (100°C)

Incubator (37°C)
Sterile 1.5-mL screw-cap microcentrifuge tubes (with O-rings)
Glass test tube
Inoculating loop or sterile toothpicks
Floating rack for microcentrifuge tubes (plastic or Styrofoam)
Scissors or razor blade

REAGENTS
Sterile ddH$_2$0 (double-distilled water)
Petri plates with Tryptic Soy Agar (TSA)
MacFarland Standard (*see* Appendix B)
Toxigenic *V. cholerae* control strain (*ctx*+)
Mineral oil

1. Using an inoculating loop, resuspend a loopful of a toxigenic *V. cholerae* control strain in 1–2 mL of ddH$_2$0 in a glass test tube.
2. Compare the suspension with McFarland's standard and adjust to match the turbidity of MacFarland's standard number 1 or 2.
3. Dilute the suspension 1:10 in sterile ddH$_2$0 in a 1.5-mL screw-cap microcentrifuge tube.
4. Boil the microcentrifuge tube in a 100°C water bath for 15 minutes.
5. Use 2 μL for the PCR amplification.

II. Amplification

A. Preparation of PCR Master Mix and Reaction Tubes: **White Area**

REAGENTS
10X Buffer A (100 m*M* Tris [pH 9.0)], 500 m*M* KCl, 1% Triton® X-100)
dNTPs (dATP, dCTP, dGTP, dTTP; 10 m*M* each in separate vials)[34]
Digoxigenin-11-dUTP, alkali-labile, 1 m*M* (Boehringer Mannheim #1 573 152)
Primers (10 m*M*)
  CTX2:   5′-CGG GCA GAT TCT AGA CCT CCT G
  CTX3:   5′-CGA TGA TCT TGG AGC ATT CCC AC
MgCl$_2$ (25 m*M*)
ddH$_2$0
Taq polymerase (5 U/μL)
Mineral oil
Positive control (toxigenic *V. cholerae* DNA or lysed toxigenic *V. cholerae*)

Note: Before preparing the PCR Master Mix, go to the **Black Area** to enter the appropriate program in the thermocycler. If the program has already been entered, review it to ensure no changes have been inadvertently introduced; if so, correct the program and store it for later use. If the PCR will be manually amplified, prepare three water baths at the following temperatures: 55°C, 72°C, and 95°C, and ensure that these temperatures are stably maintained.

1. Calculate the amount of PCR Master Mix that will be necessary for the desired number of reactions, each containing 98 μL of Master Mix.
2. Fill out the PCR Worksheet according to the following table.

---

34. A mixture of nucleotides that includes the four dNTPs in addition to alkali-labile digoxigenin-11–dUTP is also available from Boerhinger Mannheim (PCR DIG Probe Synthesis Mix, # 1 636 090). This mixture contains 2 m*M* dATP, 2 m*M* dCTP, 2 m*M* dGTP, 1.3 mM dTTP, and 0.7 m*M* DIG-11–dUTP.

3.

Ingredient	Description	Stock conc.	Vol/100 µL rxn	Final conc.
Buffer 10X	Buffer B	10X	10 µL	1X
dNTPs	dATP	10 m*M*	2.0 µL	0.2 m*M*
	dCTP	10 m*M*	2.0 µL	0.2 m*M*
	dGTP	10 m*M*	2.0 µL	0.2 m*M*
	dTTP	10 m*M*	1.3 µL	0.13 m*M*
	DIG–11–dUTP	1.0 m*M*	7.0 µL	0.07 m*M*
Primer 1	CTX2	10 µ*M*	10 µL	1 µ*M*
Primer 2	CTX3	10 µ*M*	10 µL	1 µ*M*
MgCl$_2$		25 m*M*	6.0 µL	1.5 m*M*
H$_2$O	ddH$_2$O		46.7 µL	
Taq	*Taq*	5 U/µL	1.0 µL	0.05 U/µL

Vol. of Master Mix	98 µL
Vol. of sample (to be added in step 13)	2 µL
Total reaction volume	100 µL

4. Label the appropriate tubes (0.5-mL or 0.2-mL tubes for thermocyclers; 1.5-mL screw-cap tubes for manual amplification).
5. Thaw aliquot(s) of each reagent. Vortex each thawed solution well and briefly spin the tubes (pulse spin) in a microcentrifuge to collect all the liquid at the bottom of the tubes.

Keep all the ingredients and tubes on ice at all times.

6. In the **White Area**, using a **white** color-coded pipettor, prepare the PCR Master Mix with all the ingredients except the *Taq* polymerase. Check off each ingredient on the Worksheet after adding it to the Master Mix.
7. Mix well using a vortex or a large pipettor.
8. Add the *Taq* polymerase and mix by pipetting carefully with a pipettor set at half the total volume of the PCR Master Mix. Be careful not to create bubbles.
9. Distribute 98 µL of the PCR Master Mix into each labeled tube.
10. Add 2 drops of mineral oil to each tube using a 1000-µL pipettor.
11. Add 2 µL of ddH$_2$O to prepare a "white area" negative control across the layer of mineral oil.
12. Transfer the tubes from the **white** ice bucket to a **grey** ice bucket.

B. Sample Addition: **Grey Area**

13. In the **Grey Area**, using a **grey** color-coded pipettor, add 2 µL of the sample or control to the appropriate tube, *across* the layer of mineral oil. Use a new pipet tip for each sample.

C. Amplification Procedure: **Black Area**

EQUIPMENT
Thermocycler or water baths at 55°C, 72°C, and 95°C
Microcentrifuge

14. Amplification profile:

95°C	30 sec		
55°C	1.5 min	40 cycles	Amplification
72°C	3 min		
72°C	10 min	1 cycle	Final extension

Product size: This amplification generates a 564-bp fragment of the *Vibrio cholerae* cholera toxin operon, *ctx*.

III. Product Analysis

Analyze 5 µL of the product using a 1.2% agarose gel and the procedure in section 5.1.2.

The product must be purified to avoid nonspecific hybridization of PCR by-products to the colony blot. Even when no by-products are visible by agarose gel electrophoresis, sufficient amounts may be present to cause nonspecific hybridization. To purify the product by agarose gel electrophoresis, *see* section 6.2.3.

5.2.2   Preparation of the Colony Blot

EQUIPMENT
Incubator (37°C)
Water bath (65°C)
Boiling water bath (100°C)
Oven at 80°C
Heat sealer (for sealing plastic bags)
Microcentrifuge
Pipettors (1000 µL, 200 µL, and 20 µL)

MATERIALS
Plastic or Pyrex trays
Beakers
Sealable plastic bags
Sterile Petri plates
Disposable gloves
Pencil
Indelible markers
Nylon membrane (Boehringer Mannheim or Magnagraph, MSI)
Sterile wooden toothpicks
Chromatographic paper (Whatman 3MM)
Filter paper
Parafilm®
Filter forceps
Graduated cylinders (100 mL and 200 mL)
Scissors

REAGENTS
Nitrotetrazolium blue (NBT)
5-bromo-4-cloro-3-indolyl-phosphate, toluidine salt (BCIP)
Buffer 1 (*see* Appendix B)
Buffer 2 (*see* Appendix B)
Buffer 3 (*see* Appendix B)
Anti-digoxigenin conjugate (Boehringer Mannheim Cat. No. 1093274)
$MgCl_2$ (50 mM)
NaOH (0.5 M)
Luria Bertani (LB) plates (very dry)
Blocking Reagent (Boehringer Mannheim Cat No. 109617650)

Sodium dodecyl sulfate (SDS; 10%)
Prehybridization Solution
Probe for cholera toxin gene labeled with digoxigenin
20X SSC (3 *M* NaCl, 300 m*M* sodium citrate, pH 7.0)
1 *M* Tris-HCl, pH 8.0
1 *M* Tris-HCl, pH 8.0/NaCl 1.5 *M*
1 *M* Tris-HCl, pH 9.5
Positive control (*V. cholerae* with the toxin gene)
Negative control (*V. cholerae* without the toxin gene)

1. To complete the procedure within one workday, start either late in the afternoon of the previous day or early in the morning. To optimize preparation of blots, it is convenient to analyze at least 48 samples at once.
2. Dry an LB agar plate in a 37°C incubator overnight.
3. Label the LB agar Petri plate with the number of the colonies to be examined, using the "colony grid" if desired (Appendix H).
4. With a sterile toothpick, pick a colony of *V. cholerae* O1 and touch the toothpick to the agar in a spot that corresponds to the number of the colony according to the grid. Make sure to include a positive control and a negative control on each plate.
5. Incubate for 1–6 hours at 37°C, until the patches of culture start to grow.
6. Cut a nylon membrane to size (or use pre-cut circular membranes). Using a lead pencil, label the membrane with the date, the number of the experiment, your initials, and an arrow in the center (to orient the membrane with respect to the Petri plate). **Never touch the membrane with ungloved hands**.
7. Wearing gloves, place the membrane over the patches on the Petri plate, letting it fall gently and slowly and being careful to avoid air bubbles. It will stick by itself.
8. Incubate the Petri plate with the membrane at 37°C for 1–5 hours. Usually, after 3 hours the patches have grown well; however, if necessary, the plate can be left overnight at ambient temperature (to avoid overgrowth).
9. Soak two sheets of 3MM chromatographic paper in one tray containing 0.5 *M* NaOH. Transfer the 3MM paper to a sheet of plastic wrap, removing the excess solution by letting it drip off the 3MM paper. Using filter forceps, remove the membrane from the Petri plate and carefully place it on the 3MM paper soaked in NaOH, with the patches facing up. Let it sit for 15 minutes at ambient temperature.
10. In another tray, wet two sheets of 3MM chromatographic paper in 1 *M* Tris-HCl, pH 8.0. Using filter forceps, transfer the membrane to this tray, again with the patches facing up, and incubate for 10 minutes at ambient temperature.
11. In a third tray, wet two sheets of 3MM chromatographic paper in 0.5 *M* Tris-HCl, pH 8.0/1.5 *M* NaCl. Using filter forceps, transfer the membrane to this tray, again with the patches facing up, and incubate for 10 minutes at ambient temperature.
12. Rinse the membrane in 40 mL of 2X SSC (in an empty Petri plate) and let it air-dry between two sheets of filter paper at ambient temperature or in the 37°C incubator.
13. Fix the *V. cholerae* DNA to the membrane by incubating the membrane in an oven at 80°C for 30 minutes and let cool. The blot is now ready for hybridization.

5.2.3 Hybridization

Prewarm the pre-hybridization solution at 65°C

1. Place the membrane blot (50 cm^2) in a sealable plastic bag and add 10 mL (0.2 mL/cm^2) of pre-hybridization solution.

2. Remove any air bubbles by rolling a pipet over the bag and forcing the bubbles through the top. Be careful not to lose any of the solution.
3. Seal the bag with a heat sealer.
4. Place the bag in a tray in a 65°C water bath and incubate for 1 hour with constant agitation.
5. Using a 20 μL pipettor, dilute 3 μL of the probe (use 2–5 μL depending on the specific activity of the probe) in 100 mL of ddH$_2$O in a 0.5-mL microcentrifuge tube.
6. Incubate the tube in a boiling water bath for 10 minutes and then place it immediately in crushed ice for several minutes. Centrifuge briefly to concentrate the probe solution at the bottom of the tube. This step should be initiated 15 minutes prior to the end of the pre-hybridization incubation.
7. Remove the bag containing the membrane from the 65°C water bath and cut one corner to pour off the pre-hybridization solution. Make sure all the solution has been removed by rolling a pipet over the bag, as in step 2.
8. Add 2.5 mL (0.05 mL/cm^2) of fresh pre-hybridization solution (pre-warmed at 65°C) to the bag and then add the 103 μL of probe. Remove the air bubbles as in step 2 and reseal the bag with a heat sealer.
9. Incubate the bag for at least 15 minutes in a tray in the 65°C water bath, with constant agitation, as in step 4. This incubation step can be conducted overnight.
10. Prepare the wash solution (500 mL/probe) and pre-warm it to 65°C using a microwave or the 65°C water bath (the latter requires a longer incubation).
11. Remove the membrane from the plastic bag and place it in a tray or 500-mL glass beaker.
12. Add 100 mL of the wash solution to the tray or beaker and briefly rinse the membrane (Figure 5.11). Discard the used wash solution.
13. Add another 200 mL of the wash solution and wash the membrane for 15 minutes in the 65°C water bath, with constant agitation. Discard the used wash solution.
14. Repeat step 13.
15. Air-dry the membrane on filter paper. The membrane can be used immediately for the visualization procedure, or it can be air-dried on a filter paper and stored dry for later detection.

Note: If the membrane is dried, it cannot be stripped and re-probed later.

5.2.4   Colorimetric Detection

The following steps are conducted at ambient temperature.

1. In a Petri plate, incubate the membrane in development Buffer 1 for 1 minute, then discard the solution.
2. Next, add 20 mL of Buffer 2 (blocking buffer) and incubate the membrane for 1 hour. Discard the solution.
3. Add 10 mL of fresh Buffer 2 to which 3 μL of anti-digoxigenin–alkaline phosphatase conjugate has been added.[35] Incubate the membrane for 30 minutes with constant agitation to ensure that the membrane is always covered. Discard the solution.
4. Wash the membrane with 20 mL of Buffer 1 for 15 minutes and discard the wash solution.
5. Repeat step 4.
6. Incubate the membrane in 20 mL of Buffer 3 for 2 minutes.
7. Add 45 μL of NBT and 35 μL of BCIP to 10 mL of Buffer 3 in another Petri plate. Transfer the blot to the solution using filter forceps. Seal the Petri plate with Parafilm® or masking tape and let the color develop in a dark place (e.g., in a drawer) for 1–16 hours.

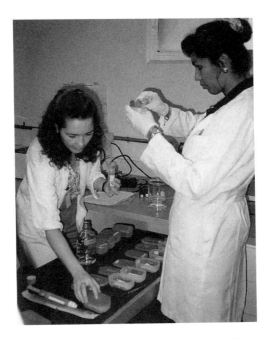

Fig. 5.11. Course instructor Josefina Coloma and participant Ana Vargas washing blots after hybridization with a nonradioactively labeled probe.

Interpretation of Results

Positive: A purple color is produced due to the alkaline phosphatase, which reacts with the substrates NBT and BIP to form a purple-blue precipitate.

Negative: No color is produced.

5.2.5   Chemiluminescent Detection

ADDITIONAL EQUIPMENT
Darkroom

ADDITIONAL MATERIALS
Clear plastic sheets
Plastic trays for photochemicals
Wooden or plastic tongs for handling photograph film
Lightproof film cassettes

ADDITIONAL REAGENTS
Chemiluminescent substrate for alkaline phosphatase (e.g., Lumi-phos 530®, Lumigen, Inc., Southfield, MI)
GBX developer and fixer (Eastman Kodak Co., Rochester, NY)
X-ray film

Steps 1–6 are the same as in section 5.2.4.

7. Cut two clear plastic sheets to the desired size. Place the blot faceup on the lower sheet. With a sterile pipet, add 0.5 mL/100 cm^2 of Lumi-phos 530$^®$ to the membrane and rock it to distribute the Lumi-phos over the entire surface.

8. Lower the upper plastic sheet over the membrane and push the bubbles off the blot by passing a paper towel over the plastic sheet. Seal with tape.

9. In the darkroom, cut a piece of X-ray film to size and cut the upper right hand corner to orient the film. Expose the blot (faceup) to a sheet of X-ray film in a light-proof film cassette for 1–5 minutes at ambient temperature. Mark the borders of the blot on the film.

10. To develop the film, incubate it for 2 minutes in GBX developer at 20°C.

11. Rinse the film in water for at least 30 seconds (16–24°C) in running water, if possible. If not, rinse the film in a tray of water with agitation.

12. Incubate the film in GBX fixer for 5 minutes (16–24°C) with agitation.

13. Rinse the film in running water for 30 minutes.

14. Hang the film to air dry.

Interpretation of Results

Positive: A dark spot is produced on the film due to the light emitted as alkaline phosphatase reacts with its chemiluminescent substrate (Figure 5.12). The spots on the film correspond to positive samples on the blot.

Negative: No specific dark spot is produced on the film.

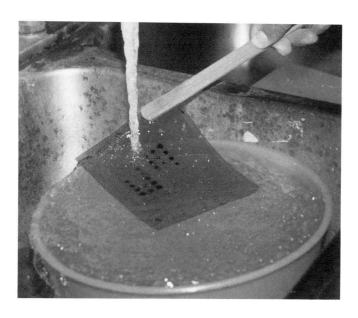

Fig. 5.12. Chemiluminscent detection of a nonradioactive probe hybridized to a dot blot of PCR products during the Phase I workshop in Ecuador.

References

5.1.2 Equipment, Materials, Controls and Procedures Common to All PCR Protocols

Desai, U.J., and Pfaffle, P.K. (1995) Single-step purification of a thermostable DNA polymerase expressed in *Escherichia coli. BioTechniques*, 19:780–784.

Engelke, D.R., Krikos, A., Bruck, M.E., and Ginsburg, D. (1990) Purification of *Thermus aquaticus* DNA polymerase expressed in *E. coli. Anal. Biochem.*, 191:396–400.

Grimm, E., and Arbuthnot, P. (1995) Rapid purification of recombinant *Taq* DNA polymerase by freezing and high temperature thawing of bacterial expression cultures. *Nucleic Acids Res.*, 23:4518–4519.

Pluthero, F.G. (1993) Rapid purification of high-activity *Taq* DNA polymerase. *Nucleic Acids Res.*, 21:4850–4851.

Sambrook, J., Fritsch, E.F., and Maniatis, T. (1989) *Molecular Cloning: A Laboratory Manual.* New York, Cold Spring Harbor Laboratory Press.

5.1.3 Dengue Virus

Chan, S.-Y., Kautner, I.M., and Lam, S.-K. (1994) The influence of antibody levels in dengue diagnosis by polymerase chain reaction. *J. Virol. Meth.*, 49:315–322.

Chungue, E., Roche, C., Lefevre, M.-F., Barbazan, P., and Chanteau, S. (1993) Ultra-rapid, simple, sensitive, and economical silica method for extraction of dengue viral RNA from clinical specimens and mosquitoes by reverse transcriptase-polymerase chain reaction. *J. Med. Virol.*, 40:142–145.

Deubel, V., Laille, M., Hugnot, J.P., Chungue, E., Guesdon, J.L., Drouet, M.T., Bassot, S., and Chevrier, D. (1990) Identification of dengue sequences by genomic amplification: Rapid diagnosis of dengue virus serotypes in peripheral blood. *J. Virol. Meth.*, 30:41–54.

Farfan, J.A., Olson, K.E., Black, W.C., Gubler, D.J., and Beaty, B.J. (1997) Rapid characterization of genetic diversity among twelve dengue-2 isolates by single-strand conformation polymorphism analysis. *Am. J. Trop. Med. Hyg.*, 57:416–422.

Halstead, S.B. (1988) Pathogenesis of dengue: Challenges to molecular biology. *Science*, 239:476–481.

Harris, E., Roberts, T.G., Smith, L., Selle, J., Kramer, L.D., Valle, S., Sandoval, E., and Balmaseda, A. (1998b) Typing of dengue viruses in clinical specimens and mosquitoes by single-tube multiplex reverse transcriptase-PCR. *J. Clin. Microbiol.*, 36:2634–2639.

Harris, E., Sandoval, E., Xet, A. M., Johnson, M., and Riley, L. W. Rapid subtyping of dengue viruses by restriction site specific (RSS)-PCR. In press.

Henchal, E., Polo, S., Vorndam, V., Yaemsiri, C., Innis, B., and Hoke, C. (1991) Sensitivity and specificity of universal primer set for the rapid diagnosis of dengue virus infections by polymerase chain reaction and nucleic acid hybridization. *Am. J. Trop. Med. Hyg.*, 45:418–428.

Lanciotti, R., Calisher, C., Gubler, D., Chang, G., and Vorndam, A. (1992) Rapid detection and typing of dengue viruses from clinical samples by using reverse transcriptase-polymerase chain reaction. *J. Clin. Microbiol.*, 30:545–551.

Meiyu, F., Huosheng, C., Cuihua, C., Xiaodong, T., Lianhua, J., Yifei, P., Weijun, C., and Huiyu, G. (1997) Detection of flaviviruses by reverse transcriptase-polymerase chain reaction with the universal primer set. *Microbiol. Immunol.*, 41:209–213.

Monath, T.P. (1994) Dengue: The risk to developed and developing countries. *Proc. Natl. Acad. Sci. USA*, 91:2395–2400.

Morens, D.M. (1994) Antibody-dependent enhancement of infection and the pathogenesis of viral disease. *Clin. Infect. Dis.*, 19:500–512.

Morita, K., Maemoto, T., Honda, S., Onishi, K., Misako, M., Tanaka, M., and Igarashi, A. (1994) Rapid detection of virus genome from imported dengue fever and dengue hemorrhagic fever patients by direct polymerase chain reaction. *J. Med. Virol.*, 44:54–58.

Morita, K., Tanaka, M., and Igarashi, A. (1991) Rapid identification of dengue virus serotypes by using polymerase chain reaction. *J. Clin. Microbiol.*, 29:2107–2110.

Pan American Health Organization (1994) *Dengue and Dengue Hemorrhagic Fever in the Americas: Guidelines for Prevention and Control.* Scientific Publication #548.

Pierre, V., Drouet, M.-T., and Deubel, V. (1994) Identification of mosquito-borne flavivirus sequences using universal primers and reverse transcriptase/polymerase chain reaction. *Res. Virol.*, 145:93–104.

Seah, C.L.K., Chow, V.T.K., Tan, H.C., and Chan, Y.C. (1995) Rapid, single-step RT-PCR typing of dengue viruses using five NS3 gene primers. *J. Virol. Meth.*, 51:193–200.

Vorndam, V., Kuno, G., and Rosado, N. (1994a) A PCR-restriction enzyme technique for determining dengue virus subgroups within serotypes. *J. Virol. Meth.*, 48:237–244.

Yenchitsomanus, P.T., Sricharoen, P., Jaruthasana, I., Pattanakitsakul, S.N., Nitayaphan, S., Mongkolsapaya, J., and Malasit, P. (1996) Rapid detection and identification of dengue viruses by polymerase chain reaction (PCR). *Southeast Asian J. Trop. Med. Pub. Health*, 27:228–236.

5.1.4 New World *Leishmania*

Adhya, S., Chatterjee, M., Hassan, M.Q., Mukherjee, S., and Sen, S. (1995) Detection of *Leishmania* in the blood of early kala-azar patients with the aid of the polymerase chain reaction. *Trans. R. Soc. Trop. Med. Hyg.*, 89:622–624.

Armijos, R.X., Chico, M.E., Cruz, M.E., Guderian, R.H., Kreutzer, R.D., Berman, J.D., Rogers, M.D., and Grögl, M. (1990) Human cutaneous leishmaniasis in Ecuador: Identification of parasites by enzyme electrophoresis. *Am. J. Trop. Med. Hyg.*, 42:424–428.

Ashford, R.W., Desjeux, P., and Deraadt, P. (1992) Estimation of populations at risk of infection with leishmaniasis. *Parasitol. Today*, 8:104–105.

Badaro, R., Reed, S.G., Barral, A., Orge, G., and Jones, T.C. (1986) Evaluation of the micro enzyme-linked immunosorbant assay (ELISA) for antibodies in American visceral leishmaniasis: Antigen selection for detecion of infection-specific responses. *Am. J. Trop. Med. Hyg.*, 35:72–78.

Barral, A., Badaro, R., Barral-Netto, M., Grimaldi, G., Jr., Momen, H., and Carvalho, E.M. (1986) Isolation of *Leishmania mexicana amazonensis* from the bone marrow in a case of American visceral leishmaniasis. *Am. J. Trop. Med. Hyg.*, 35:732–734.

Barral, A., Pedral-Sampaio, D., Grimaldi, G.J., Momen, H., McMahon-Pratt, D., Ribeiro de Jesus, A., Almeida, R., Badaro, R., Barral-Netto, M., Carvalho, E.M., and Johnson, W.D. (1991) Leishmaniasis in Bahia, Brazil: Evidence that *Leishmania amazonensis* produces a wide spectrum of clinical disease. *Am. J. Trop. Med Hyg.*, 44:536–546.

Belli, A., Rodriguez, B., Avilés, H., and Harris, E. (1998) Simplified PCR detection of New World *Leishmania* from clinical specimens. *Am. J. Trop. Med. Hyg.* 58:102–109.

Belli, A., Garcia, D., Palacios, X., Rodriguez, B., Videa, E., Valle, S., Tinoco, E., Marin, F., and Harris, E. *Leishmania chagasi* causes visceral disease and widespread atypical cutaneous leishmaniasis. Submitted for publication.

Bhattacharyya, R., Das, K., Sen, S., Roy, S., and Majumder, H.K. (1996) Development of a genus specific primer set for detectin of *Leishmania* parasites by polymerase chain reaction. *FEMS Microbiol. Letts.*, 135:195–200.

Bozza, M., Fernandes, O., Degrave, W.M., and Lopes, U.G. (1995) Characterization of "Old World" *Leishmania* species using amplified minicircle variable regions as molecular probes. *Trans. R. Soc. Trop. Med. Hyg.*, 89:333–334.

Camargo, M.E., and Rebonato, C. (1969) Cross-reactivity in immunofluorescence test for *Trypanosoma* and *Leishmania* antibodies. A simple inhibition procedure to ensure specific results. *Am. J. Top. Med. Hyg.*, 18:500–505.

Costa, J.-M., Durand, R., Deniau, M., Rivollet, D., Izri, M., Houin, R., Vidaud, M., and Bretagne, S. (1996) PCR enzyme-linked immunosorbant assay for diagnosis of leishmaniasis in human immunodeficiency virus-infected patients. *J. Clin. Microbiol.*, 34:1831–1833.

de Brujin, M.H., and Barker, D.C. (1992) Diagnosis of New World leishmaniasis: Specific detection of species of the *Leishmania braziliensis* complex by amplification of kinetoplast DNA. *Acta Trop.*, 52:45–58.

Eresh, S., McCallum, S.M., and Barker, D.C. (1994) Identification and diagnosis of *Leishmania mexicana* complex isolates by polymerase chain reaction. *Parasitology*, 109:423–433.

Grimaldi, G., Jr., David, J.R., and McMahon-Pratt, D. (1987) Identification and distribution of New World *Leishmania* species characterized by serodeme analysis using monoclonal antibodies. *Am. J. Trop. Med. Hyg.*, 36:270–287.

Grimaldi, G., and McMahon-Pratt, D. (1996) Monoclonal antibodies for the identification of New World *Leishmania* species. *Mem. Inst. Oswaldo Cruz*, 91:37–42.

Grimaldi, G., Jr., and Tesh, R.B. (1993) Leishmaniasis of the New World: Current concepts and implications for future research. *Clin. Microbiol. Rev.*, 6:230–250.

Guevara, P., Alonso, G., da Silveira, J.F., de Mello, M., Scorza, J.V., Anez, N., and Ramirez, J.L. (1992) Identification of new world *Leishmania* using ribosomal gene spacer probes. *Mol. Biochem. Parasitol.*, 56:15–26.

Harris, E., Kropp, G., Belli, A., Rodriguez, B., and Agabian, N. (1998a) Single-step multiplex PCR assay for characterization of New World *Leishmania* complexes. *J. Clin. Microbiol.* 36:1989–1995.

Hassan, M.Q., Ghosh, A., Ghosh, S.S., Gupta, M., Basu, D., Mallik, K.K., and Adhya, S. (1993) Enzymatic amplification of mini-exon-derived RNA gene spacers of *Leishmania donovani*: Primers and probes for DNA diagnosis. *Parasitology*, 107:509–517.

Hernandez, D.E., Rodriguez, N., Wessolossky, M., and Convit, J. (1991) Visceral leishmaniasis due to a *Leishmania* variant that shares kinetoplast DNA sequences with *Leishmania braziliensis* and *Leishmania mexicana* in a patient infected with human immunodeficiency virus: Identification of the *Leishmania* species with use of the polymerase chain reaction. *Clin. Infect. Dis.*, 21:701–702.

Kreutzer, R.D., and Christensen, H.A. (1980) Characterization of *Leishmania* spp. by isozyme electrophoresis. *Am. J. Trop. Med. Hyg.*, 29:199–208.

López, M., Inga, R., Cangalaya, M., Echevarria, J., Llanos-Cuentas, A., Orrego, C., and Arévalo, J. (1993) Diagnosis of *Leishmania* using the polymerase chain reaction: A simplified procedure for field work. *Am. J. Trop. Med. Hyg.*, 49:348–356.

Mathis, A., and Deplazes, P. (1995) PCR and in vitro cultivation for detection of *Leishmania* spp. in diagnostic samples from humans and dogs. *J. Clin. Microbiol.*, 33:1145–1149.

Meredith, S.E., Zijlstra, E.E., Schoone, G.J., Kroon, C.C., van Eys, G.J., Schaeffer, K.U., el-Hassan, A.M., and Lawyer, P.G. (1993) Development and application of the polymerase chain reaction for the detection and identification of *Leishmania* parasites in clinical material. *Arch. Inst. Pasteur Tunis*, 70:419–431.

Neva, F., and Sacks, D. (1990) Leishmaniasis. In *Tropical and Geographical Medicine*, K.S. Warren and A.A.F. Mahmoud, eds., New York, McGraw-Hill Information Services Co.

Noyes, H.A., Belli, A.A., and Maingon, R. (1996) Appraisal of various random amplified polymorphic DNA-polymerase chain reaction primers for *Leishmania* identification. *Am. J. Trop. Med. Hyg.*, 55:98–105.

Nuzum, E., White, F., Thakur, C., Dietze, R., Wages, J., Grogl, M., and Berman, J. (1995) Diagnosis of symptomatic visceral leishmaniasis by use of the polymerase chain reaction on patient blood. *J. Infect. Dis.*, 171:751–754.

Ponce, C., Ponce, E., Morrison, A., Cruz, A., Kreutzer, R., McMahon-Pratt, D., and Neva, F. (1991) *Leishmania donovani chagasi*: New clinical variant of cutaneous leishmaniasis in Honduras. *Lancet*, 337:67–70.

Qiao, Z., Miles, M.A., and Wilson, S.M. (1995) Detection of parasites of the *Leishmania donovani*-complex by a polymerase chain reaction-solution hybridization enzyme-linked immunoassay (PCR-SHELA). *Parasitology*, 110:269–275.

Ramos, A., Maslov, D.A., Fernandes, O., Campbell, D.A., and Simpson, L. (1996) Detection and identification of human pathogenic *Leishmania* and *Trypanosoma* species by hybridization of PCR-amplified mini-exon repeats. *Exp. Parasitol.*, 82:242–250.

Ravel, S., Cuny, G., Reynes, J., and Veas, F. (1995) A highly sensitive and rapid procedure for direct PCR detection of *Leishmania infantum* within human peripheral blood mononuclear cells. *Acta Trop.*, 59:187–196.

Rodgers, M.R., Popper, S.J., and Wirth, D.F. (1990) Amplification of kinetoplast DNA as a tool in the detection and diagnosis of *Leishmania*. *Exp. Parasitol.*, 71:267–275.

Smyth, A.J., Ghosh, A., Hassan, M.Q., de Brujin, M.H.L., Adhya, S., Mallik, K.K., and Barker, D.C. (1992) Rapid and sensitive detection of *Leishmania* kinetoplast DNA from spleen and blood samples of kala-azar patients. *Parasitology*, 105:183–192.

Uliana, S.R.B., Nelson, K., Beverley, S.M., Camargo, E.P., and Floeter-Winter, L.M. (1994) Discrimination amongst *Leishmania* by polymerase chain reaction and hybridization with small subunit ribosomal DNA derived oligonucleotides. *J. Eukaryot. Microbiol.*, 41:324–330.

van Eys, G.J.J.M., Schoone, G.J., Kroon, N.C.M., and Ebeling, S.B. (1992) Sequence analysis of small subunit ribosomal RNA genes and its use for detection and identification of *Leishmania* parasites. *Mol. Biochem. Parasitol.*, 51:133–142.

Wilson, S.M. (1995) DNA-based methods in the detection of *Leishmania* parasites: Field applications and practicalities. *Ann. Trop. Med. Parasitol.*, 89:95–100.

5.1.5   *Mycobacterium tuberculosis*

Afghani, B., and Stutman, H.R. (1997) Quantitative-competitive polymerase chain reaction for rapid susceptibility testing of *Mycobacterium tuberculosis* to isoniazid. *Biochem. Mol. Med.*, 60:182–186.

Amicosante, M., Richeldi, L., Trenti, G., Paone, G., Campa, M., Bisetti, A., and Saltini, C. (1995) Inactivation of polymerase inhibitors for *Mycobacterium tuberculosis* DNA amplification in sputum by using capture resin. *J. Clin. Microbiol.*, 33:629–630.

Andersen, A.B., Thybo, S., Godfrey-Faussett, P., and Stoker, N.G. (1993) Polymerase chain reaction for detection of *Mycobacterium tuberculosis* in sputum. *Eur. J. Clin. Microbiol. Infect. Dis.*, 12:922–927.

Brisson-Noel, A., Gicquel, B., Lecossier, D., Levy-Frebault, V., Nassif, X., and Hance, A.J. (1989) Rapid diagnosis of tuberculosis by amplification of mycobacterial DNA in clinical samples. *Lancet*, 2:1069–1071.

Clarridge, J.E., Shawar, R.M., Shinnick, T.M., and Plikaytis, B.B. (1993) Large-scale use of polymerase chain reaction for detection of *Mycobacterium tuberculosis* in a routine mycobacteriology laboratory. *J. Clin. Microbiol.*, 31:2049–2056.

Cormican, M., Glennon, M., Riain, U.N., and Flynn, J. (1995) Multiplex PCR for identifying mycobacterial isolates. *J. Clin. Pathol.*, 48:203–205.

Cousins, D., Francis, B., and Dawson, D. (1996) Multiplex PCR provides a low-cost alternative to DNA probe methods for rapid identification of *Mycobacterium avium* and *Mycobacterium intracellulare*. *J. Clin. Microbiol.*, 34:2331–2333.

Daniel, T.M. (1996) Immunodiagnosis of tuberculosis. In *Tuberculosis*, W.N. Rom and S.M. Garay, eds., Boston, Little, Brown and Company.

De Wit, D., Steyn, L., Shoemaker, S., and Sogin, M. (1990) Direct detection of *Mycobacterium tuberculosis* in clinical specimens by DNA amplification. *J. Clin. Microbiol.*, 28:2437–2441.

Del Portillo, P., Murillo, L.A., and Patarroyo, M.E. (1991) Amplification of a species-specific DNA fragment of *Mycobacterium tuberculosis* and its possible use in diagnosis. *J. Clin. Microbiol.*, 29:2163–2168.

Del Portillo, P., Thomas, M.C., Martinez, E., Maranon, C., Valladares, B., Patarroyo, M.E., and Carlos Lopez, M. (1996) Multiprimer PCR system for differential identification of mycobacteria in clinical samples. *J. Clin. Microbiol.*, 34:324–328.

Eisenach, K.D., Cave, M.D., Bates, J.H., and Crawford, J.T. (1992) Polymerase chain reaction amplification of a repetitive DNA sequence specific for *Mycobacterium tuberculosis*. *J. Infect. Dis.*, 161:977–981.

Forbes, B., and Hicks, K. (1993) Direct detection of *Mycobacterium tuberculosis* in respiratory specimens in a clinical laboratory by polymerase chain reaction. *J. Clin. Microbiol.*, 31:1688–1694.

Forbes, B.A. (1997) Critical assessment of gene amplification approaches on the diagnosis of tuberculosis. *Immunol. Invest.*, 26:105–116.

Forbes, B.A. and Hicks, K.E. (1996) Substances interfering with direct detection of *Mycobacterium tuberculosis* in clinical specimens by PCR: Effects of bovine serum albumin. *J. Clin. Microbiol.*, 34:2125–2128.

Fox, E. (1991) Mycobacterial infections. In *Hunter's Tropical Medicine*, G. T. Strickland, ed., Philadelphia, W. B. Saunders.

Friedman, C.R., Stoeckle, M.Y., Johnson, W.D., Jr., and Riley, L.W. (1995) Double-repetitive-element PCR method for subtyping *Mycobacterium tuberculosis* clinical isolates. *J. Clin. Microbiol.*, 33:1383–1384.

Groenen, P.M., Bunschoten, A.E., van Soolingen, D., and van Embden, J.D. (1993) Nature of DNA polymorphism in the direct repeat cluster of *Mycobacterium tuberculosis*: Application for strain differentiation by a novel typing method. *Mol. Microbiol.*, 10:1057–1065.

Haas, D.W., and Des Prez, R.M. (1995) Mycobacterium tuberculosis. In *Principles and Practice of Infectious Diseases*, G.L. Mandell, J.E. Bennett, and R. Dolin, eds., New York, Churchill Livingstone.

Haas, W.H., Butler, W.R., Woodley, C.L., and Crawford, J.T. (1993) Mixed-linker polymerase chain reaction: A new method for rapid fingerprinting of isolates of the *Mycobacterium tuberculosis* complex. *J. Clin. Microbiol.*, 31:1293–1298.

Hermans, P.W., Schuitema, A.R., Van Soolingen, D., Verstynen, C.P., Bik, E.M., Thole, J.E., Kolk, A.H., and van Embden, J.D. (1990) Specific detection of *Mycobacterium tuberculosis* complex strains by polymerase chain reaction. *J. Clin. Microbiol.*, 28:1204–1213.

Jacobs, W.R., Jr., Barletta, R.G., Udani, R., Chan, J., Kalkut, G., Sosne, G., Kieser, T., Sarkis, G.J., Hatfull, G.F., and Bloom, B.R. (1993) Rapid assessment of drug susceptibilities of *Mycobacterium tuberculosis* by means of luciferase reporter phages. *Science*, 260:819–822.

Jou, N.T., Yoshimori, R.B., Mason, G.R., Louie, J.S., and Liebling, M.R. (1997) Single-tube, nested, reverse transcriptase PCR for detection of viable *Mycobacterium tuberculosis*. *J. Clin. Microbiol.*, 35:1161–1165.

Kaltwasser, G., Garcia, S., Salinas, A.M., and Montiel, F. (1993) Enzymatic DNA amplification (PCR) in the diagnosis of extrapulmonary *Mycobacterium tuberculosis* infection. *Mol. Cell. Probes*, 7:465–470.

Kamerbeek, J., Schouls, L., Kolk, A., van Agterveld, M., van Soolingen, D., Kuijper, S., Bunschoten, A., Molhuizen, H., Shaw, R., and Goyal, M. (1997) Simultaneous detection and strain differentiation of *Mycobacterium tuberculosis* for diagnosis and epidemiology. *J. Clin. Microbiol.*, 35:907–914.

Kennedy, N., Gillespie, S.H., Saruni, A.O., Kisyombe, G., McNerney, R., Ngowi, F.I., and Wilson, S. (1994) Polymerase chain reaction for assessing treatment response in patients with pulmonary tuberculosis. *J. Infect. Dis.*, 170:713–716.

Lee, T.Y., Lee, T.J., and Kim, S.K. (1994) Differentiation of *Mycobacterium tuberculosis* strains by arbitrarily primed polymerase chain reaction-based DNA fingerprinting. *Yonsei Med. J.*, 35:286–294.

Levee, G., Glaziou, P., Gicquel, B., and Chanteau, S. (1994) Follow-up of tuberculosis patients undergoing standard anti-tuberculosis chemotherapy by using a polymerase chain reaction. *Res. Microbiol.*, 145:5–8.

Linton, C.J., Jalal, H., Leeming, J.P., and Millar, M.R. (1994) Rapid discrimination of *Mycobacterium tuberculosis* strains by random amplified polymorphic DNA analysis. *J. Clin. Microbiol.*, 32:2169–2174.

Mustafa, A.S., Ahmed, A., Abal, A.T., and Chugh, T.D. (1995) Establishment and evaluation of a multiplex polymerase chain reaction for detection of mycobacteria and specific identification of *Mycobacterium tuberculosis* complex. *Tubercle Lung Dis.*, 76:336–343.

Neimark, H., Barg, M.A., and Carleton, S. (1996) Direct identification and typing of *Mycobacterium tuberculosis* by PCR. *J. Clin. Microbiol.*, 34:2454–2459.

Nolte, F.S., Metchock, B., McGowan, J.E.J., Edwards, A., Okwumabua, O., Thurmond, C., Mitchell, P.S., Plikaytis, B., and Shinnick, T. (1993) Direct detection of *Mycobacterium tuberculosis* in sputum by polymerase chain reaction and DNA hybridization. *J. Clin. Microbiol.*, 31:1777–1782.

Noordhoek, G.T., Kolk, A.H., Bjune, G., Catty, D., Dale, J.W., Fine, P.E., Godfrey-Faussett, P., Cho, S.N., Shinnick, T., Svenson, S.B., Wilson, S., and van Embden, J.D.A. (1994) Sensitivity and specificity of PCR for detection of *Mycobacterium tuberculosis*: A blind comparison study among seven laboratories. *J. Clin. Microbiol.*, 32:277–284.

Noordhoek, G.T., van Embden, J.D., and Kolk, A.H. (1996) Reliability of nucleic acid amplification for detection of *Mycobacterium tuberculosis*: An international collaborative quality control study among 30 laboratories. *J. Clin. Microbiol.*, 34:2522–2525.

Oggioni, M.R., Fattorini, L., Li, B., De Milito, A., Zazzi, M., Pozzi, G., Orefici, G., and Valensin, P.E. (1995) Identification of *Mycobacterium tuberculosis* complex, *Mycobacterium avium* and *Mycobacterium intracellulare* by selective nested polymerase chain reaction. *Mol. Cell. Probes*, 9:321–326.

Pao, C.C., Yen, T.S.B., You, J.-B., Maa, J.-S., Fiss, E.H., and Chang, C.-H. (1990) Detection and identification of *Mycobacterium tuberculosis* by DNA amplification. *J. Clin. Microbiol.*, 28:1877–1880.

Patel, S., Wall, S., and Saunders, N.A. (1996) Heminested inverse PCR for IS6110 fingerprinting of *Mycobacterium tuberculosis* strains. *J. Clin. Microbiol.*, 34:1686–1690.

Plikaytis, B.B., Crawford, J.T., Woodley, C.L., Butler, W.R., Eisenach, K.D., Cave, M.D., and Shinnick, T.M. (1993) Rapid, amplification-based fingerprinting of *Mycobacterium tuberculosis*. *J. Gen. Microbiol.*, 139:1537–1542.

Plikaytis, B.B., Marden, J.L., Crawford, J.T., Woodley, C.L., Butler, W.R., and Shinnick, T.M. (1994) Multiplex PCR assay specific for the multidrug-resistant strain W of *Mycobacterium tuberculosis*. *J. Clin. Microbiol.*, 32:1542–1546.

Riley, L.W., and Harris, E. Double Repetitive Element-Polymerase Chain Reaction method for subtyping *Mycobacterium tuberculosis* strains. In *Basic Techniques in Mycobacterial and Nocardial Molecular Biology*, R. Ollar and N. Connell, eds., Philadelphia, Raven Publishers, in press.

Ross, B., and Dwyer, B. (1993) Rapid, simple method for typing isolates of *Mycobacterium tuberculosis* by using the polymerase chain reaction. *J. Clin. Microbiol.*, 31:329–334.

Scarpellini, P., Racca, S., Cinque, P., Delfanti, F., Gianotti, N., Terreni, M.R., Vago, L., and Lazzarin, A. (1995) Nested polymerase chain reaction for diagnosis and monitoring treatment response in AIDS patients with tuberculous meningitis. *Aids*, 9:895–900.

Schluger, N.W., Condos, R., Lewis, S., and Rom, W.N. (1994) Amplification of DNA of *Mycobacterium tuberculosis* from peripheral blood of patients with pulmonary tuberculosis. *Lancet*, 344:232–233.

Scorpio, A., Lindholm-Levy, P., Heifets, L., Gilman, R., Siddiqi, S., Cynamon, M., and Zhang, Y. (1997) Characterization of *pncA* mutations in pyrazinamide-resistant *Mycobacterium tuberculosis*. *Antimicrob. Agents Chemother.*, 41:540–543.

Sepkowitz, K.A., Raffalli, J., Riley, L., Kiehn, T.E., and Armstrong, D. (1995) Tuberculosis in the AIDS era. *Clin. Microbiol. Rev.*, 8:180–199.

Sougakoff, W., Lemaitre, N., Cambau, E., Szpytma, M., Revel, V., and Jarlier, V. (1997) Nonradioactive single-strand conformation polymorphism analysis for detection of fluoroquinolone resistance in mycobacteria. *Eur. J. Clin. Microbiol. Infect. Dis.*, 16:395–398.

Suffys, P.N., de Araujo, M.E.I., and Degrave, W.M. (1997) The changing face of the epidemiology of tuberculosis due to molecular strain typing-A review. *Mem. Inst. Oswaldo Cruz*, 92:297–316.

Tan, M.F., Ng, W.C., Chan, S.H., and Tan, W.C. (1997) Comparative usefulness of PCR in the detection of *Mycobacterium tuberculosis* in different clinical specimens. *J. Med. Microbiol.*, 46:164–169.

Telenti, A., Imboden, P., Marchesi, F., Schmidheini, T., and Bodmer, T. (1993) Direct, automated detection of rifampin-resistant *Mycobacterium tuberculosis* by polymerase chain reaction and single-strand conformation polymorphisn analysis. *Antimicrob. Agents Chemother.*, 37:2054–2058.

Temesgen, Z., Satoh, K., Uhl, J.R., Kline, B.C., and Cockerill, F.R., 3rd. (1997) Use of polymerase chain reaction single-strand conformation polymorphism (PCR-SSCP) analysis to detect a point mutation in the catalase-peroxidase gene (katG) of *Mycobacterium tuberculosis*. *Mol. Cell. Probes*, 11:59–63.

Thierry, D., Brisson-Noel, A., Vincent-Levy-Frebault, V., Nguyen, S., Guesdon, J.L., and Gicquel, B. (1990) Characterization of a *Mycobacterium tuberculosis* insertion sequence, IS6110, and its application in diagnosis. *J. Clin. Microbiol.*, 28:2668–2673.

Van Embden, J.D., Cave, M.D., Crawford, J.T., Dale, J.W., Eisenach, K.D., Gicquel, B., Hermans, P., Martin, C., McAdam, R., Shinnick, T.M., and Small, P.M. (1993) Strain identification of *Mycobacterium tuberculosis* by DNA fingerprinting: Recommendations for a standardized methodology. *J. Clin. Microbiol.*, 31:406–409.

van Vollenhoven, P., Heyns, C.F., de Beer, P.M., Whitaker, P., van Helden, P.D., and Victor, T. (1996) Polymerase chain reaction in the diagnosis of urinary tract tuberculosis. *Urol. Res.*, 24:107–111.

Wilson, S., McNerney, R., Nye, P., Godfrey-Faussett, P., Stoker, N., and Voller, A. (1993) Progress toward a simplified polymerase chain reaction and its application to diagnosis of tuberculosis. *J. Clin. Microbiol.*, 31:776–782.

Yuen, K.Y., Chan, K.S., Chan, C.M., Ho, P.L., and Ng, M.H. (1997) Monitoring the therapy of pulmonary tuberculosis by nested polymerase chain reaction assay. *J. Infect.*, 34:29–33.

5.1.6 *Plasmodium falciparum* and *P. vivax*

Arai, M., Mizukoshi, C., Kubochi, F., Kakutani, T., and Wataya, Y. (1994) Detection of *Plasmodium falciparum* in human blood by a nested polymerase chain reaction. *Am. J. Trop. Med. Hyg.*, 51:617–626.

Barker, R.H., Banchongaksorn, T., Courval, J.M., Suwonkerd, W., Rimwungtragoon, K., and Wirth, D.W. (1992) A simple method to detect *Plasmodium falciparum* directly from blood samples using the polymerase chain reaction. *Am. J. Trop. Med. Hyg.*, 46:416–426.

Barker, R.H.J., Banchongaksorn, T., Courval, J.M., Suwonkerd, W., Rimwungtragoon, K., and Wirth, D.F. (1994) *Plasmodium falciparum* and *P. vivax*: Factors affecting sensitivity and specificity of PCR-based diagnosis of malaria. *Exp. Parasitol.*, 79:41–49.

Bouare, M., Sangare, D., Bagayoko, M., Toure, A., Toure, Y.T., and Vernick, K.D. (1996) Short report: Simultaneous detection by polymerase chain reaction of mosquito species and *Plasmodium falciparum* infection in *Anopheles gambiae* sensu lato. *Am. J. Trop. Med. Hyg.*, 54:629–631.

Brown, A.E., Kain, K.C., Pipithkul, J., and Webster, H.K. (1992) Demonstration by the polymerase chain reaction of mixed *Plasmodium falciparum* and *P. vivax* infections undetected by conventional microscopy. *Trans. R. Soc. Trop. Med. Hyg.*, 86:609–612.

Carcy, B., Bonnefoy, S., Schrevel, J., and Mercereau-Puijalon, O. (1995) *Plasmodium falciparum*: Typing of malaria parasites based on polymorphism of a novel multigene family. *Exp. Parasitol.*, 80:463–472.

Contamin, H., Fandeur, T., Rogier, C., Bonnefoy, S., Konate, L., Trape, J.F., and Mercereau-Puijalon, O. (1996) Different genetic characteristics of *Plasmodium falciparum* isolates collected during successive clinical malaria episodes in Senegalese children. *Am. J. Trop. Med. Hyg.*, 54:632–643.

Das, A., Holloway, B., Collins, W.E., Shama, V.P., Ghosh, S.K., Sinha, S., Hasnain, S.E., Talwar, G.P., and Lal, A.A. (1995) Species-specific 18S rRNA gene amplification for the detection of *P. falciparum* and *P. vivax* malaria parasites. *Mol. Cell. Probes*, 9:161–165.

Eldin de Pecoulas, P., Abdallah, B., Dje, M.K., Basco, L.K., le Bras, J., and Mazabraud, A. (1995a) Use of a semi-nested PCR diagnosis test to evaluate antifolate resistance of *Plasmodium falciparum* isolates. *Mol. Cell. Probes*, 9:391–397.

Eldin de Pecoulas, P., Basco, L.K., Abdallah, B., Dje, M.K., Le Bras, J., and Mazabraud, A. (1995b) *Plasmodium falciparum*: Detection of antifolate resistance by mutation-specific restriction enzyme digestion. *Exp. Parasitol.*, 80:483–487.

Felger, I., Tavul, L., Kabintik, S., Marshall, V., Genton, B., Alpers, M., and Beck, H.P. (1994) *Plasmodium falciparum*: Extensive polymorphism in merozoite surface antigen 2 alleles in an area with endemic malaria in Papua New Guinea. *Exp. Parasitol.*, 79:106–116.

Frean, J.A., el Kariem, F.M., Warhurst, D.C., and Miles, M.A. (1992) Rapid detection of *pfmdr1* mutations in chloroquine-resistant *Plasmodium falciparum* malaria by polymerase chain reaction analysis of blood spots. *Trans. R. Soc. Trop. Med. Hyg.*, 86:29–30.

Humar, A., Ohrt, C., Harrington, M.A., Pillai, D., and Kain, K.C. (1997) Parasight F test compared with the polymerase chain reaction and microscopy for the diagnosis of *Plasmodium falciparum* malaria in travelers. *Am. J. Trop. Med. Hyg.*, 56:44–48.

Jelinek, T., Proll, S., Hess, F., Kabagambe, G., von Sonnenburg, F., Loscher, T., and Kilian, A.H. (1996) Geographic differences in the sensitivity of a polymerase chain reaction for the detection of *Plasmodium falciparum* infection. *Am. J. Trop. Med. Hyg.*, 55:647–651.

Kain, K.C., Brown, A.E., Lanar, D.E., Ballou, W.R., and Webster, H.K. (1993a) Response of *Plasmodium vivax* variants to chloroquine as determined by microscopy and quantitative polymerase chain reaction. *Am. J. Trop. Med. Hyg.*, 49:478–484.

Kain, K.C., Brown, A.E., Mirabelli, L., and Webster, H.K. (1993b) Detection of *Plasmodium vivax* by polymerase chain reaction in a field study. *J. Infect. Dis.*, 168:1323–1326.

Kain, K.C., Craig, A.A., and Ohrt, C. (1996) Single-strand conformational polymorphism analysis differentiates *Plasmodium falciparum* treatment failures from re-infections. *Mol. Biochem. Parasitol.*, 79:167–175.

Kain, K.C., Keystone, J., Franke, E.D., and Lanar, D.E. (1991) Global distribution of a variant of the circumsporozoite gene of *Plasmodium vivax*. *J. Infect. Dis.*, 164:208–210.

Kain, K.C., Kyle, D.E., Wongsrichanalai, C., Brown, A.E., Webster, H.K., Vanijanonta, S., and Looareesuwan, S. (1994) Qualitative and semiquantitative polymerase chain reaction to predict *Plasmodium falciparum* treatment failure. *J. Infect. Dis.*, 170:1626–1630.

Kain, K.C., and Lanar, D.E. (1991) Determination of genetic variation within *Plasmodium falciparum* by using enzymatically amplified DNA from filter paper disks impregnated with whole blood. *J. Clin. Microbiol.*, 29:1171–1174.

Kaneko, O., Kimura, M., Kawamoto, F., Ferreira, M.U., and Tanabe, K. (1997) *Plasmodium falciparum*: Allelic variation in the merozoite surface protein 1 gene in wild isolates from southern Vietnam. *Exp. Parasitol.*, 86:45–57.

Kawamoto, F. (1991) Rapid diagnosis of malaria by fluorescence microscopy with light microscope and interference filter. *Lancet*, 337:200–202.

Kimura, M., Miyake, H., Kim, H.S., Tanabe, M., Arai, M., Kawai, S., Yamane, A., and Wataya, Y. (1995) Species-specific PCR detection of malaria parasites by microtiter plate hybridization: Clinical study with malaria patients. *J. Clin. Microbiol.*, 52:2342–2346.

Krogstad, D.J. (1995) *Plasmodium* species (Malaria). In *Principles and Practice of Infectious Diseases*, G.L. Mandell, J.E. Bennett, and R. Dolin, eds., New York, Churchill Livingstone.

Long, G.W., Fries, L., Watt, G.H., and Hoffman, S.L. (1995) Polymerase chain reaction amplification from *Plasmodium falciparum* on dried blood spots. *Am. J. Trop. Med. Hyg.*, 52:344–346.

Mercereau-Puijalon, O., Fandeur, T., Bonnefoy, S., Jacquemot, C., and Sarthou, J.L. (1991) A study of the genomic diversity of *Plasmodium falciparum* in Senegal. 2. Typing by the use of the polymerase chain reaction. *Acta Trop.*, 49:293–304.

Moleón-Borodowsky, I., Altamirano, F., Plaza, L.E., Mite, P., Jurado, H., and Harris, E. Utilización de la técnica de la reacción en cadena de la polimerasa para la detección de *P. falciparum* y *P. vivax* en el Servicio Nacional de Control de la Malaria del Ecuador. Manuscript in preparation.

Oliveira, D.A., Shi, Y.P., Oloo, A.J., Boriga, D.A., Nahlen, B.L., Hawley, W.A., Holloway, B.P., and Lal, A.A. (1996) Field evaluation of a polymerase chain reaction-based nonisotopic liquid hybridization assay for malaria diagnosis. *J. Infect. Dis.*, 173:1284–1287.

Plowe, C.V., Djimde, A., Bouare, M., Doumbo, O., and Wellems, T.E. (1995) Pyrimethamine and proguanil resistance-conferring mutations in *Plasmodium falciparum* dihydrofolate reductase: Polymerase chain reaction methods for surveillance in Africa. *Am. J. Trop. Med. Hyg.*, 52:565–568.

Reeder, J.C., Rieckmann, K.H., Genton, B., Lorry, K., Wines, B., and Cowman, A.F. (1996) Point mutations in the dihydrofolate reductase and dihydropteroate synthetase genes and in vitro susceptibility to pyrimethamine and cycloguanil of *Plasmodium falciparum* isolates from Papua New Guinea. *Am. J. Trop. Med. Hyg.*, 55:209–213.

Rickman, L.S., Long, G.W., Oberst, R., Cabanban, A., Sangalang, R., Smith, J.I., Chulay, J.D., and Hoffman, S.L. (1989) Rapid diagnosis of malaria by acridine orange staining of centrifuged parasites. *Lancet*, 1:68–71.

Robert, F., Ntoumi, F., Angel, G., Candito, D., Rogier, C., Fandeur, T., Sarthou, J.L., and Mercereau-Puijalon, O. (1996) Extensive genetic diversity of *Plasmodium falciparum* isolates collected from patients with severe malaria in Dakar, Senegal. *Trans. R. Soc. Trop. Med. Hyg.*, 90:704–711.

Rojas, M.O., De-Castro, J., Marino, G., and Wasserman, M. (1996) Detection of genomic polymorphism in *Plasmodium falciparum* using an arbitrarily primed PCR assay. *J. Eukaryot. Microbiol.*, 43:323–326.

Roper, C., Elhassan, I.M., Hviid, L., Giha, H., Richardson, W., Babiker, H., Satti, G.M., Theander, T.G., and Arnot, D.E. (1996) Detection of very low level *Plasmodium falciparum* infections using the nested polymerase chain reaction and a reassessment of the epidemiology of unstable malaria in Sudan. *Am. J. Trop. Med. Hyg.*, 54:325–331.

Schriefer, M.E., Sacci, J.B., Jr., Wirtz, R.A., and Azad, A.F. (1991) Detection of polymerase chain reaction-amplified malarial DNA in infected blood and individual mosquitoes. *Exp. Parasitol.*, 73:311–316.

Sethabutr, O., Brown, A.E., Panyim, S., Kain, K.C., Webster, H.K., and Echeverria, P. (1992) Detection of *Plasmodium falciparum* by polymerase chain reaction in a field study. *J. Infect. Dis.*, 166:145–148.

Singh, B., Cox-Singh, J., Miller, A.O., Abdullah, M.S., Snounou, G., and Rahman, H.A. (1996) Detection of malaria in Malaysia by nested polymerase chain reaction amplification of dried blood spots on filter papers. *Trans. R. Soc. Trop. Med. Hyg.*, 90:519–521.

Snewin, V.A., Khouri, E., Wattavidanage, J., Perera, L., Premawansa, S., Mendis, K.N., and David, P.H. (1995) A new polymorphic marker for PCR typing of *Plasmodium vivax* parasites. *Mol. Biochem. Parasitol.*, 71:135–138.

Snounou, G., Pinheiro, L., Goncalves, A., Fonseca, L., Dias, F., Brown, K.N., and do Rosario, V.E. (1993a) The importance of sensitive detection of malaria parasites in the human and insect hosts in epidemiological studies, as shown by the analysis of field samples from Guinea Bissau. *Trans. R. Soc. Trop. Med. Hyg.*, 87:649–653.

Snounou, G., Viriyakosol, S., Jarra, W., Thaithong, S., and Brown, K.N. (1993b) Identification of the four human malaria parasite species in field samples by the polymerase chain reaction and detection of a high prevalence of mixed infections. *Mol. Biochem. Parasitol.*, 58:283–292.

Stoffels, J.A., Docters van Leeuwen, W.M., and Post, R.J. (1995) Detection of *Plasmodium* sporozoites in mosquitoes by polymerase chain reaction and oligonucleotide rDNA probe, without dissection of the salivary glands. *Med. Vet. Entomol.*, 9:433–437.

Strickland, G.T. (1991) Malaria. In *Hunter's Tropical Medicine*, G. T. Strickland, ed., Philadelphia, W. B. Saunders.

Su, X.Z., and Wellems, T.E. (1997) *Plasmodium falciparum*: A rapid DNA fingerprinting method using microsatellite sequences within var clusters. *Exp. Parasitol.*, 86:235–236.

Tassanakajon, A., Boonsaeng, V., Wilairat, P., and Panyim, S. (1993) Polymerase chain reaction detection of *Plasmodium falciparum* in mosquitoes. *Trans. R. Soc. Trop. Med. Hyg.*, 87:273–275.

Tirasophon, W., Ponglikitmongkol, M., Wilairat, P., Boonsaeng, V., and Panyim, S. (1991) A novel detection of a single *Plasmodium falciparum* in infected blood. *Biochem. Biophys. Res. Commun.*, 175:179–184.

Tirasophon, W., Rajkulchai, P., Ponglikitmongkol, M., Wilairat, P., Boonsaeng, V., and Panyim, S. (1994) A highly sensitive, rapid, and simple polymerase chain reaction-based method to detect human malaria (*Plasmodium falciparum* and *Plasmodium vivax*) in blood samples. *Am. J. Trop. Med. Hyg.*, 51:308–313.

Viriyakosol, S., Siripoon, N., Petcharapirat, C., Petcharapirat, P., Jarra, W., Thaithong, S., Brown, K.N., and Snounou, G. (1995) Genotyping of *Plasmodium falciparum* isolates by the polymerase chain reaction and potential uses in epidemiological studies. *Bull. WHO*, 73:85–95.

Walliker, D. (1994) The role of molecular genetics in field studies on malaria parasites. *Int. J. Parasitol.*, 24:799–808.

Wooden, J., Gould, E.E., Paull, A.T., and Sibley, C.H. (1992) *Plasmodium falciparum*: A simple polymerase chain reaction method for differentiating strains. *Exp. Parasitol.*, 75:207–212.

Zalis, M.G., Ferreira-da-Cruz, M.F., Balthazar-Guedes, H.C., Banic, D.M., Alecrim, W., Souza, J.M., Druilhe, P., and Daniel-Ribeiro, C.T. (1996) Malaria diagnosis: Standardization of a polymerase chain reaction for the detection of *Plasmodium falciparum* parasites in individuals with low-grade parasitemia. *Parasitol. Res.*, 82:612–616.

Zindrou, S., Dao, L.D., Xuyen, P.T., Dung, N.P., Sy, N.D., Skold, O., and Swedberg, G. (1996) Rapid detection of pyrimethamine susceptibility of *Plasmodium falciparum* by restriction endonuclease digestion of the dihydrofolate reductase gene. *Am. J. Trop. Med. Hyg.*, 54:185–188.

5.1.7   Vibrio cholerae

Bej, A., Mahbubani, M., Dicesare, J., and Atlas, R. (1991) Polymerase chain reaction-gene probe detection of microorganisms by using filter-concentrated samples. *Appl. Environ. Microbiol.*, 57:3529–3534.

Coelho, A., Vicente, A.C., Baptista, M.A., Momen, H., Santos, F.A., and Salles, C.A. (1995) The distinction of pathogenic *Vibrio cholerae* groups using arbitrarily primed PCR fingerprints. *Res. Microbiol.*, 146:671–683.

DePaola, A., and Hwang, G.C. (1995) Effect of dilution, incubation time, and temperature of enrichment on cultural and PCR detection of *Vibrio cholerae* obtained from the oyster *Crassostrea virginica. Mol. Cell. Probes*, 9:75–81.

Falklind, S., Stark, M., Albert, M.J., Uhlen, M., Lundeberg, J., and Weintraub, A. (1996) Cloning and sequence of a region of *Vibrio cholerae* O139 Bengal and its use in PCR-based detection. *J. Clin. Microbiol.*, 34:2904–2908.

Fields, P.I., Popovic, T., Wachsmuth, K., and Olsvik, O. (1992) Use of polymerase chain reaction for detection of toxigenic *Vibrio cholerae* O1 strains from the Latin American cholera epidemic. *J. Clin. Microbiol.*, 30:2118–2121.

Holmgren, J. (1981) Actions of cholera toxin and the prevention and treatment of cholera. *Nature*, 292:413–417.

Karunasagar, I., Sugumar, G., Karunasagar, I., and Reilley, A. (1995) Rapid detection of *Vibrio cholerae* contamination of seafood by polymerase chain reaction. *Mol. Marine Biol. Biotech.*, 4:365–368.

Koch, W.H., Payne, W.L., Wentz, B.A., and Cebula, T.A. (1993) Rapid polymerase chain reaction method for detection of *Vibrio cholerae* in foods. *Appl. Environ. Microbiol.*, 59:556–560.

Lee, H.F., Yeh, H.L., Hsiao, H.L., Wang, T.K., and Liu, C.H. (1993) Detection and identification of toxigenic *Vibrio cholerae* O1 strains by a simplified polymerase chain reaction method. *Chin. J. Microbiol. Immunol.*, 26:6–14.

Nalin, D.R., and Morris, J.G., Jr. (1991) Cholera and other vibrioses. In *Hunter's Tropical Medicine*, G. T. Strickland, ed., Philadelphia, W.B. Saunders.

Ramamurthy, T., Bhattacharya, S.K., Uesaka, Y., Horigome, K., Paul, M., Sen, D., Pal, S.C., Takeda, T., Takeda, Y., and Nair, G.B. (1992) Evaluation of the bead enzyme-linked immunoabsorbent assay for detection of cholera toxin directly from stool specimens. *J. Clin. Microbiol.*, 30:1783–1786.

Ramamurthy, T., Pal, A., Bag, P.K., Bhattacharya, S.K., Nair, G.B., Kurozano, H., Yamasaki, S., Shirai, H., Takeda, T., Uesaka, Y., Horigome, K., and Takeda, Y. (1993) Detection of cholera toxin gene in stool specimens by polymerase chain reaction: Comparison with bead enzyme-linked immunosorbent assay and culture method for laboratory diagnosis of cholera. *J. Clin. Microbiol.*, 31:3068–3070.

Rivera, I.G., Chowdhury, M.A., Huq, A., Jacobs, D., Martins, M.T., and Colwell, R.R. (1995) Enterobacterial repetitive intergenic consensus sequences and the PCR to generate finger-prints of genomic DNAs from *Vibrio cholerae* O1, O139, and non-O1 strains. *Appl. Environ. Microbiol.*, 61:2898–2904.

Shangkuan, Y.H., Show, Y.S., and Wang, T.M. (1995) Multiplex polymerase chain reaction to detect toxigenic *Vibrio cholerae* and to biotype *Vibrio cholerae* O1. *J. Appl. Bacteriol.*, 79:264–273.

Shears, P. (1994) Cholera. *Ann. Trop. Med. Parasitol.*, 88:109–122.

Shirai, H., Nishibuchi, M., Ramamurthy, T., Bhattacharya, S., Pal, S., and Takeda, Y. (1991) Polymerase chain reaction for detection of the cholera enteroxin operon of *Vibrio cholerae*. *J. Clin. Microbiol.*, 29:2517–2521.

Varela, P., Pollevick, G.D., Rivas, M., Chinen, I., Binsztein, N., Frasch, A.C., and Ugalde, R.A. (1994) Direct detection of *Vibrio cholerae* in stool samples. *J. Clin. Microbiol.*, 32:1246–1248.

Varela, P., Rivas, M., Binsztein, N., Cremona, M.L., Herrmann, P., Burrone, O., Ugalde, R.A., and Frasch, A.C.C. (1993) Identification of toxigenic *Vibrio cholerae* from the Argentine outbreak by PCR for ctx A1 and ctx A2–B. *Febs Lett.*, 315:74–76.

Vaughan, M. (1982) Cholera and cell regulation. *Hosp. Practice*, 17:145–152.

5.1.8   Diarrheagenic *E. coli* and *Shigella*

Abe, A., Obata, H., Matsushita, S., Yamada, S., Kudoh, Y., Bangtrakulnonth, A., Ratchtrachenchat, O.A., and Danbara, H. (1992) A sensitive method for the detection of enterotoxigenic *Escherichia coli* by the polymerase chain reaction using multiple primer pairs. *Int. J. Med. Microbiol. Virol. Parasitol. Infect. Dis.*, 277:170–178.

Acheson, D.W.K. and Keusch, G.T. (1995) *Shigella* and enteroinvasive *E. coli*. In *Infections of the Gastrointestinal Tract*, M.J. Blaser, P.D. Smith, J.I. Ravdin, H.B. Greenberg, and R.L. Guerrant, eds., New York, Raven Press, Ltd.

Candrian, U., Furrer, B., Hofelein, C., Meyer, R., Jermini, M., and Luthy, J. (1991) Detection of *Escherichia coli* and identification of enterotoxigenic strains by primer-directed enzymatic amplification of specific DNA sequences. *Int. J. Food Microbiol.*, 12:339–351.

Deng, M.Y., Cliver, D.O., Day, S.P., and Fratamico, P.M. (1996) Enterotoxigenic *Escherichia coli* detected in foods by PCR and an enzyme-linked oligonucleotide probe. *Int. J. Food Microbiol.*, 30:217–229.

Eisenstein, B.I. (1995) Enterobacteriaceae. In *Principles and Practice of Infectious Diseases*, G.L. Mandell, J.E. Bennett, and R. Dolin, eds., New York, Churchill Livingstone.

Franke, J., Franke, S., Schmidt, H., Schwarzkopf, A., Wieler, L.H., Baljer, G., Beutin, L., and Karch, H. (1994) Nucleotide sequence analysis of enteropathogenic *Escherichia coli* (EPEC) adherence factor probe and development of PCR for rapid detection of EPEC har-boring virulence plasmids. *J. Clin. Microbiol.*, 32:2460–2463.

Frankel, G., Giron, J.A., Valmassoi, J., and Schoolnik, G.K. (1989) Multi-gene amplification: Simultaneous detection of three virulence genes in diarrhoeal stool. *Mol. Microbiol.*, 3:1729–1734.

Frankel, G., Riley, L., Giron, J.A., Valmassoi, J., Friedmann, A., Strockbine, N., Falkow, S., and Schoolnik, G.K. (1990) Detection of *Shigella* in feces using DNA amplification. *J. Infect. Dis.*, 161:1252–1256.

Gunzburg, S.T., Tornieporth, N.G., and Riley, L.W. (1995) Identification of enteropathogenic *Escherichia coli* by PCR-based detection of the bundle-forming pilus gene. *J. Clin. Microbiol.*, 33:1375–1377.

Houng, H.S., Sethabutr, O., and Echeverria, P. (1997) A simple polymerase chain reaction technique to detect and differentiate *Shigella* and enteroinvasive *Escherichia coli* in human feces. *Diag. Microbiol. Infect. Dis.*, 28:19–25.

Islam, D., and Lindberg, A.A. (1992) Detection of *Shigella dysenteriae* type 1 and *Shigella flexneri* in feces by immunomagnetic isolation and polymerase chain reaction. *J. Clin. Microbiol.*, 30:2801–2806.

Lang, A.L., Tsai, Y.L., Mayer, C.L., Patton, K.C., and Palmer, C.J. (1994) Multiplex PCR for detection of the heat-labile toxin gene and shiga-like toxin I and II genes in *Escherichia coli* isolated from natural waters. *Appl. Environ. Microbiol.*, 60:3145–3149.

Levine, M.M. (1991) Diarrhea caused by *Escherichia coli*. In *Hunter's Tropical Medicine*, G. T. Strickland, ed., Philadelphia, W. B. Saunders.

Lou, Q., Chong, S.K., Fitzgerald, J.F., Siders, J.A., Allen, S.D., and Lee, C.H. (1997) Rapid and effective method for preparation of fecal specimens for PCR assays. *J. Clin. Microbiol.*, 35:281–283.

Olive, D.M. (1989) Detection of enterotoxigenic *Escherichia coli* after polymerase chain reaction amplification with a thermostable DNA polymerase. *J. Clin. Microbiol.*, 27:261–265.

Oyofo, B.A., Mohran, Z.S., el-Etr, S.H., Wasfy, M.O., and Peruski, L.F., Jr. (1996) Detection of enterotoxigenic *Escherichia coli*, *Shigella* and *Campylobacter* spp. by multiplex PCR assay. *J. Diar. Dis. Res.*, 14:207–210.

Schultsz, C., Pool, G.J., van Ketel, R., de Wever, B., Speelman, P., and Dankert, J. (1994) Detection of enterotoxigenic *Escherichia coli* in stool samples by using nonradioactively labeled oligonucleotide DNA probes and PCR. *J. Clin. Microbiol.*, 32:2393–2397.

Seigel, R.R., Santana, C., Salgado, K., and Jesus, P. (1996) Acute diarrhea among children from high and low socioeconomic communities in Salvador, Brazil. *Int. J. Infect. Dis.*, 1:28–34.

Sethabutr, O., Venkatesan, M., Murphy, G.S., Eampokalap, B., Hoge, C.W., and Echeverria, P. (1993) Detection of *Shigellae* and enteroinvasive *Escherichia coli* by amplification of the invasion plasmid antigen H DNA sequence in patients with dysentery. *J. Infect. Dis.*, 167:458–461.

Stacy-Phipps, S., Mecca, J.J., and Weiss, J.B. (1995) Multiplex PCR assay and simple preparation method for stool specimens detect enterotoxigenic *Escherichia coli* DNA during course of infection. *J. Clin. Microbiol.*, 33:1054–1059.

Tamanai-Shacoori, Z., Jolivet-Gougeon, A., Pommepuy, M., Cormier, M., and Colwell, R.R. (1994) Detection of enterotoxigenic *Escherichia coli* in water by polymerase chain reaction amplification and hybridization. *Can. J. Microbiol.*, 40:243–249.

Tornieporth, N.G., John, J., Salgado, K., de Jesus, P., Latham, E., Melo, M.C., Gunzburg, S.T., and Riley, L.W. (1995) Differentiation of pathogenic *Escherichia coli* strains in Brazilian children by PCR. *J. Clin. Microbiol.*, 33:1371–1374.

Victor, T., du Toit, R., van Zyl, J., Bester, A.J., and van Helden, P.D. (1991) Improved method for the routine identification of toxigenic *Escherichia coli* by DNA amplification of a conserved region of the heat-labile toxin A subunit. *J. Clin. Microbiol.*, 29:158–161.

Wang, G., Whittam, T.S., Berg, C.M., and Berg, D.E. (1993) RAPD (arbitrary primer) PCR is more sensitive than multilocus enzyme electrophoresis for distinguishing related bacterial strains. *Nucleic Acids Res.*, 21:5930–5933.

Yavzori, M., Cohen, D., Wasserlauf, R., Ambar, R., Rechavi, G., and Ashkenazi, S. (1994) Identification of *Shigella* species in stool specimens by DNA amplification of different loci of the *Shigella* virulence plasmid. *Eur. J. Clin. Microbiol. Infect. Dis.*, 13:232–237.

Ye, L.Y., Lan, F.H., Zhu, Z.Y., Chen, X.M., and Ye, X.L. (1993) Detection of *Shigella* and enteroinvasive *Escherichia coli* using polymerase chain reaction. *J. Diar. Dis. Res.*, 11:38–40.

5.1.9   *Chlamydia trachomatis* and *Neisseria gonorrhoeae*

An, Q., Liu, J., O'Brien, W., Radcliffe, G., Buxton, D., Popoff, S., King, W., Vera-Garcia, M., Lu, L., Shah, J., Klinger, J., and Olive, D.M. (1995) Comparison of characteristics of Q beta replicase-amplified assay with competitive PCR assay for *Chlamydia trachomatis*. *J. Clin. Microbiol.*, 33:58–63.

An, Q., Radcliffe, G., Vassallo, R., Buxton, D., O'Brien, W.J., Pelletier, D.A., Weisburg, W.G., Klinger, J.D., and Olive, D.M. (1992) Infection with a plasmid-free variant chlamydia related to *Chlamydia trachomatis* identified by using multiple assays for nucleic acid detection. *J. Clin. Microbiol.*, 30:2814–2821.

Bell, T.A., and Perine, P.L. (1991) Gonococcal infections. In *Hunter's Tropical Medicine*, G. T. Strickland, ed.,. Philadelphia, W. B. Saunders.

Black, C.M. (1997) Current methods of laboratory diagnosis of *Chlamydia trachomatis* infections. *Clin. Microbiol. Rev.*, 10:160–184.

Bobo, L., Coutlee, F., Yolken, R.H., Quinn, T., and Viscidi, R.P. (1990) Diagnosis of *Chlamydia trachomatis* cervical infection by detection of amplified DNA with an enzyme immunoassay. *J. Clin. Microbiol.*, 28:1968–1973.

Claas, H.C., Melchers, W.J., de Bruijn, I.H., de Graaf, M., van Dijk, W.C., Lindeman, J., and Quint, W.G. (1990) Detection of *Chlamydia trachomatis* in clinical specimens by the polymerase chain reaction. *Eur. J. Clin. Microbiol. Infect. Dis.*, 9:864–868.

Claas, H.C., Wagenvoort, J.H., Niesters, H.G., Tio, T.T., Van Rijsoort Vos, J.H., and Quint, W.G. (1991) Diagnostic value of the polymerase chain reaction for *Chlamydia* detection as determined in a follow-up study. *J. Clin. Microbiol.*, 29:42–45.

Dean, D., Oudens, E., Bolan, G., Padian, N., and Schachter, J. (1995) Major outer membrane protein variants of *Chlamydia trachomatis* are associated with severe upper genital tract infections and histopathology in San Francisco. *J. Infect. Dis.*, 172:1013–1022.

Dean, D., Pant, C.R., and O'Hanley, P. (1989) Improved sensitivity of a modified polymerase chain reaction amplified DNA probe in comparison with serial tissue culture passage for detection of *Chlamydia trachomatis* in conjunctival specimens from Nepal. *Diag. Microbiol. Infect. Dis.*, 12:133–137.

Dean, D., Schachter, J., Dawson, C.R., and Stephens, R.S. (1992) Comparison of the major outer membrane protein variant sequence regions of B/Ba isolates: A molecular epidemiologic approach to *Chlamydia trachomatis* infections. *J. Infect. Dis.*, 166:383–392.

Dean, D., Shama, A., Schachter, J., and Dawson, C.R. (1993) Molecular identification of an avian strain of *Chlamydia psittaci* causing severe keratoconjunctivitis in a bird fancier. *Clin. Infect. Dis.*, 20:1179–1185.

Dean, D., and Stephens, R.S. (1994) Identification of individual genotypes of *Chlamydia trachomatis* from experimentally mixed serovars and mixed infections among trachoma patients. *J. Clin. Microbiol.*, 32:1506–1510.

Dutilh, B., Bebear, C., Rodriguez, P., Vekris, A., Bonnet, J., and Garret, M. (1989) Specific amplification of a DNA sequence common to all *Chlamydia trachomatis* serovars using the polymerase chain reaction. *Res. Microbiol.*, 140:7–16.

Frost, E.H., Deslandes, S., Bourgaux-Ramoisy, D., and Bourgaux, P. (1995) Quantitation of *Chlamydia trachomatis* by culture, direct immunofluorescence and competitive polymerase chain reaction. *Genitourin. Med.*, 71:239–243.

Frost, E.H., Deslandes, S., Veilleux, S., and Bourgaux-Ramoisy, D. (1991) Typing *Chlamydia trachomatis* by detection of restriction fragment length polymorphism in the gene encoding the major outer membrane protein. *J. Infect. Dis.*, 163:1103–1107.

Gaydos, C.A., Bobo, L., Welsh, L., Hook, E.W.I., Viscidi, R., and Quinn, T.C. (1992) Gene typing of *Chlamydia trachomatis* by polymerase chain reaction and restriction endonuclease digestion. *Sex. Transm. Dis.*, 19:303–308.

Griffais, R., and Thibon, M. (1989) Detection of *Chlamydia trachomatis* by the polymerase chain reaction. *Res. Microbiol.*, 140:139–141.

Handsfield, H.H., and Sparling, P.F. (1995) *Neisseria gonorrhoeae*. In *Principles and Practice of Infectious Diseases*, G.L. Mandell, J.E. Bennett, and R. Dolin, eds., New York, Churchill Livingstone.

Herrmann, B., Nystrom, T., and Wessel, H. (1996) Detection of *Neisseria gonorrhoeae* from air-dried genital samples by single-tube nested PCR. *J. Clin. Microbiol.*, 34:2548–2551.

Ho, B.S.W., Feng, W.G., Wong, B.K.C., and Egglestone, S.I. (1992) Polymerase chain reaction for the detection of *Neisseria gonorrhoeae* in clinical samples. *J. Clin. Pathol.*, 45:439–442.

Holland, S.M., Gaydos, C.A., and Quinn, T.C. (1990) Detection and differentiation of *Chlamydia trachomatis*, *Chlamydia psittaci*, and *Chlamydia pneumoniae* by DNA amplification. *J. Infect. Dis.*, 162:984–987.

Lan, J., Ossewaarde, J.M., Walboomers, J.M., Meijer, C.J., and van den Brule, A.J. (1994) Improved PCR sensitivity for direct genotyping of *Chlamydia trachomatis* serovars by using a nested PCR. *J. Clin. Microbiol.*, 32:528–530.

Lan, J., Walboomers, J.M., Roosendaal, R., van Doornum, G.J., MacLaren, D.M., Meijer, C.J., and van den Brule, A.J. (1993) Direct detection and genotyping of *Chlamydia trachomatis* in cervical scrapes by using polymerase chain reaction and restriction fragment length polymorphism analysis. *J. Clin. Microbiol.*, 31:1060–1065.

Loeffelholz, M.J., Lewinski, C.A., Silver, S.R., Purohit, A.P., Herman, S.A., Buonagurio, D.A., and Dragon, E.A. (1992) Detection of *Chlamydia trachomatis* in endocervical specimens by polymerase chain reaction. *J. Clin. Microbiol.*, 30:2847–2851.

Lucotte, G., Petit, M.C., Francois, M.H., and Reveilleau, S. (1992) Detection of *Chlamydia trachomatis* by use of polymerase chain reaction. *Mol. Cell. Probes*, 6:89–92.

Mahony, J.B., Luinstra, K.E., Sellors, J.W., and Chernesky, M.A. (1993) Comparison of plasmid- and chromosome-based polymerase chain reaction assays for detecting *Chlamydia trachomatis* nucleic acids. *J. Clin. Microbiol.*, 31:1753–1758.

Mahony, J.B., Luinstra, K.E., Sellors, J.W., Jang, D., and Chernesky, M.A. (1992) Confirmatory polymerase chain reaction testing for *Chlamydia trachomatis* in first-void urine from asymptomatic and symptomatic men. *J. Clin. Microbiol.*, 30:2241–2245.

Mahoney, J.B., Luinstra, K.E., Tyndall, M., Sellors, J.W., Krepel, J., and Chernesky, M. (1995) Multiplex PCR for detection of *Chlamydia trachomatis* and *Neisseria gonorrheoae* in genitourinary specimens. *J. Clin. Microbiol.*, 33:3049–3053.

Murallidhar, B., and Steinman, C.R. (1994) Design and characterization of PCR primers for detection of pathogenic *Neisseriae*. *Mol. Cell. Probes*, 8:55–61.

Naher, H., Drzonek, H., Wolf, J., von Knebel Doeberitz, M., and Petzoldt, D. (1991) Detection of *C. trachomatis* in urogenital specimens by polymerase chain reaction. *Genitourin. Med.*, 67:211–214.

Ossewaarde, J.M., Rieffe, M., Rozenberg-Arska, M., Ossenkoppele, P.M., Nawrocki, R.P., and van Loon, A.M. (1992) Development and clinical evaluation of a polymerase chain reaction test for detection of *Chlamydia trachomatis*. *J. Clin. Microbiol.*, 30:2122–2128.

Ostergaard, L., Birkelund, S., and Christiansen, G. (1990) Use of polymerase chain reaction for detection of *Chlamydia trachomatis*. *J. Clin. Microbiol.*, 28:1254–1260.

Palmer, H.M., Gilroy, C.B., Thomas, B.J., Hay, P.E., Gilchrist, C., and Taylor-Robinson, D. (1991) Detection of *Chlamydia trachomatis* by the polymerase chain reaction in swabs and urine from men with non-gonococcal urethritis. *J. Clin. Pathol.*, 44:321–325.

Pecharatana, S., Pickett, M.A., Watt, P.J., and Ward, M.E. (1993) Genotyping ocular strains of *Chlamydia trachomatis* by single-tube nested PCR. *PCR Meth. Appl.*, 3:200–204.

Peterson, E.M., Markoff, B.A., Schachter, J., and de la Maza, L.M. (1990) The 7.5–kb plasmid present in *Chlamydia trachomatis* is not essential for the growth of this microorganism. *Plasmid*, 23:144–148.

Ratti, G., Moroni, A., and Cevenini, R. (1991) Detection of *Chlamydia trachomatis* DNA in patients with non-gonococcal urethritis using the polymerase chain reaction. *J. Clin. Pathol.*, 44:564–568.

Rodriguez, P., Vekris, A., de Barbeyrac, B., Dutilh, B., Bonnet, J., and Bebear, C. (1991)

Typing of *Chlamydia trachomatis* by restriction endonuclease analysis of the amplified major outer membrane protein gene. *J. Clin. Microbiol.*, 29:1132–1136.

Roosendaal, R., Walboomers, J.M., Veltman, O.R., Melgers, I., Burger, C., Bleker, O.P., MacClaren, D.M., Meijer, C.J., and van den Brule, A.J. (1993) Comparison of different primer sets for detection of *Chlamydia trachomatis* by the polymerase chain reaction. *J. Med. Microbiol.*, 38:426–433.

Sayada, C., Denamur, E., Orfila, J., Catalan, F., and Elion, J. (1991) Rapid genotyping of the *Chlamydia trachomatis* major outer membrane protein by the polymerase chain reaction. *FEMS Microbiol. Lett.*, 83:73–78.

Schachter, J. (1997) DFA, EIA, PCR, LCR and other technologies: What tests should be used for diagnosis of chlamydia infections? *Immunol. Invest.*, 26:157–161.

Scieux, C., Grimont, F., Regnault, B., Bianchi, A., Kowalski, S., and Grimont, P.A.D. (1993) Molecular typing of *Chlamydia trachomatis* by random amplification of polymorphic DNA. *Res. Microbiol.*, 144:395–404.

Tabrizi, S.N., Chen, S., Borg, A.J., Lees, M.I., Fairley, C.K., Jackson, H.D., Gust, C.H., Migliorini, G., and Garland, S.M. (1996) Patient-administered tampon-collected genital cells in the assessment of *Chlamydia trachomatis* infection using polymerase chain reaction. *Sex. Transm. Dis.*, 23:494–497.

Tabrizi, S.N., Paterson, B., Fairley, C.K., Bowden, F.J., and Garland, S.M. (1997) A self-administered technique for the detection of sexually transmitted diseases in remote communities. *J. Infect. Dis.*, 176:289–292.

Taylor, H.R., and Bell, T.A. (1991) Chlamydial infections: General principles. In *Hunter's Tropical Medicine*, G. T. Strickland, ed., Philadelphia, W. B. Saunders.

Taylor-Robinson, D., Gilroy, C.B., Thomas, B.J., and Keat, A.C. (1992) Detection of *Chlamydia trachomatis* DNA in joints of reactive arthritis patients by polymerase chain reaction. *Lancet*, 340:81–82.

Watson, M.W., Lambden, P.R., and Clarke, I.N. (1991) Genetic diversity and identification of human infection by amplificatioin of the chlamydial 60–kilodalton cysteine-rich outer membrane protein gene. *J. Clin. Microbiol.*, 29:1188–1193.

Welch, D., Lee, C.H., and Larsen, S.H. (1990) Detection of plasmid DNA from all *Chlamydia trachomatis* serovars with a two-step polymerase chain reaction. *Appl. Environ. Microbiol.*, 56:2494–2498.

Wong, K.C., Ho, B.S., Egglestone, S.I., and Lewis, W.H. (1995) Duplex PCR system for simultaneous detection of *Neisseria gonorrhoeae* and *Chlamydia trachomatis* in clinical specimens. *J. Clin. Pathol.*, 48:101–104.

World Health Organization (1995) *Bridging the Gaps. The World Health Report 1995.* Geneva, World Health Organization.

Zhu, X., Kong, F., Zhang, G., and Chen, S. (1995) Identification and classification of *Neisseria gonorrhoeae* by RAPD fingerprinting. *Chin. Med. J.*, 108:269–272.

5.1.10   Leptospira

Bal, A.E., Gravecamp, C., Hartskeeri, R.A., de Meza-Brewster, J., Korver, H., and Terpstra, W.J. (1994) Detection of leptospires in urine by PCR for early diagnosis of leptospirosis. *J. Clin. Microbiol.*, 32:1894–1898.

Boom, R., Sol, C.J.A., Heijtink, R., Wertheim-van Dillen, P.M.E., and van der Norrdaa, J. (1991) Rapid purification of hepatitis B virus DNA from serum. *J. Clin. Microbiol.*, 29:1804–1811.

Boom, R., Sol, C.J.A., Salimans, M.M.M., Jansen, C.L., Wertheim-van Dillen, P.M.E., and van der Norrdaa, J. (1990) Rapid and simple method for purification of nucleic acids. *J. Clin. Microbiol.*, 28:495–503.

Brown, P.D., Gravecamp, C., Carrington, D.G., van de Kemp, H., Hartskeeri, R.A., Edwards, C.N., Everard, C.O.R., Terpstra, W.J., and Levett, P.N. (1995) Evaluation of the polymerase chain reaction for early diagnosis of leptospirosis. *J. Med. Microbiol.*, 43:110–114.

Brown, P.D., and Levett, P.N. (1997) Differentiation of *Leptospira* species and serovars by

PCR-restriction endonuclease analysis, arbitrarily primed PCR and low-stringency PCR. *J. Med. Microbiol.*, 46:173–181.

Corney, B.G., Colley, J., Djordjevic, S.P., Whittington, R., and Graham, G.C. (1993) Rapid identification of some *Leptospira* isolates from cattle by random amplified polymorphic DNA fingerprinting. *J. Clin. Microbiol.*, 31:2927–2932.

de Caballero, O.L.S.D., Neto, E.D., Koury, M.C., Romanha, A.J., and Simpson, A.J.G. (1994) Low-stringency PCR with diagnostically useful primers for identification of *Leptospira* serovars. *J. Clin. Microbiol.*, 32:1369–1372.

Gerritsen, M.A., Smits, M.A., and Olyhoek, T. (1995) Random amplified polymorphic DNA fingerprinting for rapid identification of leptospiras of serogroup Sejroe. *J. Med. Microbiol.*, 42:336–339.

Gravecamp, C., van de Kemp, H., Franzen, M., Carrington, D., Schoone, G.J., Van Eys, G.J.J.M., Everard, C.O.R., Hartskeerl, R.A., and Terpstra, W.J. (1993) Detection of seven species of pathogenic leptospires by PCR using two sets of primers. *J. Gen. Microbiol.*, 139:1691–1700.

Kee, S.-H., Kim, I.-K., Choi, M.-S., and Chang, W.-H. (1994) Detection of leptospiral DNA by PCR. *J. Clin. Microbiol.*, 32:1035–1039.

Masri, S.A., Nguyen, P.T., Gale, S.P., Howard, C.J., and Jung, S.C. (1997) A polymerase chain reaction assay for the detection of *Leptospira* spp. in bovine semen. *Can. J. Vet. Res.*, 61:15–20.

Merien, F., Amouriaux, P., Perolat, P., Baranton, G., and Saint Girons, I. (1992) Polymerase chain reaction for detection of *Leptospira* spp. in clinical samples. *J. Clin. Microbiol.*, 30:2219–2224.

Merien, F., Baranton, G., and Perolat, P. (1995) Comparison of polymerase chain reaction with microagglutination test and culture for diagnosis of leptospirosis. *J. Infect. Dis.*, 172:281–285.

Ralph, D., McClelland, M., Welsh, J., Baranton, G., and Perolat, P. (1993) *Leptospira* species categorized by arbitrarily primed polymerase chain reaction (PCR) and by mapped restriction polymorphisms in PCR-amplified rRNA genes. *J. Bacteriol.*, 175:973–981.

Savio, M.L., Rossi, C., Fusi, P., Tagliabue, S., and Pacciarini, M.L. (1994) Detection and identification of *Leptospira interrogans* serovars by PCR coupled with restriction endonuclease analysis of amplified DNA. *J. Clin. Microbiol.*, 32:935–941.

Terpstra, W., Schoone, G.J., and ter Schegget, J. (1986) Detection of leptospiral DNA by nucleic acid hybridization with 32P- and biotin-labelled probes. *J. Med. Microbiol.*, 22:23–28.

van Eys, G.J.J.M., Gravecamp, C., Gerritsen, M.J., Quint, W., Cornelissen, M.T.E., ter Schegget, J., and Terpstra, W.J. (1989) Detection of leptospires in urine by polymerase chain reaction. *J. Clin. Microbiol.*, 27:2258–2262.

Wagenaar, J.A., Segers, R.P.A.M., and van de Zeijst, B.A.M. (1994) Rapid and specific detection of pathogenic *Leptospira* species by amplification of ribosomal sequences. *Mol. Biotech.*, 2:1–15.

Watt, G. (1991) Leptospirosis. In *Hunter's Tropical Medicine*, G. T. Strickland, ed., Philadelphia, W. B. Saunders.

White, F.H., and Ristic, M. (1959) Detection of *Leptospira pomona* in guinea pig and bovine urine with fluorescein-labeled antibody. *J. Infect. Dis.*, 105:118–123.

Woo, T.H., Smythe, L.D., Symonds, M.L., Norris, M.A., Dohnt, M.F., and Patel, B.K. (1997) Rapid distinction between *Leptospira interrogans* and *Leptospira biflexa* by PCR amplification of 23S ribosomal DNA. *Fems Microbiol. Lett.*, 150:9–18.

Woodward, M.J., and Redstone, J.S. (1993) Differentiation of leptospira serovars by the polymerase chain reaction and restriction fragment length polymorphism. *Vet. Rec.*, 132:325–326.

Yasuda, P.H., Steigerwalt, A.G., Sulzer, K.R., Kaufman, A.F., Rogers, F., and Brenner, D.J. (1987) Deoxyribonucleic aid relatedness between serogroups and serovars in the family *Leptospiracae* with proposals for seven new *Leptospira* species. *Int. J. Syst. Bacteriol.*, 37:407–415.

Zuerner, R.L., Alt, D., and Bolin, C.A. (1995) IS*1533*–based PCR assay for identification of *Leptospira interrogans* sensu lato serovars. *J. Clin. Microbiol.*, 33:3284–3289.

5.1.11   *Trypanosoma cruzi*

Avila, H.A., Pereira, J.B., Thiemann, O., de Paiva, E., Degrave, W., Morel, C.M., and Simpson, L. (1993) Detection of *Trypanosoma cruzi* in blood specimens of chronic chagasic patients by polymerase chain reaction amplification of kinetoplast minicircle DNA: Comparison with serology and xenodiagnosis. *J. Clin. Microbiol.*, 31:2421–2426.

Avila, H.A., Sigman, D.S., Cohen, L.M., Millikan, R.C., and Simpson, L. (1991) Polymerase chain reaction amplification of *Trypanosoma cruzi* kinetoplast minicircle DNA isolated from whole blood lysates: Diagnosis of chronic Chagas' disease. *Mol. Biochem. Parasitol.*, 48:211–222.

Black, W.C. (1993) PCR with arbitrary primers: Approach with care. *Insect Mol. Biol.*, 2:1–6.

Breniere, S.F., Bosseno, M.F., Telleria, J., Carrasco, R., Vargas, F., Yaksic, N., and Noireau, F. (1995) Field application of polymerase chain reaction diagnosis and strain typing of *Trypanosoma cruzi* in Bolivian triatomines. *Am. J. Trop. Med. Hyg.*, 53:179–184.

Britto, C., Cardoso, M.A., Moneiro Vanni, C.M., Hasslocher-Moreno, A., Xavier, S.S., Oelemann, W., Santoro, A., Pirmez, C., Morel, C.M., and Wincker, P. (1995) Polymerase chain reaction detection of *Trypanosoma cruzi* in human blood samples as a tool for diagnosis and treatment evaluation. *Parasitology*, 110:241–247.

Britto, C., Cardoso, M.A., Wincker, P., and Morel, C.M. (1993) A simple protocol for the physical cleavage of *Trypanosoma cruzi* kinetoplast DNA present in blood samples and its use in polymerase chain reaction (PCR)-based diagnosis of chronic Chagas' disease. *Mem. Inst. Oswaldo Cruz*, 88:171–172.

Diaz, C., Nussenzweig, V., and Gonzalez, A. (1992) An improved polymerase chain reaction assay to detect *Trypanosoma cruzi* in blood. *Am. J. Trop. Med. Hyg.*, 46:616–623.

Gonzalez, N., Galindo, I., Guevara, P., Novak, E., Scorza, J.V., Añez, N., da Silveira, J.F., and Ramirez, J.L. (1994) Identification and detection of *Trypanosoma cruzi* by using a DNA amplification fingerprint obtained from the ribosomal intergenic spacer. *J. Clin. Microbiol.*, 32:153–158.

Kirchhoff, L.V. (1995) *Trypanosoma* species (American trypanosomiasis, Chagas disease): Biology of trypanosomes. In *Principles and Practice of Infectious Diseases*, G.L. Mandell, J.E. Bennett, and R. Dolin, eds., New York, Churchill Livingstone.

Moser, D.R., Kirchhoff, L.V., and Donelson, J.E. (1989) Detection of *Trypanosoma cruzi* by DNA amplification using the polymerase chain reaction. *J. Clin. Microbiol.*, 27:1477–1482.

Novak, E., de Mello, M.P., Gomes, H.B.M., Galindo, I., Guevara, P., Ramirez, J.L., and da Silveira, J.F. (1993) Repetitive sequences in the ribosomal intergenic spacer of *Trypansoma cruzi*. *Mol. Biochem. Parasitol.*, 60:273–280.

Requena, J.M., Jimenez-Ruiz, A., Soto, M., Lopez, M.C., and Alonso, C. (1992) Characterization of a highly repeated interspersed DNA sequence of *Trypanosoma cruzi*: Its potential use in diagnosis and strain classification. *Mol. Biochem. Parasitol.*, 51:271–280.

Revollo, S., Oury, B., Laurent, J.P., Barnabe, C., Quesney, V., Noel, S., and Tibayrenc, M. (1998) *Trypanosoma cruzi*: Impact of clonal evolution of the parasite on its biological and medical properties. *Exp. Parasitol.* 89:30–39.

Russomando, G., Rojas de Arias, A., Almiron, M., Figueredo, A., Ferreira, M.E., and Morita, K. (1996) *Trypanosoma cruzi*: Polymerase chain reaction-based detection in dried feces of *Triatoma infestans*. *Exp. Parasitol.*, 83:62–66.

Shikanai-Yasuda, M.A., Ochs, D.E., Tolezano, J.E., and Kirchhoff, L.V. (1996) Use of the polymerase chain reaction for detecting *Trypanosoma cruzi* in triatomine vectors. *Trans. R. Soc. Trop. Med. Hyg.*, 90:649–651.

Silber, A.M., Bua, J., Porcel, B.M., Segura, E.L., and Ruiz, A.M. (1997) *Trypanosoma cruzi*: Specific detection of parasites by PCR in infected humans and vectors using a set of primers (BP1/BP2) targeted to a nuclear DNA sequence. *Exp. Parasitol.*, 85:225–32.

Souto, R.P., Fernandes, O., Macedo, A.M., Campbell, D.A., and Zingales, B. (1996) DNA markers define two major phylogenetic lineages of *Trypanosoma cruzi*. *Mol. Biochem. Parasitol.*, 83:141–152.

Souto, R.P., and Zingales, B. (1993) Sensitive detection and strain classification of *Trypanosoma cruzi* by amplification of a ribosomal RNA sequence. *Mol. Biochem. Parasitol.*, 62:45–52.

Steindel, M., Dias Neto, E., de Menezes, C.L., Romanha, A.J., and Simpson, A.J. (1993) Random amplified polymorphic DNA analysis of *Trypanosoma cruzi* strains. *Mol. Biochem. Parasitol.*, 60:71–79.

Sturm, N.R., Degrave, W., Morel, C., and Simpson, L. (1989) Sensitive detection and schizodeme classification of *Trypansoma cruzi* cells by amplificaon of kinetoplast mini-circle DNA sequences: Use in diagnosis of Chagas' disease. *Mol. Biochem. Parasitol.*, 33:205–214.

Tibayrenc, M., Neubauer, K., Barnabe, C., Guerrini, F., Skarecky, D., and Ayala, F.J. (1993) Genetic characterization of six parasitic protozoa: Parity between random-primer DNA typing and multilocus enzyme electrophoresis. *Proc. Natl. Acad. Sci. USA*, 90:1335–1339.

WHO Expert Committee (1991) *Control of Chagas disease.* Geneva, World Health Organization.

Wincker, P., Bosseno, M.-F., Britto, C., Yaksic, N., Cardoso, M.A., Morel, C.M., and Breniere, S.F. (1994a) High correlation between Chagas' disease serology and PCR-based detection of *Trypanosoma cruzi* kinetoplast DNA in Bolivian children living in an endemic area. *FEMS Microbiol. Lett.*, 124:419–424.

Wincker, P., Britto, C., Pereira, J.B., Cardoso, M.A., Oelemann, W., and Morel, C.M. (1994b) Use of a simplified polymerase chain reaction procedure to detect *Trypanosoma cruzi* in blood samples from chronic chagasic patients in a rural endemic area. *Am. J. Trop. Med. Hyg.*, 51:771–777.

5.1.2 Nonradioactive DNA Probes: *V. cholerae* Colony Blot

Boehringer Mannheim. *The DIG System User's Guide for Filter Hybridization.* Mannheim, Germany: Boehringer Mannheim GmbH, Biochemica, 1995.

Fields, P.I., Popovic, T., Wachsmuth, K., and Olsvik, O. (1992) Use of polymerase chain reaction for detection of toxigenic *Vibrio cholerae* O1 strains from the Latin American cholera epidemic. *J. Clin. Microbiol.*, 30:2118–2121.

Olsvik, O., Popovic, T., and Fields, P.I. (1993) PCR detection of toxin genes in strains of *Vibrio cholerae* O1. In *Diagnostic Molecular Microbiology: Principles and Applications*, D.H. Persing, T.F. Smith, F.C. Tenover, and T.J. White, eds., Washington DC, ASM Press.

Sambrook, J., Fritsch, E.F., and Maniatis, T. (1989) *Molecular Cloning: A Laboratory Manual.* New York, Cold Spring Harbor Laboratory Press.

6

Rapid Cloning of PCR Products

PCR products can be visualized directly or cloned by ligating the amplified product into the vector of choice. Cloning of PCR products is useful for many purposes; for instance, the cloned fragment can then be sequenced, modified, expressed, labeled, or used as a DNA probe. While PCR methods have been described to perform many of these functions without cloning, it is often useful to have a cloned stock of PCR product (modified or unmodified) as a permanent source of the material. PCR products can be notoriously difficult to clone, and numerous PCR cloning strategies have been developed and are commercially available. One simple and effective in-house approach, which will be described in this chapter, is the introduction of restriction endonuclease sites into the PCR product, followed by classical cloning procedures.

6.1   Primer Design

One approach to facilitating the cloning of PCR products is to incorporate restriction enzyme sites into the 5' end of the amplification primers, ideally using a different "sticky" (3' or 5' overhang) site for each primer. It is critical to include several extra nucleotides after the restriction site, before the end of the primer. This allows adequate space for the restriction enzyme to "sit" on the PCR product in order to cleave the DNA at the restriction site. Generally, 2–3 extra nucleotides are sufficient. The number of additional nucleotides necessary for cleavage by particular enzymes is presented in a table in the New England Biolabs yearly catalog.[1] Amplification with these modified primers should be conducted according to the standard protocol. When calculating the annealing temperature (T_{ann}), only the nucleotides that hybridize to the genomic target sequence should be taken into consideration (thus excluding the nucleotides that comprise the restriction enzyme cleavage site from the calculation).

---

1. "Cleavage close to the end of DNA fragments (oligonucleotides)," pp. 238–239, 1996/97 catalog.

6.2   Preparation of PCR Products for Cloning

6.2.1   Digestion of the Vector and PCR Products

EQUIPMENT
Refrigerator (4°C)
Freezer (-20°C)
Incubator or water bath at 37°C
Water bath at 80°C
Vortex
Microcentrifuge
Adjustable pipettors (1000 µL, 200 µL, 20 µL)
Metal block for microcentrifuge tubes (pre-cooled to -20°C)

MATERIALS
Beaker with bleach
Sterile yellow and blue pipet tips
Sterile 1.5-mL microcentrifuge tubes
Plastic racks for microcentrifuge tubes
Colored laboratory tape
Scissors or razor blade
Permanent markers (indelible ink)
Gloves (disposable latex or vinyl)
Ice buckets with ice

REAGENTS
Proteinase K (10 mg/mL)
Restriction Enzyme 1 (XX U/µL)
Restriction Enzyme 2 (XX U/µL)
Appropriate Buffer
100 mM EDTA, pH 8.0
Sterile ddH$_2$O
PCR products
Cloning vector (e.g., Bluescript, 100 ng/µL)

1. Calculate the concentration of each PCR product, comparing the intensity of the fragment with that of the DNA marker bands.
   _____ ng/µL product #1
   _____ ng/µL product #2
2. Label the tubes and prepare the reaction with Proteinase K:
   40 µL of DNA
   10 µl Proteinase K (10 mg/mL)
   50 µL total volume
   The final concentration of product is 80% of the inital DNA concentration. Calculate the new concentration of product:
   _____ ng/µL product #1
   _____ ng/µL product #2
3. Mix well by pipetting.
4. Incubate the reaction at 37°C for 2 hours.
5. Incubate for another 10 minutes at 80°C to inactivate the Proteinase K and terminate the reaction.

6. Calculate the volume of the mixture (product + Proteinase K) that contains ~1.5 μg of DNA.

_____ μL product #1

_____ μL product #2

Restriction enzymes are very labile; remove from the − 20°C freezer only when necessary and for as short a time as possible. Maintain in a pre-cooled metal block on ice at all times.

7. Prepare the restriction enzyme digestion as follows: Calculate the amount of enzyme required using the formula below. Verify the concentration of the restriction enzyme stock and determine the volume that contains the desired units of enzyme activity. Select the optimal buffer for the double digestion by referring to the appropriate charts supplied by the restriction enzyme manufacturer. The volume of buffer in the reaction should be 1/10 of the total volume. The volume of enzyme used should never exceed 1/10 of total volume because the glycerol in the concentrated enzyme stock can interfere with the activity of the restriction enzymes. This type of interference is referred to as "star activity."

A. PCR products

        μL of DNA digested with Proteinase K (~1.5 μg)

        μL Restriction Enzyme 1 (XX U/μL)

        μL Restriction Enzyme 2 (XX U/μL)

  9 μL Appropriate Buffer

_____ μl ddH$_2$O

 90 μL total volume

B. Vector

 40 μL vector (100 ng/μL) = 4 μg

        μL Restriction Enzyme 1 (XX U/μL)

        μL Restriction Enzyme 2 (XX U/μL)

  7 μL Appropriate Buffer

_____ μl ddH$_2$O

 70 μL total volume

C. Controls: Vector digested with one enzyme

Control #1:

  5 μL vector (100 ng/μL) = 500 ng

        μL Restriction Enzyme 1 (XX U/μL)

  2 μL Appropriate Buffer

_____ μl ddH$_2$O

 20 μL total volume

Control #2

  5 μL vector (100 ng/μL) = 500 ng

        μL Restriction Enzyme 2 (XX U/μL)

  2 μL Appropriate Buffer

_____ μl ddH$_2$O

 20 μL total volume

8. Mix well by pipetting.

9. Incubate all reactions at 37°C for 1 hour.

10. Add 100 mM EDTA, pH 8.0, to a final concentration of 10 mM to completely stop all reactions.

Calculations to Determine the Amount of Enzyme Required

The following formula can be used to determine the amount of enzyme necessary for a digestion.

Units of enzyme required = g • λ/n$_\lambda$ • n$_x$/x• f

where	g	=	micrograms of DNA to be digested
	λ	=	size of phage λ
	n$_\lambda$	=	number of restriction sites in λ
	n$_x$	=	number of restriction sites in DNA X
	x	=	size of DNA X
	f	=	multiplication factor for vectors[2]

Example: cloning a 306-bp product of dengue-3 into the vector Bluescript using restriction enzymes *Eco*RI and *Bam* HI.

DNA	Size (bp)	# of *Eco*RI sites	# of *Bam*HI sites
λ phage	40,000	5	5
Bluescript	2960	1	1
Den-3RE product	306	1	1

EcoRI Digestion of 1 μg of Dengue-3 PCR Product

g	=	1 μg
λ	=	40,000 bp
n$_\lambda$	=	5
v$_x$	=	1
x	=	306 bp
f	=	1 (the multiplication factor does not apply to PCR products)

$$\text{Units of } Eco\text{RI required} = g \cdot \lambda/n_\lambda \cdot n_x/x \cdot f$$
$$= 1 \cdot 40{,}000/5 \cdot 1/306 \cdot 1$$
$$= 26.1 \text{ U}$$

EcoRI Digestion of 4 μg of the Bluescript Vector

g	=	4 μg
λ	=	40,000 bp
n$_\lambda$	=	5
n$_x$	=	1
x	=	2960 bp
f	=	2.5-fold more *Eco*RI required to digest the pUC19 vector (the progenitor of Bluescript) than λ

---

2. It takes more enzyme to completely digest certain supercoiled plasmids than to digest phage λ; this "multiplication" factor is presented in the New England Biolabs annual catalog ("Cleavage of pBR322, pUC19, and LITMUS™", p. 240, 1996/97 catalog) and does not apply to PCR products.

$$\begin{aligned}
\text{Units of } EcoRI \text{ required} &= g \cdot \lambda/n_\lambda \cdot n_x/x \cdot f \\
&= 4 \cdot 40{,}000/5 \cdot 1/2960 \cdot 2.5 \\
&= 27.0 \text{ U}
\end{aligned}$$

*Bam*HI *Digestion of 1 μg of Dengue-3 PCR Product*

$$\begin{aligned}
g &= 1\ \mu g \\
\lambda &= 40{,}000 \text{ bp} \\
n_\lambda &= 5 \\
n_x &= 1 \\
x &= 306 \text{ bp} \\
f &= 1 \text{ (the multiplication factor does not apply to PCR products)}
\end{aligned}$$

$$\begin{aligned}
\text{Units of } BamHI \text{ required} &= g \cdot \lambda/n_\lambda \cdot n_x/x \cdot f \\
&= 1 \cdot 40{,}000/5 \cdot 1/306 \cdot 1 \\
&= 26.1 \text{ U}
\end{aligned}$$

*Bam*HI *Digestion of 4 μg of the Bluescript Vector*

$$\begin{aligned}
g &= 4\ \mu g \\
\lambda &= 40{,}000 \text{ bp} \\
n_\lambda &= 5 \\
n_x &= 1 \\
x &= 2960 \text{ bp} \\
f &= 1 \text{ (equivalent amount of } BamHI \text{ required to digest the pUC19 vector and l}
\end{aligned}$$

$$\begin{aligned}
\text{Units of } BamHI \text{ required} &= g \cdot \lambda/n_\lambda \cdot n_x/x \cdot f \\
&= 4 \cdot 40{,}000/5 \cdot 1/2960 \cdot 1 \\
&= 10.8 \text{ U}
\end{aligned}$$

6.2.2 Preparative Agarose Gel

EQUIPMENT
Microcentrifuge
Balance (for weighing ~1 g)
Microwave or Bunsen burner to melt agarose
Power supply
UV transilluminator
Plexiglass shield (high-grade UV-transmitting Plexiglass)
Camera (preferably Polaroid)
Orange filter
Hood or darkroom
Gel box
Adjustable pipettors (200 μL, 20 μL)

MATERIALS
Gel tray
Combs
250-mL Erlenmeyer flask
100-mL, 250-mL and 1-L graduated cyclinders
Weighing paper

Sterile yellow pipet tips
Sterile 1.5-mL microcentrifuge tubes
Plastic microcentrifuge tube racks
Colored laboratory tape (or masking tape)
Transparent tape
Gloves (disposable latex or vinyl)
Permanent markers
Parafilm
UV protective eyewear (goggles or face shield)
Razor blade
Filter forceps (flat)

REAGENTS
1X TAE (Tris Acetate EDTA Running Buffer)
Agarose
Sample loading buffer (*see* Appendix B)
DNA size markers with known concentration
Ethidium bromide (10 mg/mL)
Polaroid 667 film

Note: TAE running buffer must be used when following the silica gel DNA purification procedure.

Wear gloves at all times when handling the carcinogen ethidium bromide!

A. Gel Preparation

1. For each gel, prepare a 1% agarose solution in 1X TAE. Heat the solution until the agarose melts.
2. Prepare the gel tray with combs. If a preparative comb is not available, use transparent tape to tape together several teeth of a standard 1.5-mm thick comb, so as to create wells of the desired width. If possible, leave one standard-sized well between each pair of preparative wells to minimize the risk of cross-contamination.
3. Let the agarose solution cool until it reaches ~55°C. Add 10 mg/mL ethidium bromide to a final concentration of 0.1 μg/mL (1/100,000 dilution). Pour the melted agarose into the tray, moving the bubbles to the sides with a pipet tip.
4. Add ethidium bromide at a final concentration of 0.1 μg/mL to prepare the 1X TAE Running Buffer.

*B. Gel Electrophoresis: **Black Area***

1. Prepare a Gel Chart showing the order of the samples in the gel.
2. Mix the desired amount of the digested PCR product and the vector DNA with 1/5 volume of sample loading buffer.
3. To 5 μL of the DNA size marker, add 2 μL of loading buffer and 3 μL of distilled water and load into a standard-sized well.
4. Place the gel in the gel box and cover it with 1X TAE Running Buffer.
5. Load the entire volume of each sample into the wells in the gel in the predetermined order.
6. Run the gel at ~100 V until the bromophenol blue (dark blue dye) has migrated approximately 70–80% of the length of the gel.

C. Visualization, Photography, and Excision of Gel Slice: **Black Area/Darkroom**

Appropriate eye protection must be worn in the presence of UV light!

1. Place the gel on a UV transilluminator and turn the transilluminator on in order to visualize the DNA fragments, which should appear orange in color. **It is critical to minimize exposure of the gel to UV light**, since the UV light nicks the DNA, gradually destroying it. This can be done by using longer-wave UV light, lowering the intensity of the UV light (in variable-intensity transilluminators), using a plexiglass shield over the UV transilluminator, and exposing the gel for as short a time as possible.

2. If a camera is available, take a photograph using the UV transilluminator and the camera with an orange filter. A Polaroid camera with Polaroid 667 film is preferable; first try 1/2 second with an 5.6 or 8 aperture and adjust as necessary. If an instant Polaroid is not available, use a 35-mm camera with standard settings.

It is imperative to use a Plexiglass shield when making incisions in the gel with a razor blade to prevent damage to the glass filter on the UV transilluminator. Be careful not to bring your face into close proximity to the gel and the UV light.

3. Briefly illuminate the gel with UV light and make incisions with a razor blade on all four sides of the band of interest **as close to the band as possible to minimize the size of the gel slice**. Turn the UV light off after use.

4. Use filter forceps to transfer the excised gel slice to the appropriately labeled tube. Wash the forceps and razor blade with water and 95% ethanol between different samples.

5. Repeat the procedure to excise the next band.

6. **Do not re-use Running Buffer** for other preparative gels, since DNA cross-contamination may occur.

7. Dispose of the gel in an ethidium bromide solid waste container. To dispose of the ethidium bromide-containing Running Buffer, the solution should be treated with activated charcoal (*see* section 5.1.2).

6.2.3   Purification of the Excised DNA Fragments Using Silica Particles

The following protocol describes the purification of DNA from an agarose gel by using silica particles, originally described by Vogelstein and Gillespie (1979). The principle underlying the purification process is the ability of negatively-charged DNA to bind to glass through charge interactions. The agarose is dissolved by heating in the presence of sodium iodide, and then the DNA is captured by incubating the solution with silica particles (fine glass beads). Next, the silica particle-bound DNA is washed several times and then eluted in distilled water or Tris-EDTA solution by heating to 45–55°C (Ausubel et al., 1995). The yield is highest for DNA fragments 500 bp to 5 kb in length; smaller fragments may remain attached to the particles to a greater degree. The silica particle method is also effective at purifying nucleic acids away from potential inhibitors of PCR amplifications. Silica particles can be prepared in-house at low cost (*see* Appendix B); several formulations are also commercially available at much higher cost. Various alternative methods for purification of DNA fragments from agarose gels have been reported, such as (1) electroelution of the DNA fragment from an excised gel slice inside dialysis membranes, followed by organic extraction and ethanol precipitation; (2) electroelution of the

DNA onto nitrocellulose membranes followed by elution from the membrane, organic extraction, and ethanol precipitation; and (3) use of low-melting point agarose (Ausubel et al., 1995). PCR products can also be purified away from primers and nucleotides simply by centrifuging the amplification reaction over a "spin column" containing resin of the appropriate mesh. However, this technique, known as spin dialysis, purifies all the products of the PCR reaction, including amplified nonspecific contaminants. The advantage of purifying PCR products using gel electrophoresis is that the specific fragment of interest can be selected and then purified.

For purification of fragments using glass beads, the preparative gel must be run in 1X TAE.

EQUIPMENT
Water bath at 50–55°C
Vortex
Microcentrifuge
Adjustable pipettors (1000 µL, 200 µL, 20 µL)

MATERIALS
Sterile yellow and blue pipet tips
Sterile microcentrifuge tubes (1.5 mL)
Floating rack for microcentrifuge tubes (plastic or Styrofoam)
Plastic racks for microcentrifuge tubes
Razor blade
Flat forceps
Colored laboratory tape
Paper towels
Permanent markers
Gloves (disposable latex or vinyl)
Parafilm

REAGENTS
6 M sodium iodide (NaI)
Silica particles (*see* Appendix C)
Sodium-ethanol wash, stored at −20°C
Tris-EDTA (TE), pH 8.0
1X TAE

1. Weigh the excised gel slice. If it weighs less than 0.4 g, use one microcentrifuge tube for the following steps. (Note that 1.0 g is equivalent to 1.0 mL.)
2. With a razor blade, cut the piece of gel in cubes of 1–2 mm^3 and place them in a labeled tube using clean forceps.
3. Add 3 volume equivalents of NaI (e.g., if the piece of gel weighs 0.1 g, add 0.3 mL NaI).
4. Incubate the tube in the 50–55°C water bath for 5 minutes, mixing the contents every 1 to 2 minutes, until the agarose has melted.
5. Vortex the silica particles to completely resuspend them. Add the silica particles to the DNA in the following amounts: for less than 5 µg of DNA, add 5 µL of the fully resuspended silica particle suspension; for each additional 0.5 µg of DNA over 5 µg, add 1 µL of the silica particle suspension.
6. Mix well and incubate for 5 minutes at ambient temperature or on ice, mixing every 1–2 minutes by inversion.

7. Centrifuge for 1 minute in a microcentrifuge.
8. Pipet off and discard the supernatant, taking care not to remove the silica particles.
9. Add between 200 and 700 μL of sodium-ethanol wash (10–50 times the volume of glass beads) and resuspend completely, using the point of the pipet tip to break up the pellet if necessary.
10. Centrifuge for 5–10 seconds only and discard the supernatant.
11. Repeat steps 9 and 10 two more times.
12. Resuspend the pellet in 15 μL of TE or ddH$_2$O.
13. Incubate the tubes at 50–55°C for 5 minutes to elute the DNA from the silica particles.
14. Centrifuge the tubes for 30–45 seconds.
15. Transfer the supernatant to a sterile microcentrifuge tube.
16. Resuspend the pellet in 10 μL of TE or ddH$_2$O.
17. Incubate the tubes at 50–55°C for another 5 minutes to ensure complete elution of the DNA.
18. Centrifuge the tubes for 30–45 seconds.
19. Transfer the supernatant to the same microcentrifuge tube containing the first eluate from step 15.

6.3   Ligation

In order to prepare the ligation reaction, the quantities of purified vector and insert fragments must be determined. The simplest method is to analyze an aliquot of the stock solution of each fragment by agarose gel electrophoresis and estimate the concentration by comparing the intensity of the resulting band with that of a DNA standard of known concentration. With this information, the ligation reaction can be prepared, using the worksheet provided in Appendix H.

6.3.1 Checking DNA Fragment Concentration by Agarose Gel Electrophoresis

1. Prepare a 1.5% agarose gel with ethidium bromide at a final concentration of 0.1 μg/mL (1/100,000 dilution).
2. Select a DNA size marker with bands of known concentration, e.g., Amplisize DNA marker (Bio-Rad Laboratories, Richmond, CA). Use sufficient DNA marker such that each band contains approximately 50 ng of DNA.
3. Prepare a gel chart showing the order of the samples in the gel.
4. Prepare a gel sample loading stage using Parafilm® and a microcentrifuge tube rack as described in section 5.1.2. Add 2 μL of each fragment to 2 μL loading buffer and 6 μL H$_2$0 in each well of the sample loading stage. Mix by pipetting the solution up and down.
5. Load the entire volume of each sample into the corresponding well according to the order on the gel chart.
6. Run the gel at ~100 V until the bromophenol blue dye has migrated 60–70% of the length of the gel.
7. Visualize the gel using a UV transilluminator and take a photograph as described previously.
8. Estimate the amount of DNA in each sample band by visually comparing the intensity to the bands of the DNA marker (50 ng/band).

Note: Since each band of DNA fragments contains 2 µL of DNA solution, the concentration of the initial solution in nanograms per microliter can be calculated by dividing the amount of DNA estimated (in nanograms) by 2 µL. For example, if the vector fragment appears roughly three times more intense than the DNA marker band closest to it in size (50 ng/band), then it can be estimated that the vector fragment represents approximately 150 ng of DNA. Since 2 µL of the vector DNA solution were analyzed in the gel, the concentration of the DNA solution is 150 ng/2 µL, or 75 ng/µL.

6.3.2 Ligation Reaction

The objective is to prepare a reaction that contains the vector, the insert, and the enzyme ligase. Typically, the reaction contains a 2:1 to 10:1 molar ratio of insert to vector. The molar ratio depends on the size of the vector and the insert. In addition, it depends on the type of ends (sticky or blunt) resulting from the digestion. More insert is used when the ends are blunt. The amount of each fragment in the ligation reaction should be in the range of 25–250 ng. The ligase reaction should be carried out in a small volume (10–20 µL, as necessary). The following example shows the calculation of the amount of DNA required for a ligation reaction with a 4:1 ratio of insert to vector.

	Insert (den-3)	**Vector**
Fragment size	306 bp	2960 bp
Size ratio	1	9.7
Required molar ratio of insert to vector (4:1)	4	1
Ratio of insert to vector DNA	4	9.7
Equivalent ratio of insert to vector DNA	1	~2.5 (9.7/4)
Total fragment/reaction in nanograms	50 ng	125 ng
Initial fragment concentration	10 ng/µL	50 ng/µL
Volume/reaction	5 µL	2.5 µL

The following controls should be included:

1. *Ligation reaction minus insert*: Although the vector has been digested with two restriction enzymes, incomplete digestion can occur. This control reveals the amount of vector that has been cut with only one enzyme. Under these conditions, the vector can still recircularize in the presence of ligase, even in the absence of insert. If the vector is completely digested with both enzymes, the resulting ends are incompatible, and the vector cannot be recircularized. Note that bacteria can only be successfully transformed with circularized plasmids; if the plasmid (vector) is linear, no transformation will be possible.
2. *Ligation reaction minus ligase*: This control measures the amount of intact vector (uncut by either enzyme). Intact plasmids stay circularized, even in the absence of ligase and insert.
3. *Ligase control*: This control verifies that the ligase is functioning. The reaction contains ligase and the vector that has been digested with one restriction enzyme. If the ligase is functioning, it should recircularize the plasmid, and the transformation should yield a large number of colonies.

ADDITIONAL EQUIPMENT
Water bath at 16°C

REAGENTS
Purified DNA fragments (vector and inserts)
T4 DNA Ligase
10X T4 DNA Ligase Buffer
Sterile ddH$_2$O

1. Calculate the required amount and volume of vector and insert.
2. Fill out the work table (Appendix H) and label the appropriate microcentrifuge tubes.
3. Add each component of the reaction to the labeled tubes. Add the enzyme last.
4. Mix the solution well by pipetting up and down, taking care not to introduce air bubbles.
5. Centrifuge the tubes rapidly to concentrate the liquid at the bottom of the tube.
6. Incubate at 16°C overnight.

The ligation reactions are now ready to be used in the transformation protocol (section 6.4.2). One-half of the ligation reaction should be used to transform the competent cells, and the remaining half should be stored at −20°C.

6.4   Preparation of Competent Cells and Transformation

The following section describes the preparation of cells that will be transformed with the ligation reaction mixtures (adapted from Chung et al. [1988]). There are other published protocols for preparing competent cells, including calcium chloride and electroporation (Ausubel et al., 1995). The following method includes a built-in color selection for plasmids that contain inserts from successful ligations. The color selection is possible using the pBluescript cloning vector (Stratagene Cloning Systems) and overlaying the LB-Amp plates with IPTG and X-Gal. If a different vector is used, the transformation procedure is identical, except that the LB-Amp plates are *not* overlayed with IPTG and X-Gal, and there is no color selection. The pBluescript blue/white selection system is based on the principle that the polylinker region in this vector, into which the inserts are cloned, is located within the N-terminal coding region of the *lacZ* gene. This gene codes for β-galactosidase, an enzyme that converts the substrates IPTG and X-Gal into a product with a blue color. Thus, when there is no insert in the vector, the *lacZ* gene is transcribed and β-galactosidase is expressed, and *E. coli* colonies transformed with the plasmid appear blue when grown on medium containing IPTG and X-Gal. However, if an insert is successfully ligated into the polylinker region, this interrupts the expression of the *lacZ* gene, so that no β-galactosidase is made and the *E. coli* colonies appear white.

EQUIPMENT
Incubator (37°C)
Centrifuge with 3500 rpm capability
Spectrophotometer measuring optical density at 600-nm wavelength
Plate spinner, if available
Bunsen burner
Adjustable pipettors (1000 µL, 200 µL, 20 µL)
Air shaker (37°C)

MATERIALS
Plate spreader (i.e., made from a glass rod)
Erlenmeyer flasks (100 mL)
Sterile yellow and blue pipet tips
Sterile test tubes (13 X 100 mm)
Sterile plastic tubes (50 mL)
Inoculating loop or sterile wooden sticks
Ice bucket

STERILE REAGENTS
Luris Broth (LB)
TSB
1 *M* glucose
Ampicillin (100 mg/mL)
LB-Amp plates
IPTG (Isopropyl β-D-Thiogalactopyranoside)
X-Gal (5-Bromo-4-chloro-3-indolyl-D-galactopyranoside)
Dimethyl formamide (DMF)
95% ethanol

6.4.1   Preparation of Competent Cells

1. Inoculate a colony of a laboratory strain of *E. coli* (e.g., DH5-α) in 3 mL of LB in a 13 X 100-mm test tube.
2. Culture the *E. coli* at 37°C with constant shaking (225 rpm) overnight (12–18 hours).
3. Inoculate 25 mL of LB in a flask or 50-mL plastic tube with 100 μL of saturated *E.coli* culture.
4. Grow the bacteria at 37°C for 2–3 hours, until an OD_{600} of ~0.5 (0.3–0.6) is obtained.
5. Transfer the culture to a sterile 50-mL tube.
6. Centrifuge at 3500 rpm at 4°C for 10 minutes.
7. Discard the supernatant.
8. Resuspend in 1/10 volume of TSB (at 4°C) and place the tube on ice for 10 minutes.

This suspension of competent cells is now ready to be used for transformation.

6.4.2   Transformation

1. Distribute 100 μL of the competent cells into cold, labeled microcentrifuge tubes.
2. To each 100 μL of the competent cells (referred to as a "transformation"), add the following DNA in the order given and mix by pipetting:

Negative control (nothing)
Half of the "ligation reaction minus ligase" control
Half of the "ligation reaction minus insert" control
Vector digested with restriction enzyme 1
Vector digested with restriction enzyme 2
Half of each ligation reaction
Half of the "ligase" control
Positive control (30 ng of the undigested vector)

3. Incubate the tubes for 30 minutes on ice.

4. Prepare a solution of TSB with 20 mM glucose, allowing 1 mL per transformation to calculate the required amount.

5. Add 0.9 mL of the TSB/glucose solution to each tube and mix.

6. Shake the tubes at 37°C for 30–60 minutes.

7. Prepare a 200-mg/ml solution of IPTG in ddH$_2$O (20 mg in 100 μL of ddH$_2$O) *and* a 20-mg/ml solution of X-Gal in DMF (20 mg in 1 mL of DMF).

8. Prepare two LB-Amp plates for each transformation. Spread each LB-Amp plate with 40 μL of X-Gal and 4 μL of IPTG.

9. Plate 100 μL of each transformation on labeled Petri plates containing LBA + IPTG + X-Gal.

10. Centrifuge the microcentrifuge tubes containing the rest (900 μL) of the transformation for 1 minute in a microcentrifuge.

11. Discard most of the supernatant, leaving approximately 100 μL to resuspend the pellet (referred to as the "concentrated transformation").

12. Plate 100 μL of each "concentrated transformation" on labeled plates containing LBA + IPTG + X-Gal prepared in step 8.

13. Place the plates upside down in a 37°C incubator for 12 to 18 hours until the colonies have grown sufficiently. The plates can be stored at 4°C. These colonies will be analyzed in section 6.5.

6.5   Checking Clones by PCR

Colonies resulting from the ligation and transformation procedures in sections 6.3 and 6.4 (Figure 6.1) can be analyzed by performing PCR directly on bacterial cells, which lyse at the high temperatures reached during the amplification procedure. Equipment and materials required in this section are listed in section 5.1.2, while detailed protocols for preparing and conducting a PCR amplification can be found in sections 5.1.3–5.1.11.

A. *Preparation of PCR Master Mix and Reaction Tubes:* **White Area**

1. Calculate the amount of PCR Master Mix that will be necessary for the desired number of reactions, each containing 50 μL of Master Mix. For every 20 reaction volumes, add 1 extra volume of Master Mix to compensate for volume lost during pipetting. Check your calculations.

2. Fill out the PCR worksheet.

3. Label the 0.5-mL (or 0.2-mL) tubes that will be used in the amplification. Label the tubes with the number of the colony on the side of the tube and the number of the reaction (corresponding to the PCR worksheet) on the top of the tube.

4. Prepare the PCR Master Mix. Distribute 50 μL of the mixture into each labeled reaction tube. **Do not cover with mineral oil**.

5. Using a designated **white** pipettor, add 1 μL of ddH$_2$O to prepare a "white area" negative control to tube 1.

B. *Sample Addition:* **Grey Area**

6. Label a Petri plate (LB-Amp) with the numbers of the colonies that will be checked.

7. With a sterile toothpick, pick a bacterial colony and touch the toothpick to the Petri

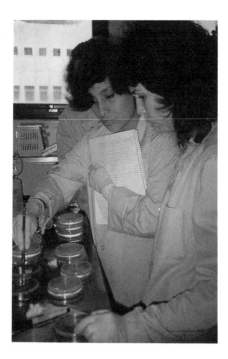

Fig. 6.1. Course instructor Adelaida Villareal and participant Betzabé Rodriguez analyzing results from the transformation of ligation reactions after cloning PCR products during an international workshop in Cuba.

plate in the spot corresponding to the number of the colony. Submerge the *same* toothpick in the appropriate PCR reaction tube that contains the PCR reaction mix, and twirl the toothpick in the solution.

8. Add 2 drops of mineral oil to each tube and close the tubes.
9. Proceed with standard amplification.
10. Analyze the PCR products by gel electrophoresis in the **Black Area**, as described in section 5.1.2.

6.6   Plasmid Purification

This procedure has been adapted from a standard plasmid purification protocol consisting of bacterial cell lysis, extraction with organic solvents, ethanol precipitation, and precipitation of plasmid DNA with polyethylene glycol (Sambrook et al., 1989). The protocol has been modified so that all of the high-speed centrifugations can be performed in a microcentrifuge, thus obviating the requirement for a high-speed floor centrifuge which may not be available. Several details are worth noting: TB medium yields 4–8 times more bacteria per milliliter of culture than LB culture medium. Adequate aeration is important; the culture should occupy no more than one-fifth of the total volume of a tube or one-fourth of the total volume of an Erlenmeyer flask. Avoid using a vortex to minimize mechanical breakage of contaminating chromosomal DNA. Precipitation with polyethylene glycol (PEG) yields "supercoiled" plasmid DNA without contamination from chromosomal DNA or RNA. This step is optional; however, it is recommended if DNA of high purity is required; for example, for sequencing.

EQUIPMENT
Refrigerator (4°C)
Freezer (-20°C)
Incubator (37°C)
Air shaker (37°C)
Vortex
Microcentrifuge
Adjustable pipettors (1000 μL, 200 μL, 20 μL)

MATERIALS
Sterile yellow and blue pipet tips
Sterile 1.5-mL microcentrifuge tubes
Sterile 50-mL plastic tubes
Erlenmeyer flasks
Glass pipets (10 mL, 25 mL) and rubber bulbs or Pipette Pumps®
Inoculating loop and Bunsen burner or sterile wooden applicators
Plastic racks for microcentrifuge tubes
Colored laboratory tape
Scissors or razor blade
Permanent markers (indelible ink)
Gloves (disposable latex or vinyl)
Ice bucket with ice

REAGENTS
GTE Buffer (50 mM glucose, 25 mM Tris [pH 8.0], 10 mM EDTA [pH 8.0]
0.2 N NaOH/1% SDS (prepare immediately before use)
Ice-cold 3.0 M potassium acetate (pH 4.8)
Phenol[3] (pH 8.0)
Chloroform[3]
Isopropanol
70% ethanol
4.0 M NaCl
RNAse (10 mg/mL)
13% PEG$_{8000}$ solution (sterilized by autoclave)
TB medium (*see* Appendix B)
Ampicillin (100 mg/mL; stored at -20°C)

A. Bacterial Culture

1. Prepare a sufficient quantity of TB containing ampicillin at 100 μg/mL. (For example, add 100 μL of ampicillin at 100 mg/mL to 100 mL of TB.)

---

3. Phenol and chloroform waste should be collected in a separate container and transferred to the organic waste container stored in the chemical fume hood.

2. Using sterile technique, distribute 15 mL of the TB-ampicillin medium into 50-mL plastic tubes.

3. Inoculate the medium with the *E. coli* colony transformed with the plasmid of interest (*see* section 6.4.2).

4. Grow the bacteria at 37°C with constant shaking (225 rpm) for 12–18 hours.

5. Centrifuge 15 mL of culture in a clinical or Sorvall centrifuge at 5000 rpm for 10 minutes.

6. Discard the supernatant and resuspend the pellet in 400 μL of GTE buffer.

7. Transfer ~250 μL of the suspension into each of two microcentrifuge tubes.

B. Bacterial Lysis

8. Prepare a solution of 0.2 N NaOH containing 1% SDS.

9. Add 300 μL of the NaOH/SDS solution to each of the two tubes containing the bacterial suspension, and mix by inversion.

10. Place the tubes on ice for 5 minutes.

11. Add 300 μL of 3.0 M potassium acetate (pH 4.8) to each tube to neutralize the pH and mix by inversion.

12. Place the tubes on ice for 5 minutes.

13. Centrifuge in a microcentrifuge for 10 minutes at ambient temperature.

14. Transfer the supernatants to two new sterile microcentrifuge tubes.

15. Add RNase A (without DNase) to each tube at a final concentration of 30 μg/mL (3 μL of a 10 mg/mL stock).

16. Incubate the tubes at 37°C for 20 minutes.

C. Extraction with Organic Solvents and Ethanol Precipitation

17. Measure the volume of the solution in each tube.

18. Add an equal volume of phenol:chloroform (1:1) to each tube, and mix by inversion for 30 seconds. Centrifuge for 2 minutes. Transfer the aqueous (upper) phase to two new microcentrifuge tubes.

19. Add an equal volume of chloroform to each tube and mix by inversion for 30 seconds. Centrifuge for 2 minutes. Transfer the aqueous (upper) phase to two new tubes.

20. Add an equal volume of 100% isopropanol to each tube in order to precipitate the DNA.

21. Centrifuge the tubes immediately at 12,000g for 10 minutes at ambient temperature.

22. Discard the supernatants carefully by using a 1000-μL pipettor.

23. Add 500 μL of 70% ethanol to each tube and centrifuge for 5 minutes at ambient temperature.

24. Using a 1000-μL pipettor (with blue tips) followed by a 200-μL pipettor (with yellow tips), carefully discard the supernatants.

25. Let the pellets air dry for 15 minutes in a horizontal position (if left to air dry in an inverted position, be careful that the pellets do not fall out).

26. Resuspend the pellets in 32 μL of ddH$_2$0.

D. PEG Precipitation (Optional)

27. Add 8 μL of 4.0 *M* NaCl followed by 40 μL of a sterile 13% PEG$_{8000}$ solution to each tube containing the resuspended pellets and mix well.

28. Incubate the tubes on ice for 20 minutes.

29. Centrifuge the tubes for 15 minutes *at 4°C*.

30. Using a 1000-μL pipettor, carefully discard the supernatants. The pellets are typically small and transparent.
31. Add 500 μL of 70% ethanol to each pellet and centrifuge for 5 minutes *at 4°C.*
32. Using a 1000-μL pipettor (with blue tips) followed by a 200-μL pipettor (with yellow tips), carefully discard the supernatants.
33. Let the pellet air dry for 15 minutes in a horizontal position as in step 25.
34. Resuspend each pellet in 20 μL of ddH$_2$O.
35. Store at −20°C.

Yield: 5–30 μg of DNA per 1.5 mL of culture.

6.7   Analysis of Clones by Restricton Enzyme Digestion

This protocol is for digesting 2 μL of the purified plasmid DNA from section 6.6. First prepare the following Master Mixture and then distribute aliquots into the labeled tubes. A control consisting of only the vector should also be included.

Note: Equipment, materials, and reagents are as in section 6.2.1.

Restriction enzymes are very labile; remove from the − 20°C freezer only when necessary and for as short a time as possible. Maintain in a pre-cooled metal block on ice at all times.

1. Complete the following worksheet and label the microcentrifuge tubes that will be needed for each digestion.
2. The Master Mixture contains:

Each digestion	# of digestions + 1	Volume
1.5 μL of the Appropriate Buffer		_____ μL Buffer
XX μL Restriction Enzyme 1		_____ μL Enzyme 1
YY μL Restriction Enzyme 2		_____ μL Enzyme 2
ZZ μL ddH$_2$O		_____ μL ddH$_2$O
13 μL Total Volume		_____ μL Total Volume

3. Add the ingredients to the Master Mixture. Add the enzyme *last* and mix well.
4. Distribute 13 μL of the Master Mixture in each labeled tube. Keep on ice.
5. Add 2 μL of the purified DNA (or vector control) to each tube as appropriate and mix well.
6. Incubate the reactions for 2 hours in an air incubator or for 1 hour in a water bath at 37°C.
7. Add EDTA to a final concentration of 10 m*M* to stop the reaction.

6.8   Agarose Gel Electrophoresis

Note: Equipment, materials, and reagents are as in section 5.1.2.

A. *Gel Electrophoresis: **Black Area***

1. Prepare a 0.8% agarose gel in 1X TBE. Let the solution cool until it reaches ~55°C. Add 10 mg/mL ethidium bromide to a final concentration of 0.5 μg/mL (1/20,000 dilution). Prepare 1X TBE buffer with ethidium bromide at a final concentration of 0.5 μg/mL.

2. Prepare a Gel Chart showing the order of the samples in the gel (digested clones, digested vector, undigested vector).
3. Cover a microcentrifuge tube rack with a piece of Parafilm.® Make shallow wells in the Parafilm over the holes in the rack. With a permanent marker, label the wells with the number of the PCR reactions in the predetermined order
4. Transfer 3 µL of sample loading buffer to each well in the Parafilm.
5. Transfer 15 µL of each PCR reaction to the appropriately labeled well in the Parafilm and mix with the loading buffer.
6. Prepare 1 µg of the DNA size marker (λ/HindIII or l/BstEII) in 10 µL in one well.
7. Place the gel in the gel box and cover it with 1X TBE Running Buffer.
8. Load the entire volume of each sample into the wells in the gel in the predetermined order.
9. Run the gel at ~100 V until the bromophenol blue (dark blue dye) has migrated approximately 70–80% of the length of the gel.

B. Visualization: **Black Area/Darkroom**

Appropriate eye protection must be worn in the presence of UV light.

1. Place the gel on a UV transilluminator and turn the transilluminator on in order to visualize the DNA fragments, which should appear orange in color. Expose the gel to UV light for as short a time as possible, since the UV light nicks the DNA, gradually destroying it. UV light is dangerous to the viewer as well.
2. If no camera is available, manually draw the size of the observed bands on the Gel Chart.
3. If a camera is available, take a photograph using the UV transilluminator and the camera with an orange filter. A Polaroid camera with Polaroid 667 film is preferable; first try 1/2 second with a 5.6 or 8 aperture and adjust as necessary. If an instant Polaroid is not available, use a 35-mm camera with standard settings.
4. Dispose of the gel in an ethidium bromide solid waste container.
5. The TBE Running Buffer can be re-used a number of times (5–8 times).
6. To dispose of the ethidium bromide-containing Running Buffer or Staining Solution, the solution should be treated with activated charcoal (*see* section 5.1.2).

Note: Because ethidium bromide is light-sensitive, the ethidium bromide stock solution and Staining Solution should be stored in a dark place, in a dark bottle, or covered with aluminum foil.

References

Ausubel, F.M., Brent, R., Kingston, R.E., Moore, D.D., Seidman, J.G., Smith, J.A., and Struhl, K., eds. (1995) *Current Protocols in Molecular Biology.* New York, John Wiley and Sons, Inc.

Chung, C.T., and Miller, R.H. (1988) A rapid and convenient method for the preparation and storage of competent bacterial cells. *Nucleic Acids. Res.,* 16:3580.

Sambrook, J., Fritsch, E.F., and Maniatis, T. (1989) *Molecular Cloning: A Laboratory Manual.* New York, Cold Spring Harbor Laboratory Press.

Vogelstein, B., and Gillespie, D. (1979) Preparative and analytical purification of DNA from agarose. *Proc. Natl. Acad. Sci. USA,* 76:615–619.

Appendix A

Construction of Laboratory Equipment

The designs, assembly instructions, and photographs of equipment in this section were contributed by Nataniel Mamani and T. Guy Roberts.[1] One equipment design was contributed by John F. Kennedy.

A.1 Horizontal Shaker

This piece of equipment is used for gentle agitation of liquids (Figures A.1 and A.2); for example, incubating a colony blot in antibody solution or staining an agarose gel in ethidium bromide solution. Commercial models cost $750–$850.[2]

TOOLS REQUIRED
Drill
Drill bits
Wrenches
Screwdriver
Pliers
Hacksaw

MATERIALS
An old manual record player (without an automatic on/off switch)
6 X 2″ machine screws with three nuts each
1 X 1″ machine screw or bolt with two nylon washers, one metal washer, and one nut
1 X 1.5″ machine screw or bolt with one nut
Connecting arm: a heavy metal strip, ~3″ long and greater than 1/16″ or 1.5 mm thick

---

1. Nataniel Mamani has successfully built and operated each piece of equipment in his laboratory at the Center for Molecular Biology in the Faculty of Pure and Natural Sciences, Universidad Mayor de San Andres, La Paz, Bolivia. He can be reached at bionatrol@megalink.com. T. Guy Roberts is experienced in designing and building small equipment. He is currently at the University of California, Berkeley, and can be reached at tgrobo@uclink4.berkeley.edu. John Kennedy is a mechanical engineer with experience in designing appropriate technology for situations with material constraints.
2. Approximate prices for the equipment listed in this appendix were obtained from Fisher Scientific and are given in U.S. dollars.

Plastic or metal tray or metal baking pan

Four furniture castors (wheels)

2 X 26-cm-length metal brackets with a U-shaped cross section or curtain tracks (as shown in Figure A.1)

1″ of metal tubing with an inside diameter slightly greater than the machine screws listed above

1/2″ bolt that screws tightly into the metal tube

ASSEMBLY INSTRUCTIONS

Remove the dust cover and the arm/needle assembly from the record player. Remove the rubber cover of the record platen, and drill a hole in the platen 1″ or 2.5 cm from its center point to accommodate a 3/8″ or 0.5-cm bolt. Using the metal strip, make an arm to connect the platen of the record player to the tray by drilling a hole approximately 3/8″ from one end that is slightly larger than the diameter of the machine screws so that a screw can freely rotate in the hole.

To complete the connecting arm, drill another hole of the same diameter in the metal strip 2″ or 5 cm from the center of the first hole. Put the 1.5″ machine screw through one hole and fasten it in place with a nut (as shown in Figure A.1). Attach the arm to the record player by assembling the 1″ machine screw, nut, spacer, and nylon washers as shown in the diagram. It is important that the 1″ screw be tight enough to hold the metal arm level, but loose enough to allow the arm to pivot freely. Gently tighten the nut against the platen. This nut raises the arm above the platen to prevent it from scraping and prevents the assembly from becoming loose and falling off.

At each end of the metal brackets, drill a hole slightly larger than the 2″ machine screws. Using the holes in the brackets as guides, mark the top of the record player where the brackets will be attached. Be sure to separate the two brackets by less space than the width of the top tray. Drill holes in the top of the record player that are large enough to allow the machine screws to fit tightly. Put the screws through the holes in the brackets and loosely put two of the nuts on each screw. Attach the brackets to the record player top, driving the screws into the holes to the same depth (~3/8″ or 0.5 cm). Tighten one of the nuts against the top of the record player and the other against the brackets, so that the brackets are held rigidly over the top of the record player. If the top surface of the record player is removable, place an additional nut on the protruding end of each machine screw and tighten each nut against the underneath of the record player's top surface. This will allow the apparatus to support more weight.

Attach the castors to the base of the tray, making sure that the placement allows the tray to travel greater than 2″ (twice the distance from the center of the platen to the point of attachment of the arm). In order to attach the connecting arm to the tray, push the tray to one end of the brackets. Rotate the platen and pull the arm in the same direction as far as it will go. Mark the position of the arm's upright screw on the bottom of the tray. This will be the position of the metal tube that will fit over the upright screw. Drill a hole in the tray big enough for the 1/2″ bolt. Use the bolt to attach the tube to the bottom of the tray. Fit the arm's upright screw into the metal tube and place the tray's castors on the brackets. Depending on the size of the castors, the length of the upright screw may need to be longer or shorter to fit into the tube. Before use, and periodically, lubricate the joints, castors, and brackets with light oil.

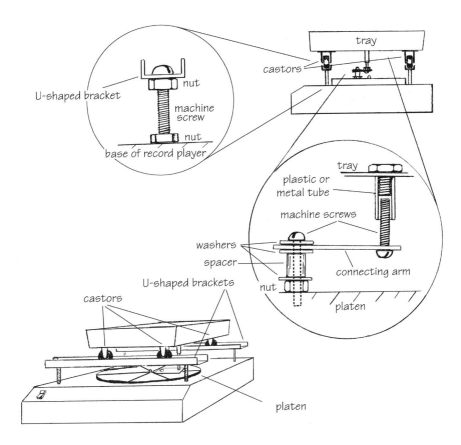

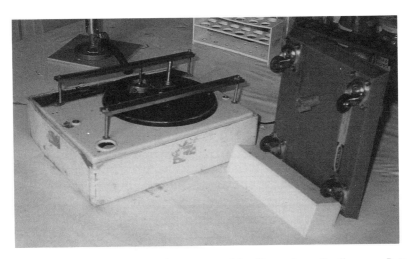

Fig. A.1. Horizontal shaker made from a turntable. *Top*, schematic diagram. *Bottom*, photograph.

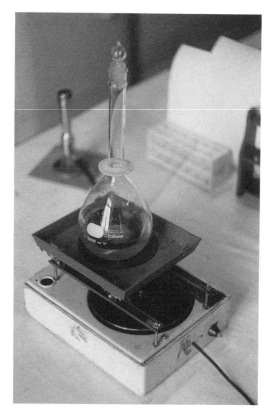

Fig. A.2. Photograph of horizontal shaker in use.

A.2   Pipet Tip Rinser

When recycling pipet tips, it is essential to completely remove the bleach and detergent used to clean the tips, since these substances can inhibit the amplification reaction. Pipet tips are often considered disposable; therefore, no commercial version of this equipment is available.

TOOLS REQUIRED
Drill
Drill bits
Pliers
Scissors

MATERIALS
Plastic bottle with a wide mouth and lid
Thin piece of rubber (cut from the inner tube of an automobile tire)
A container with a diameter greater than the lid of the bottle
A hose or surgical tubing and hose or tubing adaptor
Hose or tubing clamp
Radio or television antenna

ASSEMBLY INSTRUCTIONS

Attach the tubing adaptor to the side of the bottle near the base, and attach the tubing with the clamp. Cut a circular opening in the lid, leaving a rim of 1 cm around the edge. Cut a circle of rubber the same diameter as the inside of the lid. Make regularly spaced holes in the rubber with the metal sections from a radio or television antenna, using the section that matches most closely the size of the tip to be used (yellow or blue). Place tips of the appropriate size snugly in the holes in the rubber, assemble the lid as shown in Figure A.3, and secure the lid to the container. Attach the tube to a faucet and allow the bottle to fill and force water though the tips until they are well rinsed (Figure 3.1). Detergent may be added to the bottle before assembly to thoroughly wash the tips. Make sure that water flows through all the tips and eliminate the ones that are blocked by pushing them into the bottle. To reverse the flow of the water through the tips, submerge the bottle in a larger container and allow the tube to drop below the level of the bottle so that water siphons from the larger container, through the tips and out the tubing.

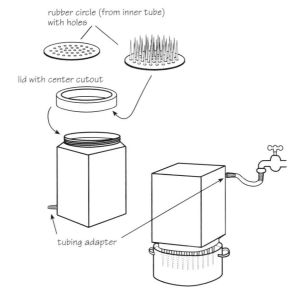

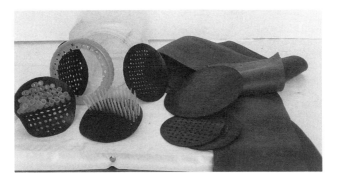

Fig. A.3. Pipet tip rinser assembly. *Top*, schematic diagram. *Bottom*, photograph.

A.3   Quick-Spin Centrifuge

This apparatus is used for quick centrifugations at fairly low speeds, e.g., for collecting liquids at the bottom of microcentrifuge tubes. Commercial models cost between $250 and $400.

TOOLS REQUIRED
Drill
Drill bits
Wrench
Screwdriver
Pliers
Ruler or tape measure
Right angles
Thread die

MATERIALS
Used kitchen blender
Small steel plate or bowl
Plastic faucet adaptors for a hose
Washers and nuts

ASSEMBLY INSTRUCTIONS
Cut the plastic rim from the motor base attached to the pitcher of the blender. This exposes the axle of the motor. Often the motor axle of the blender is threaded. If it is not, use a thread die or go to a metal worker to have threads cut in the axle.

Make the rotor out of a small steel bowl by finding the exact center of the bowl and marking the positions for the holes in the dish where the microcentrifuge tube adaptors will fit. Use a pair of carpenter's right angles to find opposing points on the rim of the bowl and measure across the bowl, marking the position halfway from rim to rim. Also mark the positions of the holes for the tubes by measuring the circumference of the bowl and dividing it by the number of tubes to be held by the rotor, an even number (8, 10, or 12 for a small bowl). The resulting number is the distance between marks made on the rim of the bowl. Measure 1 cm from each mark on the rim directly toward the center of the bowl. Punch a hole using a small, sharp nail, being careful not to create any dents in the bowl. Be precise in positioning the holes in order to insure that the rotor will be well balanced and safe to operate. Drill a hole at the center of the bowl of the same diameter as the motor axle. Drill holes along the rim of the bowl of the same diameter as the faucet adaptors.

Place the bowl, washer, and nut on the threaded axle and tighten the nut, making sure that the plate is centered on the axle. Place the faucet adaptors in the holes at the edge of the bowl (Figure A.4). These adaptors are good for 0.5-mL microcentrifuge tubes. Adapt the switch so that it only turns on while being pressed (not continuous).

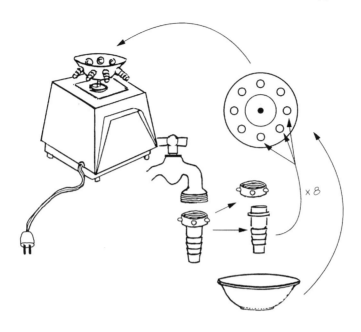

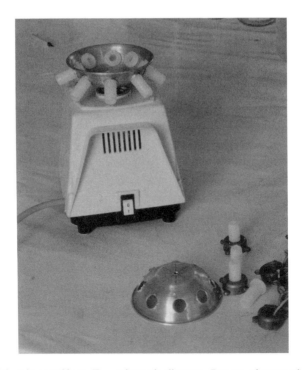

Fig. A.4. Quick-spin centrifuge. *Top*, schematic diagram. *Bottom*, photograph.

A.4   Blender Vortex Mixer

Vortex mixers are used to rapidly shake tubes in order to thoroughly mix their contents; they usually cost approximately $250.

TOOLS REQUIRED
Drill
Drill bits
Wrenches
Screwdriver

MATERIALS
Used kitchen blender (type with a plastic connecting plate)
Disk of plywood or thick plastic 1.5–2″ in diameter
Large rubber or plastic bottle lid
Machine screw (1/8″ or 3 mm diameter, 3/4″ or 2 cm long) with three nuts
Machine screw (equal in diameter to the screw holding the connecting plate on the blender, but 3/4″ or 7 mm longer)
Steel or nylon washers to fit the 1/8″ machine screws
Foam rubber (1″ thick, cut to fit inside the bottle cap)

ASSEMBLY INSTRUCTIONS
Remove the screw that attaches the connecting plate to the blender. Drill two 1/8″ holes in the wooden or plastic disk; one through the center of the disk and another 1/4″ (7 mm) from the center of the disk. Insert the screw that will attach the disk to the connecting plate through the center hole. Insert the 3/4″ machine screw through the off-center hole in the disk and secure it in place by tightening a nut against the disk. Attach the disk firmly to the connecting plate by tightening the central screw into the hole in the plate. Drill a 3/16″ hole in the center of the plastic bottle cap (slightly larger than the diameter of the machine screw, to allow the cap to freely rotate). Place a washer over the end of the machine screw, followed by the cap and another washer (see Figure A.5). Screw the nuts onto the machine screw until they hold the bottle cap in place, yet allow it to rotate freely. Tighten the two nuts securely against one another to prevent the cap from loosening during operation of the blender. Insert the foam rubber into the cap so that it prevents the test tubes from contacting the machine screw/nut assembly.

Note: Be careful not to place too much pressure on the microcentrifuge tubes while holding it in the vortex mixer. This could damage the vortex mixer and cause the vortex assembly to become loose.

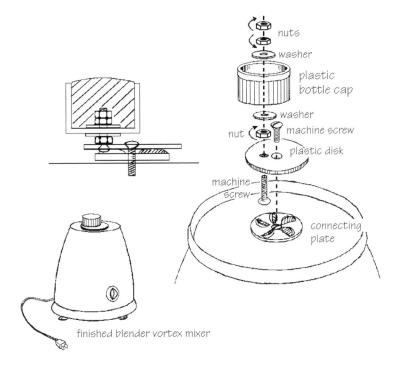

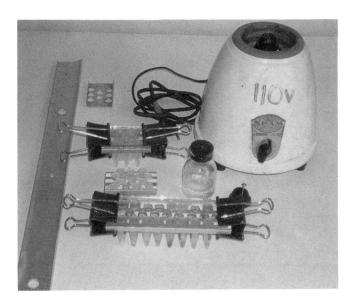

Fig. A.5. Vortex mixer made from a blender. *Top*, schematic diagram. *Bottom*, photograph.

A.5   Water Bath

General-purpose water baths can be used for incubating tubes or flasks of solutions at at a variety of temperatures. They range in cost from approximately $400 to $1000 dollars.

TOOLS REQUIRED
Sharp knife
Scissors
Metal borer

MATERIAL
Fish tank heater with thermostat
Silicone rubber sealant or glue that is flexible when set
Rubber adaptor/seal rings
Water container (plastic tub or pitcher or deep metal baking pan)
Styrofoam or foam rubber
Adhesive plastic sheets (drawer liner material)

ASSEMBLY INSTRUCTIONS
Select rubber adaptors that are large enough to slide tightly over the glass tube of the fish tank heater. Cut a hole in the side of the container (below the level of the water line) that has a diameter slightly smaller than the rubber adaptor (when on the heater). Use sandpaper to smooth the edges of the hole in the container.

Slide the rubber adaptor all the way up the heater tube. Apply a ring of glue around the rubber adaptor and insert the heater/adaptor into the hole in the container until the glue forms a seal between the adaptor and the container (Figure A.6). Allow the glue to set completely. In order to insulate the container, cut the foam rubber or styrofoam to make a box that fits it tightly. Completely cover the entire insulation box with the adhesive plastic material to protect it from abrasion. Seal the top of the insulation box with glue to prevent water from getting between the insulation and the container.

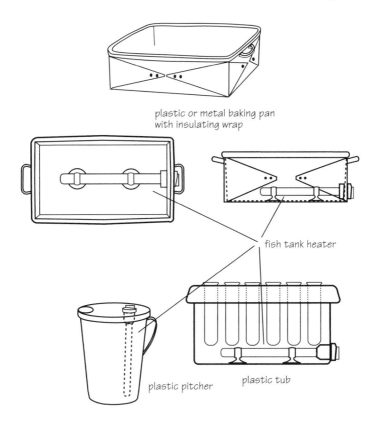

plastic or metal baking pan
with insulating wrap

fish tank heater

plastic pitcher   plastic tub

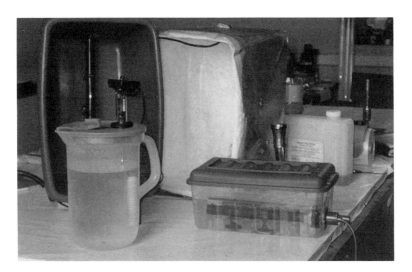

Fig. A.6. Assembled water baths. *Top*, schematic diagram. *Bottom*, photograph.

A.6   Ultraviolet Transilluminator

UV transilluminators are used to visualize ethidium bromide-stained nucleic acids, often after gel electrophoresis. Commercial models range in cost from $1300 to $2000.

EQUIPMENT REQUIRED
Saw
Hammer
Wire crimper
Sheet metal cutter
Wrenches
Screwdriver
Pliers

MATERIALS
Wooden boards
Metal sheet
Nails
2 mirrors (10 X 46 cm)
1 mirror (12 X 38 cm)
UV filter
Heavy adhesive tape
Double-sided adhesive tape
Fluorescent light fixtures
Electrical wire
Heavy-gauge insulated copper wire for internal wiring
Power cord with plug
UV tubular flourescent light bulbs (305-nm wavelength)
Black silicone rubber sealer

ASSEMBLY INSTRUCTIONS
Construct an open wooden box of the following dimensions: 12 X 31 X 49 cm. On the inside of the shorter (31-cm) sides of box, attach small pieces of wood that will serve as a support to hold the sockets of the UV tubes. Cut a piece of wood 1 cm thick and 4–15 cm wide, whose length is exactly equal to the inside width of the box. This will be the crosspiece that supports the mirrors. With the box lying on a flat surface, set the crosspiece across the center of the bottom of the box so that it connects the two longer (49 cm) sides of the box (Figure A.7). Secure the crosspiece in place with nails. The UV light fixtures should be attached to the short sides of the box so that the tubular bulbs will be positioned lengthwise in the center of the box, 1.5–2 cm below the upper edge of the box.

Connect the electric circuit for the light fixtures according to the type of bulb fixture available (ballast built into the fixture vs. ballast wired separately in the circuit). If using separate ballasts, mount them on the long sides above the crosspiece and wire one ballast to each light fixture (generally diagrammed on the ballast). Cut a small hole in one of the short sides of the box (0.5-cm diameter) for the power cord to pass through. Wire a single power cord to the circuit so that it provides power to both sockets. Cut a small hole (1-cm diameter) in one of the long sides of the box for the electrical switch. Attach the switch to the outside of the box and wire the power cord through the inside of the box to the switch.

Attach the central mirror (12 X 38 cm) to the wooden crosspiece lengthwise beneath the tubes using double-sided adhesive tape. Place the side mirrors (10 X 46 cm) in the box with one long edge adjacent to the central mirror and the other long edge against the the side of the box, so that the side mirrors are inclined and will reflect the light from the tubes to the center of the top of the box. From the bottom side of the box attach each side mirror to the central mirror and to the side of the box with strips of adhesive tape along the connecting edges of the mirrors.

From a metal (or wood) sheet, make a snugly fitting cover for the box. In the center of the cover, cut a hole to accommodate the UV filter (Figure A.7). Leave tabs in the metal that can be bent to hold the filter in place. Be sure that UV light cannot escape unfiltered from the box. Use black silicone sealer to fill any cracks that allow light to pass through.

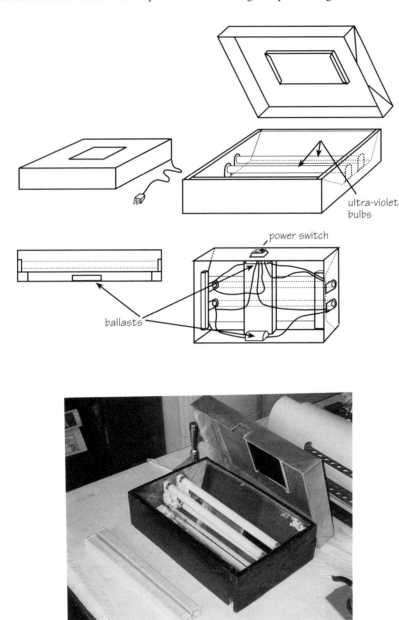

Fig. A.7. UV transilluminator. *Top*, schematic diagram. *Bottom*, photograph.

A.7   Horizontal Gel Electrophoresis Box

Horizontal gel boxes are used for electrophoresis of nucleic acids in agarose gels. Numerous commercially available models of this apparatus are available and range in cost from $250 to $500 depending on the size and the manufacturer.

Gel Box Model 1:

TOOLS REQUIRED
Table saw
Drill
Drill bits
Pliers
Heat sealer (for plastic bags)
Sanding block of 2 X 4″ wood (should be at least 1/2 the length of the finished box)
Shop clamp
T-square

MATERIALS
Acrylic sheet, at least 3/8″ in thickness
Acrylic glue
Silicone cement
Acrylic tubing (approximately 1/4″ diameter: 4 pieces, each 3/8″ long for use as guides for the electrodes)
Platinum wire (30 or 32 gauge; 0.013″ diameter)
Copper wire
Connector posts and complementary jacks *or* brass bolts and plastic-shielded alligator clips
Brass bolts of 1/8″ or 2.5 mm diameter
Electrical leads
Electrical tape or heat-shrink tubing

ASSEMBLY INSTRUCTIONS
Cut the acrylic sheet into three pieces (two side pieces and the full length of the center section with dimensions as shown in Figure A.8), and mark the lines across the sheet where it is to be folded. If a heat sealer is available, carefully heat the acrylic along each line with the bag sealer. While the sheet is very hot, fold it as shown in the diagram (along the dotted lines), making sure that the folds are precisely parallel to one another. Use the sanding block to flatten the edges so that the side pieces will fit evenly. Set the folded center piece upside down and clamp the side pieces to the center piece as shown. Apply glue evenly along the seams between the center and side pieces and allow to dry. Turn the box over and apply glue to the inside seams and allow to dry. Glue the pieces of acrylic tube in the buffer reservoirs as shown in Figure A.8.

At each end of the gel box, mark the position of the holes for the small brass bolts that will form the points for attaching the electrical leads. These holes should be ~1 cm from the top edge of each end of the box. Drill the holes through the box to fit the small brass bolts; the holes can be slightly larger than the bolts, since the acrylic is brittle and will crack if the holes are too small. For each electrode, put one end of the wire through the hole and bend it down. Screw the connector post or bolt into the hole over the electrode wire to fasten it in place. Cover the inner hole with a blob of silicone cement. It is only necessary to use platinum wire for the positive electrode (anode); the other electrode can be made from copper wire. Run the electrode wires through the two short tubes at each end. Double the wire back around the second tube and twist it around itself to hold it in place as shown in Figure A.9.

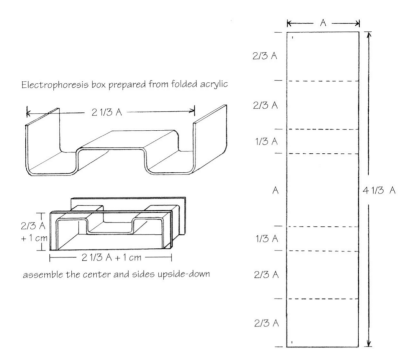

Electrophoresis box prepared from folded acrylic

2 1/3 A

2/3 A
+ 1 cm

2 1/3 A + 1 cm

assemble the center and sides upside-down

A

2/3 A

2/3 A

1/3 A

A

4 1/3 A

1/3 A

2/3 A

2/3 A

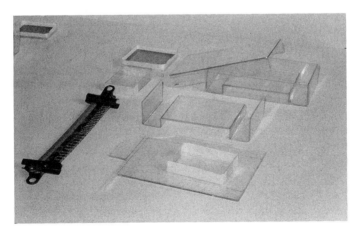

Fig. A.8. Horizontal gel electrophoresis box Model 1. *Top*, schematic diagram. *Bottom*, photograph.

Gel Box Model 2: (Contributed by John F. Kennedy)

TOOLS REQUIRED
Table saw or jigsaw
Drill
Soldering iron
Thread tap, if available

MATERIAL
Lucite or acrylic (3/16–1/4″ thick for all pieces except A and D; 1/2″ for A and D)
Acrylic tubing (approximately 1/4″ diameter: 4 pieces, each 3/8″ long for use as guides for the
    electrodes)
Acrylic glue or epoxy
Silicone cement
Platinum wire (30 or 32 gauge; 0.013″ diameter)
Connector posts and complementary jacks *or* brass bolts and plastic-shielded alligator clips
Electrical leads
Electrical tape or heat-shrink tubing

ASSEMBLY INSTRUCTIONS
Select the dimensions of the box to be constructed by using Table A.1 as a guide. Cut the
acrylic to size using a table saw or jigsaw. It is critical that the edges be smooth and that the
pieces be cut precisely to size to avoid leakage. Drill holes for electrodes and connectors in
pieces A and D according to Figure A.10. If possible, cut threads in the larger hole to match
the threads on the brass bolt or connector post. If unable to cut thread with a tap in the larger
hole, make sure that the diameter of the larger hole is the same size as the diameter of the
threaded bolt; use the bolt to pre-thread the hole prior to assembly.

Assemble the box, clamping all of the pieces together on a flat surface so that all joints are
square. Lay a bead of epoxy or acrylic glue on the inside corner of each joint and allow to set
as recommended by the glue manufacturer. Glue the acrylic tubing into place as shown in the
diagram.

After the glue is set, lead the platinum wire through the narrow hole to the outside of the
box. Allow the wire to protrude from the hole 1/8″. Apply silicone glue from the outside of
the large diameter hole in order to seal the small-diameter hole. Fill the hole until glue is
forced out the small-diameter hole, with the platinum wire in place. Before the silicone glue
sets, screw the brass bolt or connector post into the large-diameter hole over the platinum wire
at least 1/4″ (Figure A.9). Wipe off excess glue from the inside of the box and allow to dry for
the recommended period of time. Once the silicone glue is set, lead the platinum wire down
to the acrylic tubing below the connector, through this acrylic tubing and across the bottom of
the box to the second tubing, then loop the wire back and wrap it around itself to secure it.
Trim excess wire. Strip the wire of the electrical leads to clear 2 cm. Lead the wire through
the hole on the complementary jack or alligator clip and wrap it around itself to secure it. It
is recommended that this connection be soldered to avoid sparking. Wrap exposed wire with
electrical tape.

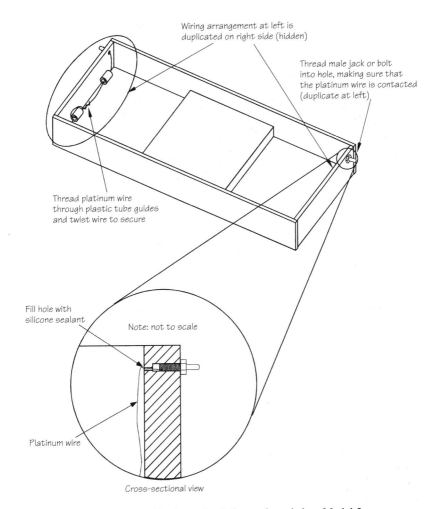

Wiring arrangement at left is
duplicated on right side (hidden)

Thread male jack or bolt
into hole, making sure that
the platinum wire is contacted
(duplicate at left)

Thread platinum wire
through plastic tube guides
and twist wire to secure

Fill hole with
silicone sealant

Note: not to scale

Platinum wire

Cross-sectional view

Fig. A.9. Schematic diagram of horizontal gel electrophoresis box Model 2.

Table A.1. Dimensions of Model 2 gel electrophoresis box components.

Component	Height	Width
B and C	2/3 X*	2 1/3 X + 1 cm
A and D	2/3 X	X
G	X	X
E and I	2/3 X	X
F and H	1/3 X	X

*X should be between 8 and 20 cm

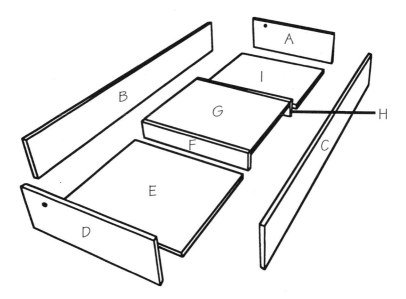

Fig. A.10. Exploded view of horizontal gel electrophoresis box Model 2.

Gel Trays

TOOLS REQUIRED
Table saw
Clamp

MATERIALS
Acrylic sheet, at least 3/8″ in thickness
Acrylic glue
Square plastic Petri plates

ASSEMBLY INSTRUCTIONS

Petri Plate Gel Tray
Use the square Petri plates for casting trays; this plastic allows UV to pass through for direct viewing of ethidium bromide-stained DNA bands. Cut opposing edges off of the Petri plates and place tape over the openings when casting gels.

Standard Gel Tray
More permanent casting trays can be made from acrylic sheet of the same type as used for the electrophoresis box, or thinner. Cut a rectangular piece with the same dimensions as the gel platform (middle section) of the electrophoresis box. Use the sanding block to shave about 3 mm from one side of the rectangle to allow it to fit loosely into the box and lie on the gel platform. Cut four side pieces from acrylic that are the length of the gel platform. The width of these pieces should be greater by a few millimeters than the depth of the gel platform (distance from the top edge of the box to the gel platform). The tray can be assembled as shown (Figure A.11) inside the electrophoresis box if the box is first lined with waxed paper.

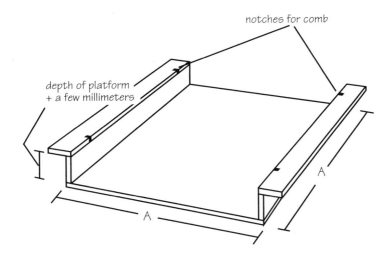

Fig. A.11. Schematic diagram of standard gel tray.

Combs

TOOLS REQUIRED
Table saw
Fine-toothed handsaw
Hammer
Razor blade

MATERIALS
Stiff plastic sheet (Teflon, nylon, PVC or acrylic) of 1/16–1/8″ or 2–3 mm
Block of wood 2″ X 4″ X 8″
Strip of wood 8″ X 2″ X <1″
Several heavy nails (1/8″ or 2 mm in diameter)
Plastic rulers

ASSEMBLY INSTRUCTIONS

Ruler Combs
Combs can be made from flat plastic rulers, using the markings as guides to cut the wells
evenly. Leave at least 2 mm between wells.

Standard Combs
Cut several rectangles from the plastic sheet with a width that is at least 1 cm greater than the
depth of the gel tray and with a length that is a few millimeters shorter than the inside width
of the gel tray. Prepare the jig for cutting the combs from the wood as shown in Figure A.12.
The guide strip is a wooden strip nailed to the block at a distance from the edge that is the
width of the plastic rectangles. The slot in the block is ~1/8″ wide (2 mm) and 3/4″ deep
(1.5–2 cm). The guide post is a nail that is spaced from the slot by the desired width of the

wells. Slide a plastic rectangle against the guides and make the first cut. It may be necessary to make two cuts in order to make the space between the comb's teeth the same as the full width of the slot (1/8″). Lift the plastic and set the first space over the guide post, then cut the next space. Repeat the process until all the spaces are cut to form the teeth of the comb.

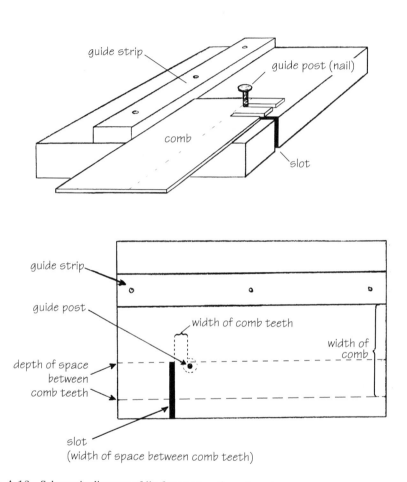

Fig. A.12. Schematic diagram of jig for construction of combs.

Appendix B

In-House Preparation of Reagents

B.1 Useful Formulas

General rules:

1. The following formulas can be used to calculate the volume (V_i) of a concentrated stock solution at an initial concentration (C_i) required to prepare a final volume (V_f) at the desired final concentration (C_f):

Version 1:

$$V_f \cdot C_f = V_i \cdot C_i$$

$$V_i = \frac{V_f \cdot C_f}{C_i}$$

Version 2:

$$\frac{C_i}{C_f} = \text{Dilution Factor (DF)} \qquad\qquad V_f = \frac{V_i}{DF}$$

Ex. What volume of a 1 M MgCl$_2$ stock is needed to prepare 100 mL of a 15 mM MgCl$_2$ solution?

$C_i = 1\ M = 1000\ \text{m}M$
$C_f = 15\ \text{m}M$
$V_f = 100\ \text{mL}$

Version 1:

$$x = V_i = \frac{V_f \cdot C_f}{C_i} = \frac{100 \cdot 15}{1000} = 1.5\ \text{mL}$$

Version 2:

$$DF = \frac{1000\ \text{m}M}{15\ \text{m}M} = 66.67 \qquad \frac{100\ \text{mL}}{66.67} = V_i = x \qquad x = 1.5\ \text{mL}$$

243

2. Solutions can be described in molarity or percentage:

Molarity:

$$1M = \frac{1 \text{ mole}}{L} \qquad 1 \text{ mole} = \frac{1 \text{ gram}}{\text{mol.wt.}} \qquad 1M = \frac{1 \text{ gram}}{\text{mol.wt.} \cdot L}$$

Percentage can refer to either weight/volume (w/v) or volume/volume (v/v):

$$1\%(\text{w/v}) = \frac{1 \text{ gram}}{100 \text{ mL}} \qquad\qquad 1\% \text{ (v/v)} = \frac{1 \text{ mL}}{100 \text{ mL}}$$

3. The following method can be used to calculate the cellular equivalents of a given amount of purified DNA or vice versa.

where

    g = g of DNA
   gen = size of organism's genome in base pairs
    A = Avogadro's number (6.02×10^{23})
# of org = number of single-cell organisms (e.g. bacteria, parasites)
   660 = the average molecular weight of a base pair (330 = the average molecular weight of single nucleotide)

$$\frac{g \cdot A}{gen \cdot 660} = \text{\# of org}$$

Ex. 1. How many *Leishmania* parasites (x) (8×10^7 bp per diploid genome) are represented by 1 pg of purified genomic DNA?

$$\frac{g \cdot A}{gen \cdot 660} = x \text{ organisms (parasites)}$$

$$\frac{(1 \times 10^{-12} \text{ g}) \cdot (6.02 \times 10^{23})}{(8 \times 10^7 \text{ bp}) \cdot 660} = x \text{ parasites}$$

$$x = 11.4 \text{ parasites}$$

Ex. 2. What amount of genomic DNA (x) represents 100 mycobacteria (2.75×10^6 base pairs per genome of *Mycobacterium tuberculosis*)?

$$\frac{x g \cdot A}{gen \cdot 660} = \text{\# of organisms (mycobacteria)}$$

$$\frac{x g \cdot (6.02 \times 10^{23})}{(2.75 \times 10^6 \text{ bp}) \cdot 660} = 100 \text{ mycobacteria}$$

$$x = 3 \times 10^{-13} \text{ g} = 300 \text{ fg}$$

4. The amount of an oligonucleotide or DNA can be described in terms of units of optical density (OD), or absorbance, usually measured at 260 nm (OD_{260}) in a spectrophotometer. 1 OD_{260} corresponds to the amount of the oligonucleotide or DNA in a volume of 1 mL, measured in a cuvette with a 1-cm path length at 260 nm, according to the following formula:

$$A = \varepsilon \cdot C \cdot L$$

where

A = absorbance, or OD
ε = the extinction coefficient (see below)
C = the concentration of the oligonucleotide in the solution, in μmol/mL
L = the path length of the cuvette, in centimeters

The extinction coefficient (ε) of an oligonucleotide can be calculated by multiplying the number of times each base is present by the extinction coefficient of each base, using the following values:

ε of dATP = 15.4 mL/μmol
ε of dCTP = 7.3 mL/μmol
ε of dGTP = 11.7 mL/μmol
ε of dTTP = 8.8 mL/μmol

Oligonucleotide sequence: CATGTTCATTGACTGGCTAG (4 X A; 4 X C; 5 X G; 7 X T)
ε of oligonucleotide = (4 X 15.4) + (4 X 7.3) + (5 X 11.7) + (7 X 8.8)
= 61.6 + 29.2 + 58.5 + 61.6 = 210.9 mL/μmol

A more approximate estimation can be derived as follows (Sambrook et al., 1989):

$$\frac{\text{total } OD_{260}}{10 \text{ X length of the oligonucleotide}} = \mu\text{mol/mL of the oligonuncleotide in the solution}$$

As a rule of thumb, an OD_{260} of 1 corresponds to approximately 33 μg/mL of single-stranded oligonucleotide or 50 μg/mL of double-stranded DNA.

B.2   Solutions

DNA/RNA Extraction

Diethyl Pyrocarbonate (DEPC)[3]-Treated Water
Carefully open the bottle of DEPC in a chemical fume hood.
Add 1 mL DEPC to 1 L of ddH$_2$0 in an Erlenmeyer flask.
Leave overnight mixing on a magnetic stirrer.
Autoclave to eliminate the DEPC.

Note: DEPC is highly toxic and carcinogenic. Wear gloves and face protection, and carry out manipulations in a chemical fume hood. Once the bottle is opened, DEPC rapidly becomes oxidized and loses activity; therefore DEPC should be purchased in small volumes and used within a month of opening the bottle.

RNA GITC Lysis Buffer

GITC	6 M (guanidine isothiocyanate)
Sodium citrate	50 mM
Sarkosyl	1%
tARN	20 µg/mL (yeast or *E. coli* tRNA, if not available use glycogen)
β-mercaptoethanol	100 mM (add immediately before use)

Guanidine Lysis Buffer (DNA/Whole Blood)

Guanidine HCl	6 M
EDTA	0.2 M

L6 Lysis Buffer

GITC	8 M
Tris-HCl, pH 6.4	100 mM
EDTA, pH 8.0	36 mM
Triton® X-100	0.2%
Do not autoclave	

L2 Washing Buffer

GITC	10 M
Tris-HCl, pH 6.4	100 mM
Do not autoclave	

Note: The solutions above contain high concentrations of guanidine isothiocyanate (GITC) or guanidine hydrochloride; thus, the chemical powder occupies a significant volume. The GITC or guanidine HCl should be added to a minimal volume of ddH$_2$O so as not to exceed the final volume of the solution. Low heat may be necessary for the GITC to dissolve completely. Dissolve the guanidine completely before adding the other ingredients of the solution. Do not autoclave these solutions.

---

3. DEPC inactivates RNases.

Dried Blood Spots (Filter Paper)[4]

EDTA	50 mM
SDS	1%
DTT	5 mM
Spermidine	0.5 mM

Adjust to volume with ddH$_2$0

Chelex® 100

Chelex® 100*	5%

Adjust to volume with ddH$_2$0

*Chelex® 100 resin, biotechnology grade, sodium form, 100–200 dry-mesh size, wet bead size (μm) 150-300 (Bio-Rad Laboratories, Richmond, CA, catalog #143-2832).

Saponin Lysis Buffer

NaCl	0.22%
Saponin	0.015%
EDTA	1 mM

NET Lysis Buffer

Tris-HCl, pH 8.0	100 mM
NaCl	400 mM
EDTA	10 mM

1 L 1X PBS, pH 7.4

To 800 mL ddH$_2$O in a 1 L beaker, add:

NaCl	8 g
KCl	0.2 g
Na$_2$HPO$_4$	1.44 g
KH$_2$PO$_4$	0.24 g

Adjust the final volume to 1L with ddH$_2$O

Autoclave

Phenol (Water-saturated)

1. Incubate an unopened bottle of phenol crystals in a 50°C water bath just until the crystals melt. Be sure not to leave the phenol in the water bath after the crystals melt.
2. Add an equal volume of RNase-free distilled water and mix well.
3. Allow the two phases to separate. Remove the aqueous phase and discard.
4. Add 0.1% 8-hydroxyquinoline to the phenol to prevent oxidation. The yellow color imparted to the phenol by the hydroxyquinoline also makes it easier to identify the organic layer during extractions.
5. Add 1/5 volume of RNase-free distilled water to form a layer over the phenol phase.
6. Store at 4°C.

---

4. M. Harvey, personal communication.

Phenol (Tris-equilibrated, pH 8.0)
1. Incubate an unopened bottle of phenol crystals in a 50°C water bath just until the crystals melt. Be sure not to leave the phenol in the water bath after the crystals melt.
2. Add an equal volume of $1M$ Tris-HCl (pH 8.0) and mix well.
3. Allow the two phases to separate. Remove the aqueous phase and discard.
4. Check the pH of the aqueous phase.
5. Repeat steps 2–4 until the pH of the aqueous phase is 8.0.
6. Remove the aqueous phase and discard.
7. Add 0.1% hydroxyquinoline to prevent oxidation. The yellow color imparted to the phenol by the hydroxyquinoline also makes it easier to identify the organic layer during extractions.
8. Add 1/5 volume Tris-EDTA (pH 8.0) to form a layer over the phenol phase.
9. Store at 4°C.

Media

Cary-Blair Transport Medium

Sodium thioglycolate	1.5 g
Disodium phosphate	1.1 g
Sodium chloride	5.0 g
Agar	5.0 g
ddH$_2$O	991.0 mL

1. Mix all the ingredients and heat with agitation until the solution becomes clear.
2. Cool to 50°C, add 9 mL of freshly prepared 1% CaCl$_2$, and adjust the pH to approximately 8.4.
3. Dispense 7 mL of the solution into previously rinsed and sterilized 9-mL screw-capped vials.
4. Steam vials for 15 minutes, cool, and tighten caps.

Alkaline Peptone Water

Peptone	10 g
NaCl	5 g
ddH$_2$O	1 L

Adjust final pH to 8.4.
Autoclave for 20 minutes at 121°C.

MacFarland's Standard 05
1. Dissolve 1.175 g of barium chloride dihydrate in 100 mL of ddH$_2$O.
2. Dilute 1 mL of sulfuric acid in 100 mL of ddH$_2$O.
3. Add 0.5 mL of the barium chloride solution to 99.5 mL of the sulfuric acid solution.

Cox Medium

Tryptose phosphate	2 g (or trypticase)
Agar	10 g

1. Dissolve 2 g of tryptose phosphate (or trypticase) and 10 g of agar in 900 mL of ddH$_2$O (pH 7.4).
2. Autoclave at 121°C for 15 minutes and let cool to 50°C.
3. Add 100 mL (10%) of rabbit serum.
4. Distribute in sterile Petri plates (30 mL/plate).

Amplification Reactions

10X Buffer A (Promega Corp.)
Tris-HCl, pH 9.0	100 mM
KCl	500 mM
Triton® X-100	1%

10X Buffer B (Perkin-Elmer Corp.)
Tris-HCl, pH 8.3	100 mM
KCl	500 mM

10X Dengue RAV-2 RT-PCR Buffer
KCl	500 mM
Tris, pH 8.5	100 mM
$MgCl_2$	15 mM
Gelatin	0.1%

Note: If the *Taq* polymerase being used does not contain detergent in its storage buffer, it is necessary to add detergent (1% Triton X-100) to the 10X PCR buffer, for a final concentration of 0.1% Triton X-100 in the PCR reactions (e.g., Buffer A).

dNTPs (nucleotides)
dATP	5 mM
dCTP	5 mM
dGTP	5 mM
dTTP	5 mM
dNTPs	20 mM total

RAV-2 Reverse Transcriptase Storage Buffer
Potassium phosphate	200 mM
DTT	2 mM
Nonidet P-40	0.2%
Glycerol	50%

Final pH should be 7.2.

Gel Electrophoresis

10X Tris Borate EDTA (TBE) Running Buffer
Tris base	108 g
Boric acid	55 g
EDTA	7.44 g (or 40 mL 0.5 M EDTA, pH 8.0)
ddH_2O	to 1 L

10X Tris Acetate EDTA (TAE) Running Buffer*
Tris base	24.2 g
Glacial acetic acid	5.71 mL
0.5 *M* EDTA, pH 8.0	10 mL
ddH_2O	to 500 mL

*for purifying DNA from agarose gels using silica particles

Sample Loading Buffer (Agarose Gels)

Glycerol	50%
EDTA	20 mM
Bromophenol blue	0.1%
Xylene cyanol	0.1%
ddH$_2$0	to volume

Cloning

Tris-EDTA (TE)

Tris-HCl, pH 8.0	10 mM
EDTA, pH 8.0	1 mM

Sodium-Ethanol Wash[5]

Tris-HCl, pH 7.4	10 mM
NaCl	50 mM
EDTA	0.5 mM
Ethanol (absolute)	50%
ddH$_2$O	to volume

Sodium Iodide

Na$_2$SO$_3$	0.75 g dissolved in 40 mL ddH$_2$O
NaI	45 g (6 M)

Stir until dissolved.
Filter through Whatman paper or nitrocellulose; store 3–4 months in the dark.
Discard if a precipitate is observed.

Luria Broth (LB)

Tryptone	10 g
Yeast extract	5 g
Sodium chloride	10 g
ddH$_2$0	to 1 L

Adjust pH to 7.5 with NaOH.
Autoclave.

LB-Amp Plates

Tryptone	10 g
Yeast extract	5 g
Sodium chloride	10 g
Agar	20 g
ddH$_2$0	to 1 L

Adjust pH to 7.5 with NaOH.
Autoclave.

When the solution cools to ~55°C, add 1 mL of ampicillin (100 mg/mL).
Pour ~25 mL per 100 X 15 mm Petri plate and allow to dry.

---

5. Commercially available as NEW wash.

Transformation and Storage Buffer (TSB)
LB	83 mL
PEG-3350	10 g (10% final concentration of polyethylene glycol, MW 3350)
DMSO	5 mL (5% final concentration of dimethyl sulfoxide)
$MgCl_2$	1 mL of a 1 M stock (10 mM final concentration)
$MgSO_4$	1 mL of a 1 M stock (10 mM final concentration)

IPTG (Isopropyl β-D-thiogalactopyranoside)
IPTG	20 mg (200 mg/mL final concentration)
ddH_2O	100 μL

X-Gal (5-Bromo-4-chloro-3-indolyl-β-D-galactopyranoside)
X-Gal	20 mg (20 mg/mL final concentration in dimethyl formamide)
DMF	1 mL

GTE Buffer
Glucose	50 mM
Tris, pH 8.0	25 mM
EDTA, pH 8.0	10 mM

TB
Prepare Solution A with
Tryptone	12 g
Yeast extract	24 g
Glycerol	4.0 mL (= 5.0 g)
dd$H_2$0	to 900 mL

Sterilize by autoclave.

Prepare Solution B (sterile) with
KH_2PO_4	0.17 M
K_2HPO_4	0.72 M
dd$H_2$0	to 100 mL

After Solution A cools, combine Solutions A and B using sterile technique.

Nonradioactive DNA Probes

20X SSC
NaCl	3 M
sodium citrate	300 mM
pH 7.0	

Buffer 1
Tris-HCl, pH 7.5	100 mM
NaCl	150 mM

Buffer 2
Nonfat milk powder 5% in Buffer 1

Buffer 3

Tris-HCl, pH 9.5	100 mM
NaCl	100 mM
MgCl$_2$	50 mM

Pre-hybridization Solution

SSC	5X
Blocking Reagent	1% (Boehringer Mannheim)
Sarkosyl	0.1%
SDS	0.02%

Note: The Blocking Reagent doesn't dissolve easily; therefore, the solution must be heated to 50–70°C for 1 hour.

Mix 250 mL of 20X SSC, 10 g of Blocking Reagent, 10 mL of 10% Sarkosyl and 2 mL of 10% SDS at 10%. Bring the volume to 1 L with ddH$_2$O and freeze aliquots of 100 mL at −20°C.

Washing Solution

SSC	1X
SDS	0.1%

B.3   Preparation of Selected Reagents

Silica particles [6]
1. Resuspend 100 g of powdered glass (325 mesh) in 100 mL distilled water using a magnetic stir plate. Stir for 1 hour.
2. Turn off the stir plate and let the slurry settle for 1 hour.
3. Pipet off the supernatant and distribute it into two 50-mL plastic centrifuge tubes.
4. Centrifuge the tubes at 3000 rpm for 3 minutes.
5. Discard the supernatant.
6. Resuspend each pellet in 50 mL RNase-free ddH$_2$O and transfer to a sterile 500-mL Erlenmeyer flask with a magnetic stir bar.
7. Add 50 mL of fuming HNO$_3$.
8. In a **chemical hood**, bring the suspension to a gentle boil on a hot plate for 1 minute with constant stirring.
9. Allow solution to cool to ambient temperature.
10. Transfer the suspension to four 50-mL plastic centrifuge tubes (if re-using the tubes, wash them extensively and then autoclave).
11. Centrifuge the tubes at 3000 rpm for 5 minutes and discard the supernatant.
12. Resuspend each pellet of powdered glass in 50 mL RNase-free ddH$_2$O (pH 7.0). It may require vigorous vortexing to resuspend the pellet.
13. Repeat steps 11 and 12 four times.
14. Check the pH of the solution.
15. Repeat steps 11 and 12 until the pH is the same as the water (~pH 7.0).
16. Add RNase-free ddH$_2$O to the pellet of powdered glass to make a 50% vol/vol slurry mixture.
17. Store the suspension at 4°C until use.

Yield: Approximately 8 g of activated silica particles (16 mL of 50% vol/vol slurry).

Notes: It is convenient to aliquot the slurry of silica particles in 1.5-mL microcentrifuge tubes.

Glycogen (Molecular Biology Grade)
1. Resuspend 1 g of chemical grade glycogen power in ddH$_2$O to a final concentration of 100 mg/mL in a 50-mL polypropylene tube.
2. Add an equal volume of phenol/chloroform (1:1), vortex thoroughly, and centrifuge at 3000g for 10 minutes.
3. Transfer the aqueous (upper) phase to a new tube and repeat step 2.
4. Transfer the aqueous upper phase to a centifuge tube.
5. Add 1/10 volume sodium acetate (pH 5.2) and 2.5 volumes of 100% ethanol.
6. Centrifuge at 12,000g for 20 minutes at 4°C.
7. Discard the supernatant.
8. Wash the pellet with 5 mL of 70% ethanol.
9. Air dry for several hours.
10. Resuspend in ddH$_2$O to a final concentrarion of 10 mg/mL.
11. Store at −20°C.

---

6. Adapted from Vogelstein and Gillespie (1979); J. Coloma, personal communication.

Wax Beads

1. Cut Parafilm® into strips.
2. Melt the Parafilm strips in a sterile glass beaker over low heat.
3. Using a 200-μL pipettor, pipet 50 μL of the melted wax and drip onto a clean surface (e.g., piece of Parafilm) so that uniform beads are formed.
4. Transfer solidified beads into plastic tubes for storage using a clean spatula.

B.4   DNA Size Markers

1. Purchase or prepare DNA from bacteriophage λ, phage φX174, or plasmid pBR322.
2. Prepare a restriction endonuclease digestion of 1 μg of λ DNA with either *Hind*III or *BstE*II or of φX174 DNA with *Hae*III or of pBR322 with *Msp*I (see sizes of resulting fragments below).
3. Prepare a working dilution of the markers that contains 1/5 volume Sample Loading Buffer, and adjust the volume with ddH2O so that the final DNA concentration is 0.2 μg/μL.
4. Use 2.5–5 μL (0.5–1 μg) per well on an agarose gel.

λ/*Hind*III	λ/*BstE*II	φX174/*Hae*III	pBR322/*Msp*I
23,130 bp	8454 bp	1353 bp	622 bp
9416	7242	1078	527
6557	6369	872	404
4361	5686	603	307
2322	4822	310	242
2027	4324	281	238
564	3675	271	217
125	2323	234	201
	1929	194	190
	1371	118	180
	1264	72	160
	702		147
	224		123
	117		110
			90
			76
			67
			34
			26
			15
			9

Appendix C

Inventory for a PCR Laboratory

The following equipment, materials and reagents are necessary for a PCR laboratory. Additional materials and reagents required for performing nonradioactive probe and cloning procedures are also listed separately. Most of the items can be purchased from standard suppliers (e.g., Fisher Scientific), although certain molecular biology reagents may need to be obtained from specialized biotechnology suppliers. When a reagent listed below should be obtained from a specific supplier, the manufaturer is listed along with the catalog number.

EQUIPMENT
Incubator (37°C)
Refrigerator (4°C)
Freezer ($-20°C$)
Freezer ($-70°C$)
Autoclave
Thermocycler
Water baths
Microcentrifuge (preferably three, one for each color-coded area; at least two are necessary, one for the Grey Area and one for the White Area)
Adjustable pipettors (at least three sets of 1000 µL, 200 µL, and 20 µL, one set for each color-coded area; if possible a 0.5–10-µL pipettor for manipulating enzymes in the White Area)
Vortex mixers
Magnetic stirrer
Rocker or rotator
Hot plates
pH meter
Vacuum pump (optional)
Microwave (preferable for melting agarose solutions; however, a hot plate or Bunsen burner can substitute for this function)
Power supplies
UV transilluminator
Polaroid camera with orange filter
Hood or camera stand and darkroom
Bunsen burner
Analytical balance

MATERIALS
Erlenmeyer flasks (100 mL, 250 mL, 1000 mL)
Graduated cylinders (100 mL, 250 mL, 500 mL, 1000 mL)
Beakers (250 mL, 500 mL, 1000 mL)
Bottles (100 mL, 500 mL)
Glass pipets (25 mL, 10 mL, 5 mL, 2 mL) and rubber bulbs or Pipette Pumps®
Sterile Pasteur pipets and rubber bulbs
Plastic racks for microcentrifuge tubes
Floating racks for microcentrifuge tubes
Thermometers
Squirt bottles for ddH$_2$O, 95% ethanol, 1.5% sodium hypochlorite (bleach)
15-mL screw-cap polypropylene tubes tubes and racks
50-mL screw-cap polypropylene tubes and racks
Sterile yellow polypropylene pipet tips (1–200 μL)
Sterile blue polypropylene pipet tips (200–1000 μL)
Sterile 1.5-mL microcentrifuge tubes
Sterile 0.5-mL microcentrifuge tubes
Sterile 0.2-mL PCR reaction tubes
1.5-mL screw-cap microcentrifuge tubes with O-rings
Parafilm®
Gloves (disposable latex or vinyl)
Colored laboratory tape
Paper towels or Kimwipes®
Magnetic stir-bars
Weigh boats
Spatulas
Scissors or razor blade
Permanent markers
Ice buckets
Sterile lancets
Vacuum-sealed blood collection tubes, e.g., Vacutainer® tubes
Collection vials
Cotton
Talc powder (for re-using gloves)
Sterile toothpicks
Inoculating loop
Petri plates
Gel trays
Gel boxes
Combs
UV protective eyewear (goggles or face shield)
Polaroid 667 film
Plexiglass shield (high-grade UV-transmitting Plexiglass)

GENERAL REAGENTS
Boric acid
EDTA
Tris base
Sodium chloride
Sodium hydroxide

Sodium acetate
Potassium chloride
Potassium acetate
Bleach (diluted to a final concentration of 1.5% sodium hypochlorite)
Hydrochloric acid
Glacial acetic acid
Triton® X-100
Glycogen
Glycerol
Gelatin
Sodium sulfate
Sodium iodide
Silica particles
Nitric acid
Chelex® 100 (Bio-Rad Laboratories, Richmond, CA, No. 143-2832)
Proteinase K
Potassium phosphate
Disodium phosphate
Sodium dodecyl sulfate (SDS)
Guanidine isothiocyanate
Sodium citrate
β-mercaptoethanol
Sarkosyl
Saponin
tRNA (yeast or *E. coli*)
Phenol (equilibrated with water for RNA and equilibrated with Tris pH 8.0 for DNA)
Isoamyl alcohol
Chloroform
Isopropanol
100% ethanol
Peptone
Tryptone
Yeast extract
Agar
Agarose
Ethidium bromide
Bromophenol blue
Xylene cyanol
DNA markers ("PCR markers"):

1. Amplisize DNA Size Standards, Bio-Rad Laboratories, Richmond, CA: 50, 100, 200, 300, 400, 500, 700, 1000, 1500, 2000 bp
2. 100 bp ladder, Gibco BRL, Grand Island, NY: 100, 200, 300, 400, 500, 600, 700, 800, 900, 1000, 1100, 1200, 1300, 1400, 1500, 2072 bp
3. φX174/*Hae*III; pBR322/*Msp*I; λ/*Bst*EII; λ/*Hind*III (New England Biolabs, Inc., Beverly, MA; Promega Corp., Madison, WI, among others; *see* Appendix B for sizes)

SPECIALTY REAGENTS
Tryptic Soy Agar (*V. cholerae*)
Barium chloride dihydrate for MacFarland's Standard (*V. cholerae*)

Sulfuric acid for MacFarland's Standard (*V. cholerae*)
Saponin (*P. falciparum/P. vivax*)
N-acetyl cysteine (*M. tuberculosis*)
Sterile phosphate buffered saline (PBS)
Sodium thioglycolate for Cary-Blair transport medium (*E. coli*)
Calcium chloride for Cary-Blair transport medium (*E. coli*)
MacConkey agar (*E. coli*)
Acetone (*Leptospira*)
Sterile Dacron®-tipped applicators (Fisherbrand #14-959-90) (*C. trachomatis/N. gonorrhoeae*)

PCR REAGENTS
Primers (Operon Technologies, Alameda, CA; New England Biolabs, Inc., Beverly, MA; Gibco BRL, Grand Island, NY; Applied Biosystems Perkin-Elmer, Foster City, CA)
Nucleotides (dNTPs: dATP, dCTP, dGTP, dTTP)
10X Buffers
$MgCl_2$
Taq polymerase (*see* section 5.1.2)
Reverse transcriptase RAV-2 (Amersham Corp., Arlington Heights, IL)
r*Tth* reverse transcriptase-polymerase (Perkin-Elmer Corp.)
Dithiothreitol (DTT)
Dimethyl sulfoxide (DMSO)
Tetramethylammonium chloride (TMAC)
Betaine (Sigma Chemical Co., St. Louis, MO, B-2629)
Bovine serum albumin (BSA)
Manganese acetate
Bicine
Nuclease-free sterile ddH_2O
Mineral oil
Wax beads

ADDITIONAL MATERIALS AND REAGENTS FOR NONRADIOACTIVE PROBES
Dot blot microfiltration apparatus
Rocker/orbital shaker
"Seal-a-meal"® for sealing hybridization bags
Plastic bags for hybridization
Plastic dishes with covers
Filter forceps
Digoxigenin-11-dUTP, alkali-labile (Boehringer Mannheim, Indianapolis, IN, No. 1573152)
Anti-digoxigenin alkaline phosphatase conjugate (Boehringer Mannheim, No. 1093274)
Nonfat milk powder
Blocking Reagent (e.g., Boehringer Mannheim, No. 1096176)
Nylon membranes (e.g., Boehringer Mannheim)
Whatman 3MM paper
Nitrotetrazolium blue (NBT)
5-bromo-4-cloro-3-indolyl-phosphate, toluidine salt (BCIP)

For chemiluminescent detection:
Darkroom setup (trays, wooden forceps, etc.) or automatic developer for X-ray film
Lumi-phos 530® (chemiluminescent substrate; Lumigen, Inc., Southfield, MI)
Plastic sheets
X-ray film

film cassettes
GBX developer and fixer

ADDITIONAL MATERIALS AND REAGENTS FOR CLONING
Metal block for microcentrifuge tubes (precooled to $-20°C$)
Centrifuge with 3500-rpm capability
Spectrophotometer measuring optical density at 600-nm wavelength
Plate spinner, if available
Air shaker (37°C)
Plate spreader (i.e., made from a glass rod)
Sterile wooden sticks
Ampicillin
Potassium acetate
Glucose
Polyethylene glycol (MW 8000)
Polyethylene glycol (MW 3350)
Magnesium sulfate
5-Bromo-4-chloro-3-indolyl-D-galactopyranoside (X-Gal)
Isopropyl β-D-thiogalactopyranoside (IPTG)
Dimethyl formamide (DMF)
Cloning vector (e.g., Bluescript, Stratagene Cloning Systems)
Restiction enzymes
Restriction enzyme buffers
T4 DNA Ligase
10X T4 DNA Ligase Buffer
RNase
Transparent tape

Appendix D

Good Lab Practice

D.1   General Tips

- Ask a knowledgeable colleague if you have questions, especially if you are unsure of how a piece of equipment functions or how to proceed in a protocol.
- Read the protocol carefully and fill out the worksheet BEFORE beginning the experiment.
- Visually check the volume of the solution in the pipet tip to ensure that the intended volume is being transferred. To familiarize yourself with how certain volumes of solution appear in the pipet tip, practice pipetting the following amounts of liquid:

  - 20-μL pipettor: 1 μL, 2.5 μL, 5 μL, 10 μL, 20 μL
  - 200-μL pipettor: 25 μL, 50 μL, 100 μL, 150 μL, 200 μL
  - 1000-μL pipettor: 100 μL, 250 μL, 500 μL, 750 μL, 1000 μL

- Always ensure that the tube you are manipulating contains what you think it does; check the label before opening the tube.
- When manipulating a series of tubes, always keep the tubes in numerical order in the tube rack (e.g., microcentrifuge tube rack, floating rack).
- Label tubes on the top and along the side. This is particularly important when using tubes with detachable caps (e.g., screw-cap microcentrifuge tubes).
- Note any mishap or irregularity that occurs in your laboratory notebook or on the PCR Worksheet or Gel Chart.
- Check off each reagent on the PCR Worksheet after adding it to the Master Mix.
- After adding a reagent to the Master Mix, replace the tube (from which the reagent was taken) in the rack or the ice bucket in a place different from its original position.
- Always keep enzymes, dNTPs, primers, and nucleic acids (samples) on ice.
- Always ensure that the centrifuge is balanced before beginning centrifugation by checking that similar tubes containing equal volumes of liquid are placed opposite each other in the rotor. For high-speed spins, tubes that are intended to balance each other should be weighed to ensure identical weight.
- Ensure that all tubes are tightly closed before centrifugation.
- Never open a centrifuge while the rotor is still spinning. Never force the timer on a centrifuge while it is running in order to reduce the length of the centrifugation.
- When preparing samples for application to an agarose gel for electrophoresis using a Parafilm®-covered microcentrifuge rack, label the wells on the Parafilm with the order of the samples, using the number of the PCR reaction and *not* the number of the well.

- Return the PCR reaction tubes to their rack in the order that they have been applied to the Parafilm-covered rack in preparation for loading the gel, then verify that the order of the samples matches the intended order as specified by the Gel Chart.
- During sample application to agarose gels, if a bubble forms at the pipet tip in the well due to mineral oil, do not continue to load the sample; withdraw the sample solution back into the pipet tip and then try re-delivering it into the gel well.

D.2   Calibration of Adjustable Pipettors

The accuracy of volume measurement should be checked after cleaning the pipettor shafts and reassembling the pipettors. If necessary, the pipettors should be recalibrated and the pipetting accuracy measured again.

To measure pipetting accuracy, weigh the following volumes of water *in triplicate* using an analytical balance. It is easiest to use a balance that can be tared easily in between each measurement. Calculate the average measurement for each volume listed below and then calculate the percentage error. Less than 10% error is generally considered acceptable. This technique is based on the fact that at sea level, 1 µL of water weighs 1 mg, 10 µL weighs 10 mg, 100 µL of water weighs 100 mg, etc.

- 1000-µL pipettor: 100 µL, 250 µL, 500 µL, 750 µL, 1000 µL
- 200-µL pipettor: 25 µL, 50 µL, 100 µL, 150 µL, 200 µL
- 20-µL pipettor: 2.5 µL, 5 µL, 10 µL, 15 µL, 20 µL

If the pipettor is inaccurate by delivering too low a volume (termed "minus" error) at both high and low volumes or by delivering too large a volume (termed "plus" error) at both high and low volumes, the pipettor can be calibrated in-house. However, if the pipettor is registering a "minus" error at high volume and a "plus" error at low volumes or vice versa, the pipettor may need to be sent to the manufacturer for repair.

Calibrating *exactly* at lower volumes generally results in a "minus" error at high volumes, whereas calibrating *exactly* at high volumes results in a "plus" error at lower volumes. Therefore, the user must decide in what approximate range the greatest accuracy is required.

Certain brands of pipettors can be calibrated in-house, depending on the model of the pipettor. With some models, the black-ribbed knobs at the top of the pipettor can be turned by removing the white cap (labeled, for example, "P1000" or "P200") and inserting a paper clip bent into a "U" shape as a lever into the holes in the upper knob (looking down along the vertical axis of the pipettor). Other models require that the knobs be loosened using an Allen wrench of the appropriate size in order to be calibrated.

If the water sample weight *exceeds* the pipettor's micrometer reading, the upper knob should be turned *clockwise* as many degrees as necessary to correct the difference between the sample weight and the micrometer reading. A 90° turn (1/4 of a full turn) of the knob on a 20-µL pipettor will decrease the volume delivered by the pipettor by approximately 0.25 µL; a full turn will decrease the volume delivered by the pipettor by approximately 1 µL. A 90° turn (1/4 of a full turn) of the knob on a 1000-µL pipettor will decrease the volume delivered by the pipettor by approximately 25 µL; a full turn will decrease the volume delivered by the pipettor by approximately 100 µL. If the water sample weight is *less* than the pipettor's micrometer reading, the upper knob should be turned *counterclockwise* as many degrees as necessary to correct the difference between the sample weight and the micrometer reading. After making an adjustment by turning the knob, the knob should be tightened with an Allen wrench (if applicable), and the pipettor should be tested by weighing specified volumes of water in triplicate as prescribed above. It is important to test both low and high volumes. If the pipettor is still not pipetting accurately, the process of adjusting the knobs and measuring the accuracy of pipetting should be repeated until the percentage of error has decreased to an acceptable level.

Appendix E

Prevention of Cross-Contamination

Once contamination has occurred in a PCR laboratory, it can be very difficult, if not impossible, to eliminate. Therefore, it is advisable to implement rigorous procedures to preclude contamination from occurring. Effective low-cost methods for carryover prevention are outlined below. Strict adherence to the following laboratory practices is critical for prevention of DNA cross-contamination.

Bleach

Use bleach (sodium hypochlorite diluted to 1.5% final concentration). The use of bleach reduces the risk of contamination by cleaving contaminating *DNA* strands so that they are no longer amplifiable. It also reduces the risk of infection by killing *pathogenic organisms.* However, be careful not to use bleach in excess, because it can also destroy the template DNA that one wishes to amplify. In addition, bleach is harmful to the environment.

- Clean work areas daily with dilute bleach (1.5% sodium hypochlorite).
- Periodically soak pipettor shafts in dilute bleach for 10 to 30 minutes, rinse thoroughly in distilled water, and dry completely. The accuracy of the pipettor should be assessed after cleaning and reassembling (*see* Appendix D).
- Clean gloves, tubes, pipet tip boxes, etc. with dilute bleach.
- Between manipulation of each sample, clean the tip of the pipettor shaft with a paper towel (or Kimwipe®) soaked in bleach, then dry completely with a clean dry paper towel.
- Always discard pipet tips into a beaker filled with dilute bleach.

Designated Color-Coded Areas

Different activities should be physically separated, ideally in different rooms. If this is not possible, then separate areas — preferably, different laminar flow hoods — must be dedicated for each activity. This minimizes the risk of contaminating one reaction with DNA or RNA sample or amplified product from another, since the reactions are set up in a separate location from where the nucleic acid template is prepared and the product is analyzed.

- "White" Area — for preparing the PCR reaction. The only reagents used in this area are the ingredients of the PCR Master Mix. If a room has been designated as the White Area, always close the door to the white room; if a laminar flow hood has been designated, lower the sash of the hood when not in use. Avoid unnecessary activities and/or traffic in the White Area.

- "Grey" Area—for preparing sample DNA or RNA and for addition of the sample to the PCR reaction tubes prior to amplification.
- "Black" Area—for amplifying and analyzing PCR products.

Different sets of pipettors must be dedicated for each color-coded work area. Designated gloves, labcoats, racks, pipet tips, tubes, tape, permanent markers, ice buckets, and other such items must also be dedicated to each work area. Reagents to be used in the different activities should be stored in the separate areas as well.

When recycling tubes or pipet tips, material from the White Area *must always* be recycled for use in the White or Grey areas only, while Grey and Black Area material *must always* be recycled for use in the Black Area only. Gloves can also be color-coded and re-used many times, as long as they remain in the designated work area. Again, gloves which originate in the White Area can be used subsequently in the Grey and then Black Areas but *never* in the opposite direction.

Controls

In order to readily identify problems due to contamination of PCR reactions (false-positive results) or inhibition of amplification (false-negative results), the following controls should be included in each amplification, in the order listed below:

- "White Area" negative control—consisting of "white" ddH$_2$O, as a control for the PCR reagents in the White Area.
- "Grey Area" negative control—consisting of "grey" ddH$_2$O, as a control for the water and pipettor used for preparation of the DNA or RNA template in the Grey Area.
- Negative extraction control—consisting of ddH$_2$O, used instead of a specimen during the extraction procedure as a control for contamination during the DNA or RNA preparation process.
- Negative specimen—as a control for specificity.
- Interspersed negative control—consisting of ddH$_2$O, used as a control every 15–20 test samples when analyzing large numbers of samples.
- Inhibition control—consisting of a representative sample(s) to which purified DNA or RNA has been added. If this control does not yield the expected product whereas the purified DNA or RNA (positive control) does, this indicates that the sample may be inhibiting the amplification.
- Positive control—consisting of purified DNA/RNA or a crude lysate of the organism of interest.
- "Final" negative control—consisting of ddH$_2$O added as the final sample in an amplification run, as a control for the process of sample addition.

Sample Manipulation

- Use sterile technique—do not pass your hand or arm over open tubes.
- Always close tubes when not in use, or at least cover them with a clean paper towel (or Kimwipe®).
- Do not put your hands inside sterile bags or jars of tubes; rather, shake several tubes out onto a clean paper towel.
- Do not touch the cap of the tube; close the tubes using the surface of the bench, covered with a clean paper towel (or Kimwipe).
- Open tubes with a clean paper towel (or Kimwipe).
- If the pipet tip touches something it is not supposed to, *always* throw away the tip. *Never* touch pipet tips with your fingers, even if your hands are gloved.
- Always manipulate the samples in the order of the most negative to the most positive.

Miscellaneous

- Reagents should be stored and used in small volumes; for example, 50-μL aliquots of *Taq* polymerase; 100-μL aliquots of dNTPs, primers, and DTT; 500-μL to 1-mL aliquots of PCR buffer, MgCl$_2$, TMAC, and betaine. By using small aliquots, if any contamination is detected, all affected solutions can immediately be disposed of without excessive loss of expensive reagents.
- Exposure of pipettors to ultraviolet light for 15 minutes prior to use reduces the risk of DNA cross-contamination since UV light destroys DNA.
- If aerosol-resistant pipet tips (ART) are available and affordable, they can be used to prevent aspiration of DNA molecules into the pipettor shaft, thereby reducing the risk of cross-contamination.

Appendix F

PCR Troubleshooting Guide and Flowchart

Problems with PCR amplification can be divided into three main categories that will be described below, i.e., chemical, physical, and thermal.

Chemical Parameters

1. If the amplification is not producing the expected results, the first step in troubleshooting is to simply repeat the amplification. It is possible that an essential ingredient was accidentally omitted from the Master Mix. If this step does not produce the expected results, then the experiment can be repeated with new aliquots of all the reagents. The user can eventually trace which reagent caused the original problem, but it is often not worth the time and trouble.

2. Make sure the PCR buffer recommended by the manufacturer for use with the particular polymerase is utilized, since the enzyme may not function optimally in other buffers.

3. It is possible that the concentration of the reaction ingredients used may be incorrect; thus, the concentration of the reagent stocks and the calculations used in the preparation of each should be verified. The concentration of magnesium is particularly critical, as a difference of only 0.25 mM in the PCR mixture can dramatically alter amplification results.

4. It is important to allow frozen reagents to thaw completely, mix them thoroughly, and centrifuge briefly prior to use. Often pockets of concentrated solution take the longest to thaw.

5. It is important to thoroughly mix the PCR Master Mix, particularly after addition of the enzyme(s). Since enzymes are stored in a buffer with high glycerol content, the enzyme solution, which is viscous and more dense than the PCR mixture, sinks to the bottom of the tube containing the Master Mix. The PCR mixture must therefore be mixed completely but carefully, since enzymes are sensitive to the physical force of vortexing and to air bubbles.

6. Solutions must be prepared with nuclease-free water that is obtained either commercially or by treatment of in-house ddH$_2$O with diethyl pyrocarbonate (DEPC), which inactivates RNases. This is especially critical for work with RNA. Water of high quality should be used in all PCR reactions. It may be worth purchasing a small stock of high-grade nuclease-free water for preparation of the PCR reaction mixture, as this can prevent many potential problems (e.g., inhibition due to contaminants such as heavy metals in the water distilled in-house).

7. Certain lots of mineral oil have been reported to be inhibitory to PCR. Therefore, a change in lot can determine whether the mineral oil is responsible for the amplification problem.

8. Certain reagents can lose activity or decompose. Therefore, it is critical to ensure proper

storage of all reagents (e.g., PCR reagents at $-20°C$, reverse transcriptase at $-70°C$, long-term storage of *Taq* polymerase at $-70°C$). It is essential that freezers be connected to an emergency generator in case of power outage. If reagents have passed their expiration dates, they may still be functional but should be tested first. Enzymes may lose activity over time, thus, their final concentration in the PCR mixture may need to be increased.

9. Samples should be processed and analyzed as quickly as possible and should always be stored frozen (DNA at $-20°C$, RNA and viral specimens at $-70°C$), as they can become degraded, especially if crude extracts have been prepared. Samples may also become contaminated with nucleases; care should be taken to always wear gloves when manipulating samples to avoid contamination with nucleases from the user's skin. It is also best to store PCR products at $-20°C$.

10. Cosolvents that aid in the denaturation of template DNA strands may be included in the PCR reaction mixture (e.g., dimethyl sulfoxide) to improve efficiency of amplification.

11. Primer integrity may be compromised. The yield may be lower than reported, or there may be a substantial amount of incomplete synthesis. The quality of the primers can be verified by analyzing a small aliquot by gel electrophoresis. Alternatively, the sequence itself may be incorrect. An error could have been made in writing out the sequence, or the reverse complement may have been accidentally synthesized. If the primers have been synthesized by a commercial source, the manufacturer may have made an error in the sequence. This can be verified by checking the sequence on the product description sheet or, as a last resort, re-synthesizing the primer. If the primers are novel, it may be necessary to try synthesizing primers with a different sequence but similar specificity, which may amplify the target more efficiently.

12. The primer sequences should be examined for regions of self-complementarity that could lead to hairpin formation (hybridization of one primer with itself instead of with the DNA target) and for regions of complementarity with the other primer(s) in the reaction (hybridization with the other primer[s] instead of with the DNA target).

13. PCR inhibitors may originate from the sample itself or from reagents used during sample preparation. Certain substances in clinical specimens are known to inhibit PCR, such as bilirubin and bile salts in feces, heavy metals in water, heme in whole blood, and nucleases in cell lysates, to name a few. Chemicals used during nucleic acid preparation can also inhibit the polymerase if subsequently they are not completely removed. These substances include guanidine isothiocyanate, sodium dodecyl sulfate (SDS), proteinase K, phenol, heparin, EDTA, and the anionic resin Chelex® 100.

14. During purification of nucleic acids using ethanol precipitation, the yield of DNA or RNA can be reduced if the sample is not subjected to sufficiently long centrifugation (30 minutes is optimal). If very small amounts of nucleic acid are being precipitated, a carrier can be added to increase the yield (e.g., salmon sperm DNA, yeast or *E. coli* tRNA[7], glycogen). It is important to completely resuspend the nucleic acid pellet in the final solution.

Physical Parameters

1. Thermocycler

• The functioning of the thermocycler should be periodically re-evaluated. If the thermocycler is designed such that a thermocouple is used to monitor the temperature in the wells, make

---

7. Nucleic acid carriers are acceptable, provided that their sequences will not amplify with the PCR primers of choice.

sure that the wire is fully submerged in the mineral oil in the well in the thermocycler block and that it is properly connected to the machine for accurate temperature readings.

- A change in thermocycler brand or model can affect amplification results. Different thermocyclers can generate different results even when they are identically programmed, due to variations in ramp time, precision in reaching and maintaining the target temperature, and efficiency of thermal transfer due to the fit of the tubes in the wells.

2. Program

It is possible that the amplification program was inadvertently changed; therefore, it is essential to review the program prior to every amplification and to observe the first few cycles to ensure that the program is being correctly executed. If possible, check the thermocycler's amplification and/or error reports after each amplification.

3. Tubes

- Certain tubes do not fit snugly into the wells in the metal block of the thermocycler. If this is the case, a drop of mineral oil should be added to the well to facilitate adequate thermal transfer. Note that mineral oil will often erase markings written with permanent markers on the side of PCR reaction tubes, so the caps of the tubes should be properly labeled.
- The thickness of the wall of the PCR reaction tube can influence the amplification. Standard thick-walled tubes may require a longer incubation at each temperature than specialty thin-walled tubes.
- According to some reports, certain tubes were made of a plastic material that contained a contaminant inhibitory to PCR amplification.

4. Pipettor

A PCR inhibitor may have been aspirated into the pipettor shaft during sample preparation. In addition, carryover from excessive use of bleach, insufficient rinsing, or inadequate drying of pipettor shafts during routine cleaning may also interfere with amplification.

5. Pipet tips

If pipet tips are being recycled, the tips must be completely rinsed so as to remove all remaining detergent and bleach, which could inhibit the polymerase. Only sterilized pipet tips should be used.

6. Gloves

The powder in certain gloves can inhibit PCR.

7. Miscellaneous

Any physical changes in the laboratory (e.g., a major cleaning or renovation, an open window that may result in the circulation of foreign particulate matter), or variation in standard laboratory practices (e.g., new cleaning products, new personnel) may affect PCR amplification results. Any change found to be temporally correlated with amplification problems should be investigated.

Thermal Cycling Parameters

1. The thermal profile can be adjusted to optimize amplification. For instance, if no product is observed:
- the annealing temperature can be lowered by 2–5°C
- the denaturation temperature can be raised by 1°C
- the extension time can be increased
- the denaturation time can be increased

The reverse modifications can be implemented to reduce nonspecific amplification products.

Table F.1 indicates what changes can be made in order to either increase the stringency of an amplification to eliminate non-specific products or to decrease stringency.

2. If a new thermocycler fails to produce the same results as those from a previous one, the new machine should be programmed so that the ramp time between each pair of temperatures is the same as in the original thermocyler, if possible.

Table F.1   Factors Affecting Stringency of an Amplification

Factor	High Stringency	Low Stringency
Annealing temperature	Increase	Reduce
Magnesium concentration	Reduce	Increase
Number of cycles	Reduce	Increase
Extension time	Reduce	Increase
Enzyme concentration	Reduce	Increase
Nucleotide concentration	Reduce	Increase
Primer concentration	Reduce	Increase
Template concentration	Reduce	Increase
Cosolvent concentration (e.g., DMSO, formamide)	Increase	Reduce

Troubleshooting Flowchart

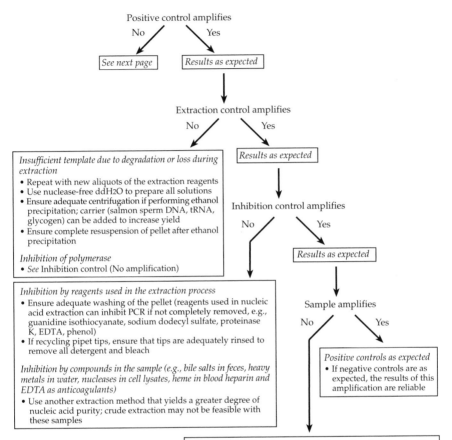

Positive control amplifies

No / Yes

See next page — Results as expected

Extraction control amplifies

No / Yes

Insufficient template due to degradation or loss during extraction
- Repeat with new aliquots of the extraction reagents
- Use nuclease-free ddH2O to prepare all solutions
- Ensure adequate centrifugation if performing ethanol precipitation; carrier (salmon sperm DNA, tRNA, glycogen) can be added to increase yield
- Ensure complete resuspension of pellet after ethanol precipitation

Inhibition of polymerase
- *See* Inhibition control (No amplification)

Results as expected

Inhibition control amplifies

No / Yes

Inhibition by reagents used in the extraction process
- Ensure adequate washing of the pellet (reagents used in nucleic acid extraction can inhibit PCR if not completely removed, e.g., guanidine isothiocyanate, sodium dodecyl sulfate, proteinase K, EDTA, phenol)
- If recycling pipet tips, ensure that tips are adequately rinsed to remove all detergent and bleach

Inhibition by compounds in the sample (e.g., bile salts in feces, heavy metals in water, nucleases in cell lysates, heme in blood heparin and EDTA as anticoagulants)
- Use another extraction method that yields a greater degree of nucleic acid purity; crude extraction may not be feasible with these samples

Results as expected

Sample amplifies

No / Yes

Positive controls as expected
- If negative controls are as expected, the results of this amplification are reliable

Insufficient template due to degradation or loss during extraction
Inhibition of polymerase
- *See* Inhibition control (No amplification)

Positive DNA control amplifies
No

"Chemical" problem
- Check that all necessary reagents were included
- Check the concentration of the reagents used to prepare the Master Mix
- Check that the calculations for preparing the reagents and the Master Mix were correctly performed
- Ensure that the correct PCR buffer is being used (e.g., the buffer recommended by the manufacturer of the *Taq* polymerase in use)
- Repeat amplification to control for the accidental omission of a key reagent
- Repeat amplification with new aliquots of reagents, especially dNTPs, primers, enzyme; if possible, repeat PCR with reagents that are being used for another amplification protocol that is yielding expected results
- Use new sterile pipet tips
- Use a new lot of mineral oil
- Increase the enzyme concentration
- Add a cosolvent such as dimethyl sulfoxide that helps denaturation
- Try a new control; the current nucleic acid control may have been degraded
- Try reducing or increasing the concentration of the DNA template
- If the primers have been manufactured by a company, check on the product description sheet that the sequence of the primers is what was intended
- Check the quality and concentration of the primers by analyzing an aliquot by gel electrophoresis (e.g., 50 ng on a 12% polyacrylamide gel); each primer should appear as a single band of the expected size and intensity (use a primer of known size and concentration as a control)
- It may be necessary to synthesize new primers; the sequence of the primers may be incorrect. If these are novel primers, try synthesizing primers with a different sequence but similar specificity

"Physical" problem
- Review the program in the thermocycler or the temperatures of the water baths
- Observe the first few cycles of the program to ensure that the thermocycler is functioning properly
- If the thermocycler has a thermocouple, ensure that the wire is completely submerged in mineral oil and that the thermocouple wire is properly connected
- If recycling pipet tips, ensure that tips are adequately rinsed to remove all detergent and bleach
- Use different gloves
- Determine whether there have been any changes in the laboratory (new cleaning products, an open window)

"Thermal" problem
- Lower the annealing temperature 2-5°C
- Increase the extension time
- Increase the denaturation time
- Raise the denaturation temperature by 1°C
- If a different thermocycler is being used, program the ramp time to be the same as in the previous thermocycler, if possible
- Add oil to the wells in the metal block in the thermocycler if the tubes do not fit perfectly in order to optimize thermal transfer

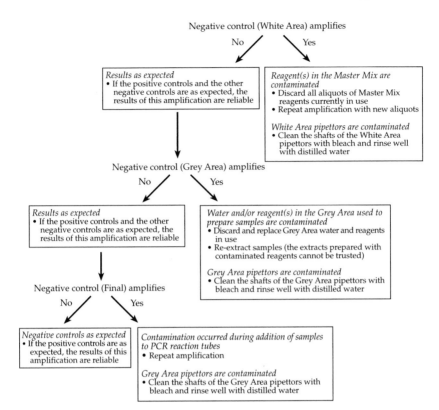

Reverse Transcriptase-PCR

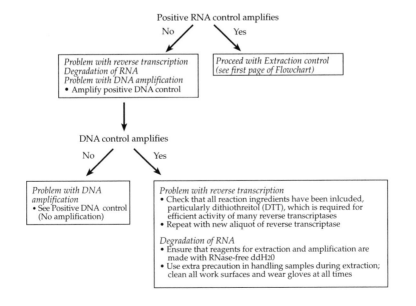

Appendix G

Workshop Organization and Teaching Tips

This section outlines certain organizational and teaching methods that have been implemented successfully in the AMB/ATT workshops.

Lectures
- Lectures should address the theoretical basis of the technique to be performed (e.g., review of molecular biology, introduction to PCR, applications of PCR, nonradioactive DNA probes). Lectures should also cover the clinical manifestations and epidemiology, classical diagnostic techniques, and molecular diagnosis and epidemiology of each disease to be investigated in the workshop. Local instructors should be invited to give as many lectures as possible.
- The lectures should be distributed throughout the workshop, with no more than 2–3 hours every morning. The first day may require a somewhat longer lecture session, since it is recommended to include one lecture presenting an overview of the workshop and another consisting of a general introduction to the laboratory, in addition to the regular morning lecture schedule.
- A coffee break should be included in both morning and afternoon sessions.
- Each laboratory session should be preceded by an introduction to the experiment and/or review of the procedure to be conducted (Figure G.1). These more informal presentations should explain the theory behind each technique; for example, the formula that describes the migration of molecules through a gel matrix; the purpose of each reagent in a DNA purification procedure. In addition, the protocol to be carried out should be reviewed with the group to point out all the relevant details. The PCR worksheet or gel chart to be used in the laboratory session should also be filled out by the participants as a group. To facilitate the latter, a master worksheet or chart can be prepared on a transparency, which is then projected during the lecture for the participants to review and copy.
- At the conclusion of each experiment, a discussion should be conducted immediately after obtaining the results in order to discuss the data and the participants' observations. As the photographs are taken of each group's results, one instructor can prepare the results for discussion, while the others prepare photocopies of each group's photograph together with the gel chart for distribution to all participants.
- During this discussion, it should be emphasized that what is important in data analysis is to have a logical scientific *explanation* of the results obtained—the results do not have to be perfect. The importance of keeping a laboratory notebook and noting any and every irregularity that may occur during a procedure should also be stressed.

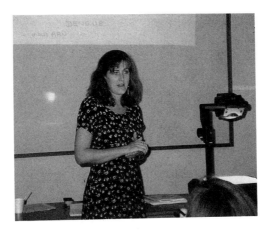

Fig. G.1. Course instructor Leïla Smith introducing the day's experiment during a workshop in Guatemala.

- For clarity, it is useful to have two dry erase boards or chalkboards in each of the three work areas, one board outlining the detailed schedule of the day and the other explaining the details of the procedure to be conducted in that area. For example, one board in the White Area should show the ingredients and composition of the PCR Master Mix; one in the Grey Area, the order in which the specimens should be extracted and the order in which the samples should be loaded into the PCR reaction tubes; and one in the Black Area, the order that the samples should be applied to the agarose gel for electrophoresis.

Instructors
- All experiments to be conducted in the workshop should be performed on-site the week preceding the course *by all instructors.* This is critical to ensure that the experiments will proceed smoothly during the workshop by resolving all of the technical problems that may arise when conducting an experiment in a new laboratory. In addition, it is essential to assure that each instructor, who will be independently leading his or her work group, is fully prepared.
- Each work group is led by an instructor who has experience with the technique and has previously performed all of the experiments to be conducted in the course. In certain instances, students or members of the host laboratory who have participated in preparation of the workshop can be included as assistant instructors.
- The instructor is responsible for explaining the procedure, answering questions, supervising the activities, and indicating when a participant's laboratory technique can be improved (Figure G.2). He or she must also ensure that all participants get equal opportunity to carry out the procedures, not just those who are most experienced or most vocal.

Work Groups
- Each work group should consist of no more than five participants. If information about the participants' background is available, assignments should be made such that each work group contains one or two participants with more experience with PCR and/or molecular techniques and others with less-specialized knowledge.

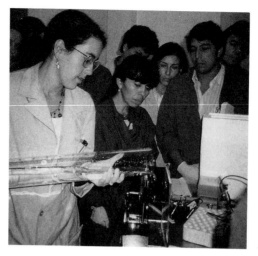

Fig. G.2. Course instructor Christine Rousseau demonstrating a laboratory procedure to her workgroup during a workshop in Cuba.

- Work groups in the Phase II course should include an epidemiologist as well as laboratory practitioners, since study design and analysis is an integral part of the Phase II course.
- As sample preparation proceeds in the Grey Area, instructors should coordinate activities of the groups that are progressing at approximately the same rate. Two groups should enter the White Area to prepare the PCR reaction tubes at the same time, return to the Grey Area to add the samples, and then load the thermocycler at the same time (assuming two groups will share each thermocycler). If one of the two groups takes longer to complete the process, the reaction tubes of the first group must be kept on ice until loaded into the thermocycler.
- The work groups should be assigned a number (1–4) and a color (e.g., blue, green, yellow, and red)—the same color of the tape used to label the material at their Grey Area work station.

Material
- For the workshop, it is highly recommended to assign separate rooms to each of the three work areas (White, Grey, and Black).
- Material in each separate work area should be labeled with different-colored tape. At least two workstations for preparing PCR reactions should be set up in the White Area, and the materials at each station should be labeled with differently colored tape (e.g., orange and pink). A workstation should be prepared for each group in the Grey Area, and all the materials at each station should be labeled with colored tape corresponding to the color assigned to each group (e.g., blue, green, yellow, and red) (Figure G.3). Within each work area, shared materials (e.g., microcentrifuge[s], gloves, extra plastic tubes, etc.) should be separated from materials for each workstation.
- Aliquots of the reagents required for each experiment should be prepared in advance for each work group, color-coded for each group, labeled with the name and concentration of the contents, and stored in small plastic bags at the appropriate temperature (e.g., $-20°C$, $4°C$). The only reagent that should not be aliquoted is the enzyme(s) (e.g., *Taq* polymerase, reverse transcriptase). When each group is ready to add the enzyme(s) to the reaction

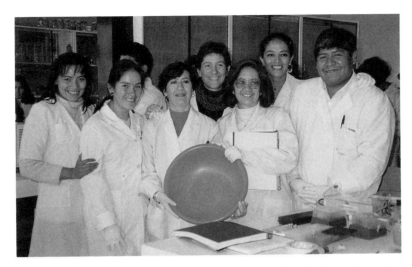

Fig. G.3. Work team ("Red Group") in the Bolivia Phase I workshop with participants. *Center back row*, instructor Deborah Lans. *Far left*, assistant instructor Maria Rosa Cortez.

mixture, the instructor should retrieve the workshop aliquot from the $-20°C$ freezer and return it immediately after use.

- Gloves can be re-used with discretion *within each work area only*. Participants should label their gloves with their names and the color of the work area.
- It is advantageous to invite technical support from students and members of the host laboratory for the preparation of the workshop materials.

Manual
- The manual should be clearly written in the local language.
- Each protocol should include all pertinent details, an introduction and references (*see* chapter 5).
- PCR Worksheets and Gel Charts should be included, with extra copies in case errors are made as they are being filled out.
- Relevant articles and reference materials should be available for participants to photocopy.
- Literature review meetings (e.g., a journal club) should be organized during the course to discuss relevant scientific articles and to serve as a model for future activities by the participants after the workshop.

Appendix H

Sample Charts and Worksheets

I.   PCR Worksheet

Title:_____ **Number:** _____ **Date:**_____

TEMPLATE				PCR MASTER MIX					
Tube #	Mix (µl)	Sample (µl)	Description	Vol. (µl)	Ingredient	Description	Conc.	µl/tube	#tubes	µl/Mix
1					10X Buffer					
2					dNTPs					
3					Primer 1					
4					Primer 2					
5					MgCl2					
6					ddH2O					
7					Other					
8					Other					
9					Other					
10					Other					
11					Other					
12					Other					
13					Other					
14					Taq					
15					**Vol. Mix**					
16					**Vol. Sample**					
17					**TOTAL**					
18										
19										
20					**CYCLING PARAMETERS**					
21										
22					Thermocycler					
23										
24						Temp. (°C)	Time	Program		
25					Initial					
26					Denaturation:					
27										
28					Denaturation:					
29					Hybridization:					
30					Extension:					
31					# of cycles					
32										
33					Denaturation:					
34					Hybridization:					
35					Extension:					
36					# of cycles					
37										
38					Final					
39					Extension:					
40										
41					Final Temp.:					
42										
43										
44										
45										
46										
47										
48										
49										
50										

II. 20-well Gel Chart

Title: _____   Date: _____

	1	2	3	4	5	6	7	8	9	10	11	12	13	14	15	16	17	18	19	20
1																				
2																				
3																				
4																				
5																				
6																				

% agarose: _____   _____ V x _____ min.   _____ µl product/well   _____ µl marker (_____)

III. 14-well Gel Chart

Title: _____   Date: _____

	1	2	3	4	5	6	7	8	9	10	11	12	13	14	15	16	17	18	19	20
1																				
2																				
3																				
4																				
5																				
6																				

% agarose: _____   ___ V x ___ min.   ___ µl product/well   ___ µl marker (___)

IV. Colony Blot Grid

Title: _____   **Date:** _____

Ligation Calculation Worksheet*

	Insert	Vector	Insert	Vector
Fragment size	bp	bp	bp	bp
Size ratio				
Required molar ratio of insert to vector				
Ratio of insert to vector DNA				
Equivalent ratio of insert to vector DNA				
Total fragment/reaction in nanograms	ng	ng	ng	ng
Initial fragment concentration	ng/μl	ng/μl	ng/μl	ng/μl
Volume/reaction	μl	μl	μl	μl

*For example, *see* section 6.3.2.

VI. Ligation Reaction Worksheet

Ligation Reactions

#	Reaction	Vector ng req'd	Vector ng / µl	**Vector** µl / Mix	Insert ng req'd	Insert ng / µl	**Insert** µl / Mix	**10X Buffer** µl / Mix	**Ligase** µl / Mix	**ddH20** µl / Mix	**Vol. Total**
1											
2											
3											
4											
5											
6											
7											
8											
9											
10											
11											
12											
13											
14											
15											
16											
17											
18											
19											
20											

Appendix I

Useful World Wide Web Sites

The World Wide Web is an excellent resource with a tremendous amount of information that can be accessed free of charge. There are also many services and information sites to which one must subscribe for access. The list of interesting and useful Web sites is continually expanding; several existing "free" sites are mentioned below.

Software Programs Available Free of Charge

National Center for Biotechnology Information (NCBI)
   http://www.ncbi.nlm.nih.gov/
Entrez
   http://www.ncbi.nlm.nih.gov/Entrez/
Primers for the World Wide Web
   http://www.williamstone.com/primers/index.html
The Institute for Genome Research
   http://www.tigr.org/
medline
   http://ncbi.nlm.nih.gov/PubMed/

Organizations

World Health Organization (WHO)
   http://www.who.ch/
World Health Organization (WHO) Division of Control of Tropical Diseases
   http://www.who.ch/programmes/ctd/ctd_home.htm
Pan American Health Organization (PAHO)
   http://www.paho.org
American Society of Tropical Medicine and Hygiene
   http://www.astmh.org/
United Nations Development Program (UNDP)
   http://www.undp.org/
National Council for International Health
   http://www.ncih.org/
Infectious Diseases Society of America
   http://www.idsociety.org/
United Nations and related organizations
   http://www.undcp.or.at/unlinks.html

United Nations Population Information Network
  http://www.undp.org/popin/popin.htm
Oxfam
  http://www.oneworld.org/oxfam/
UNICEF
  http://www.unicef.org/
Centers for Disease Control and Prevention (CDC) Home Page
  http://www.cdc.gov/
CDC, International Health Program Office
  http://www.cdc.gov/ihpo/homepage.htm#
Institute of Medicine (National Academy of Sciences)
  http://www2.nas.edu/iom/
World Bank
  http://www.worldbank.org
Doctors Without Borders USA (Medecins Sans Frontieres USA)
  http://www.tiac.net/users/dwb/
Physicians for Human Rights
  http://www.phrusa.org/
U.S. Agency for International Development
  http://www.info.usaid.gov
U.S. Department of Health and Human Services
  http://www.hhs.gov
Australian Centre for International and Tropical Health and Nutrition
  http://www.acithn.uq.edu.au/index.html

Foundations

Research funding opportunities
  http://www.grainger.uiuc.edu/iris/
The John D. and Catherine T. MacArthur Foundation
  http://www.macfdn.org/
The Wellcome Trust
  http://www.wellcome.ac.uk/
International Development Research Council
  http://www.idrc.ca
Rockefeller Foundation
  http://www.rockfound.org
Robert Wood Johnson Foundation
  http://www.rwjf.org/main.html
Ford Foundation
  http://www.fordfound.org/
Novartis Foundation for Sustainable Development
  http://foundation.novartis.com/foundtn.htm#mission

Associations

Appropriate Health Resources and Technologies Action Group
  http://www.poptel.org.uk/ahrtag/
American Society for Parasitology
  http://www-museum.unl.edu/asp_image/aspjava.html
British Society for Parasitology
  http://www.umds.ac.uk/bsp/welcome.html

Japanese Society for Parasitology
  http://crew.med.uoeh-u.ac.jp/~parasite/
Interaction: American Council for Voluntary International Action
  http://www.interaction.org/
International Federation of Medical Students' Associations
  http://www.ifmsa.org

On-Line Journals (Only Sites Where the Full Text is Available are Listed)

Memorias do Instituto Oswaldo Cruz
  http://www.dbbm.fiocruz.br/www-mem/
Emerging Infectious Diseases
  http://www.cdc.gov/ncidod/eid/eid.html/
Journal of Biological Chemistry
  http://www.jbc.org/
Technical Tips Online
  http://tto.trends.com/cgi-bin/tto/pr/pg_home.cgi
International Network for Availability of Scientific Publications
  http://www.oneworld.org/inasp/index.html
Medscape
  http://www.medscape.com/Home/About.html
Elsevier "Trends" Journals
  http://www.elsevier.com/locate/ppages
The British Medical Journal has just put on the Internet the book, "Epidemiology for the
  Uninitiated," in full text, and available for free worldwide. It is highly recommended for
  people new to the field of epidemiology:
  http://www.bmj.com/epidem/epid.html
CAB International Publication and distribution
  http://www.cabi.org/

Schools of Public Health

University of California, Berkeley, School of Public Health
  http://garnet.berkeley.edu/~sph/
Johns Hopkins University School of Public Health
  http://www.sph.jhu.edu/
Harvard School of Public Health
  http://www.hsph.harvard.edu/index.html
London School of Hygiene and Tropical Medicine
  http://www.lshtm.ac.uk/
Boston University School of Public Health
  http://www-busphbu.edu/Depts/IH/
Tulane School of Public Health International Health programs
  http://www.tulane.edu./~inhl/inhl.htm

Informative Sites

Search engine specific to health: Medexplorer
http://www.medexplorer.com/medexplr.htm
Search engine specific to medicine: HealthAtoZ
  http://www.healthatoz.com

Tropical Medicine information/search center
   http://galaxy.tradewave.com/galaxy/Medicine/Health-
      Occupations/Medicine/Tropical-Medicine.html
Networking for Tropical Diseases Research
   http://www.who.ch/programmes/tdr/kh/res_link.html
Tropical Medicine Internet Resources
   http://www.liv.ac.uk/lstm/internet.html
SatelLife
   http://www.healthnet.org/
Global Health: Making Contacts
   http://www.pitt.edu/HOME/GHNet/GHNet.html
International Healthcare Opportunities Clearinghouse
   http://library.ummed.edu/ihoc/
International Health Care Research Guide
   http://www.health.ucalgary.ca/
Population Reference Bureau (PRB)
   http://www.prb.org/prb/
Ministries of Health
   http://www.fda.gov/oia/agencies.html
Library of Congress Country Studies
   http://lcweb2.loc.gov/frd/cs/cshome.html#toc
Parasites and Parasitological Resources
   http://www.biosci.ohio-state.edu/~zoology/parasite/societies.html
Pedro's Biomolecular Research Tools
   http://cistron.sfsu.edu/Pedro/rt_1.html
BCM Search Launcher (Baylor College of Medicine) for sequence analysis
   http://kiwi.imgen.bcm.tmc.edu:8088/search-launcher/launcher.html
American Council for Voluntary International Action
   http://www.interaction.org/
UNAIDS
   http://www.unaids.org/index.html
Index of NGOs in Official Relations with WHO
   http://www.who.ch/programmes/ina/ngo/1index.htm
Health on the Net Foundation
   http://www.hon.ch/
New York On-line Access to Health (NOAH) Home Page (in Spanish as well)
   http://noah.cuny.edu/
Evidence-based information seeking site
   http://panizzi.shef.ac.uk/auracle/ed/guidelin.html
AIDS Treatment Data Network
   http://www.aidsnyc.org/network/index.html
Malaria Database
   http://www.wehi.edu.au/biology/malaria/who.htm
South Africa Essential National Health Rsearch (MRC site in Zambia)
   http://www.mrc.ac.za/enhr/enhr.htm#lys
The World Intellectual Property Organization
   http://www.wipo.org/eng/index.htm
U.S. Patent and Trademark Office
   http://patent.womplex.ibm.com

Discussion Groups

Association for Biotechnology Resource
 abrf-request@aecom.yu.edu (to subscribe)
 abrf@aecom.yu.edu

Additional Useful Resources

Topics in International Health: Educational CD-ROM series
This series of educational CD-ROMs, which is produced by The Wellcome Trust, provides students of medicine and life sciences with a new, exciting approach to learning. Each CD focuses on one disease (or group of diseases), and contains three resources:

1. Interactive tutorials—highly visual, structured learning tools
2. Image collection—searchable database of high-quality images
3. Glossary—definitions of medical and scientific terminology

The topics to be covered include: AIDS/HIV, diarrheal diseases, leprosy, malaria, nutrition, schistosomiasis, sexually transmitted diseases, sickle cell disease, trachoma, and tuberculosis. For more information, contact CAB INTERNATIONAL, Wallingford, Oxon OX10 8DE, U.K.
Tel: +44 (0)1491 832111; Fax: +44 (0)1491 826090
E-mail: publishing@cabi.org

Or for customers in North America:
CAB INTERNATIONAL, 198 Madison Avenue, New York, NY10016-4314, USA
Tel: +1 212 726 6490/6491 or Toll-free +1 800 528 4841
Fax: +1 212 686 7993
E-mail: cabi-nao@cabi.org

Books
Commission on Health Research for Development (1990) *Health Research: Essential Link to Equity in Development.* New York, Oxford University Press.
Curtis, C.F. (1991) *Control of Disease Vectors in the Community.* London, Wolfe Publishing Ltd. Galen, R.S. and Gambino, S.R. (1975) *Beyond Normality: The Predictive Value and Efficiency of Medical Diagnoses.* New York, John Wiley.
Giesecke, J. (1994) *Modern Infectious Disease Epidemiology.* London, Edward Arnold.
Glantz, S.A. (1992) *Primer of Biostatistics*, third ed. New York, McGraw-Hill, Inc.

References

Appendix A

Kadokami, Y., Takao, K., and Saigo, K. (1984) An economic power supply using a diode for agarose and polyacrylamide gel electrophoresis. *Anal. Biochem.*, 137:156-160.

Appendix B

Sambrook, J., Fritsch, E.F., and Maniatis, T. (1989) *Molecular Cloning: A Laboratory Manual.* New York, Cold Spring Harbor Laboratory Press.
Vogelstein, B. and Gillespie, D. (1979) Preparative and analytical purification of DNA from agarose. *Proc. Natl. Acad. Sci. USA*, 76:615-619.

Glossary

accessible. Making a new technique or technology available by removing barriers to implementation.

AFLP. Amplified fragment length polymorphism. Digestion of the DNA of interest with restriction enzymes followed by ligation of the resulting fragments with specific oligonucleotides called linkers. Amplification with primers complementary to the linker sequences produces a pattern of bands unique to each organism.

alkaline phosphatase. An enzyme that converts specific substrates into products that can be easily detected due to the formation of a colored precipitate or the emission of light. Alkaline phosphatase is often used in association with a DNA probe for nonradioactive detection of PCR products.

allele. One of several alternative forms of a gene that can occupy a given locus on a chromosome.

amplicon. A copy of a DNA fragment resulting from amplification.

amplification. In PCR, the exponential replication of a specific DNA fragment of a defined length by DNA polymerase to produce multiple copies.

annealing. The second step in the amplification cycle in which, at a particular temperature, two complementary single DNA strands hybridize to form a double helix. Also referred to as hybridization and renaturation. *See* **hybridization.**

appropriate. Compatible with local needs, of local relevance, and feasible under existing conditions.

autoradiography. Use of photographic film to detect radioactive isotopes on nucleic acids or proteins that have been directly radiolabeled or hybridized with a labeled probe. The labeled molecules, usually fixed to a solid support (e.g., a nylon membrane or polyacrylamide gel) are overlaid with X-ray film, and the radioactive emissions behave like photons of light such that patterns on the developed film correspond to the location of the label.

blot. A nylon or nitrocellulose membrane to which nucleic acids (DNA in a Southern blot, RNA in a Northern blot) have been transferred and fixed, using heat or ultraviolet light. The blot is incubated with a DNA probe that hybridizes to complementary sequences fixed to the membrane. A colony blot consists of DNA transferred from lysed colonies, and a dot blot or slot blot consists of DNA or RNA applied directly to the membrane. When proteins are transferred to the membrane and detected using antibodies, it is referred to as a Western blot.

blunt end. A flush double-stranded break in DNA that has been cleaved by a restriction enzyme at the center of its recognition site. *Compare with* **sticky end.**

buffer. A chemical solution that maintains the pH of a solution. A PCR buffer is a specific formulation recommended for a particular polymerase in order to stabilize the pH of the reaction during DNA amplification.

carryover. The cross-contamination of an amplification reaction with template or product from another, resulting in false-positive artifactual results. *See* **cross-contamination**.

cation. A positively charged ion.

cDNA. Complementary DNA. The DNA copy of a specific RNA generated through the action of the enzyme reverse transcriptase. RNA must be converted into cDNA before amplification by DNA polymerase during PCR can occur.

chemiluminescent. A nonradioactive detection system based on the emission of light from an enzyme-labeled probe or antibody during the enzymatic conversion of certain substrates to products. This light can be detected on photographic film much like autoradiography.

chromosome. A single uninterrupted molecule of linear or circular DNA, consisting of an end-to-end arrangement of genes and other DNA, which constitutes part (or all) of an organism's genome.

clone. Individual entities with identical genetic composition.

cloning. Isolation of a particular gene or sequence of DNA and its insertion into a vector that allows replication of the inserted fragment. Also, the process of producing genetically identical cells or molecules from a parent cell.

colony. A visible growth of cloned cells (i.e., bacteria).

colony blot. A blot performed with colonies of bacteria. The bacteria are lifted directly onto a membrane from the agar growth medium and lysed. The nucleic acids released are then fixed to the membrane and hybridized with an appropriate probe for detection. *See* **blot**.

competent cells. Cells capable of incorporating foreign DNA. Cells can be manipulated to make them competent for transformation by foreign DNA.

complementary. The alignment of one nucleic acid sequence with another such that the nucleotide adenosine pairs with thymidine or uridine (RNA) and cytidine pairs with guanosine. This interaction is mediated by hydrogen bonds formed between the paired bases (three hydrogen bonds between cytidine and guanosine and two hydrogen bonds between adenosine and thymidine [or uridine]).

conserved region. A genetic sequence with a high degree of similarity among different species in a genus or different members of a gene family. Primers directed to a constant region of the chromosome will amplify all members of the gene family, whereas primers specific to a variable region will target only a particular species or gene. *See* **variable region**.

control. A known sample included in every amplification to verify reaction conditions. A set of controls must be included in all PCR amplifications so that cross-contamination and/or inhibition can be immediately detected. Only when all controls produce the expected results can the other results of the amplification be relied on.

cross-contamination. Introduction of exogenous DNA fragments from a positive sample or from another amplification into the PCR reaction tube, leading to false-positive results. *See* **carryover.**

cycle. During PCR amplification, each cycle consists of a series of three different temperatures at which the ingredients of the reaction undergo distinct physical and biochemical processes (denaturation, annealing, and extension), resulting in the exponential replication of target molecules. In certain procedures, three-step cycles are reduced to two-step cycles consisting of only denaturation and annealing. When the product is short enough, extension can occur as the temperature rises from the annealing to the denaturation temperature.

denaturation. The disruption of the hydrogen bonds between base pairs on complementary nucleic acid strands by exposure to heat or high pH, leading to the separation of the double-stranded DNA helix into two single strands. Denaturation is the first step in the amplification cycle.

digestion. Enzymatic cleavage of nucleic acids or proteins. The process of cutting DNA using restriction enzymes.

DNA. Deoxyribonucleic acid. A covalently linked chain of deoxyribonucleotides. DNA is distinguished from RNA in that the 2′ position of the ribose sugar is linked to hydrogen, as opposed to a hydroxyl group (OH) in RNA. Two complementary strands of DNA form a double helix.

DNase I. Deoxyribonuclease I, an enzyme that degrades DNA into nucleotides. At low concentrations, this enzyme reveals nuclease-sensitive sites lacking nucleosomes. Because the enzyme does not interact intimately with DNA bases, it does not discriminate nucleotide sequences efficiently.

dNTP(s). Deoxynucleotide triphosphate(s). The building blocks of the DNA replicated during PCR. *See* **nucleotide**.

electrophoresis. The migration of charged particles through a matrix in an electric field. This method is used to separate negatively-charged fragments of DNA according to their size, since smaller fragments migrate more rapidly toward the positive pole than do larger fragments.

ELISA. Enzyme linked immunosorbent assay, a serological technique of which many variations exist. To detect a particular antigen in a sample, microtiter wells are first coated with specific antibodies. The sample is then added, and if the antigen is present, it binds to the immobilized antibody. A second antibody with an attached enzyme is then added, followed by a substrate that is converted to a colored compound by the enzyme. Alternatively, to detect an antibody in the sample, the solid support is coated with antigen, which captures the specific antibody in the samples if it is present. The subsequent steps in the assay are identical.

enhancer. A chemical used to optimize the performance and sensitivity of PCR amplification by facilitating DNA denaturation and rendering it more accessible for primer hybridization and subsequent strand replication.

epidemiology. A field of study of the causes and patterns of disease occurrence in a given population.

exonuclease. An enzyme that cleaves nucleotides one at a time from either the 5′ or 3′ end of a polynucleotide chain.

extension. The third and final step in the amplification cycle, in which the polymerase extends from the primer in the direction 5′ to 3′, replicating the template DNA strand.

extraction. Treatment of a sample with organic solvents. Also, processing specimens to obtain nucleic acids of varying purity, depending on the method of preparation.

fidelity. The degree of accuracy during the process of DNA replication by polymerases.

fingerprint. A distinct pattern of DNA fragments, separated by electrophoresis, that is characteristic of a particular strain of an organism.

5′ terminus. The end of a nucleic acid strand where the phosphate groups are located. The term 5′ refers to the fifth carbon from the base of a nucleotide where a phosphodiester binds to the ribose backbone. *See* **3′ terminus**.

fragment. A specific sequence (piece) of DNA of a given size.

gene. A sequence of DNA that is transcribed to generate mRNA, which is then translated to form a protein with a specific function.

genome. The entire database of genetic information stored in the chromosomes of a given organism.

genus. A subdivision in the classification of organisms, between family and species.

HMA. Heteroduplex mobility assay. Analysis of bands with altered mobility in a gel matrix, which are intentionally caused by electrophoresis of heteroduplex fragments. Useful for identification of mutations when compared with reference material.

heteroduplex. Double-stranded DNA formed by the denaturation and reannealing of DNA fragments from a polymorphic region containing regions of noncomplementary sequence.

homology. Similarity in nucleic acid or amino acid sequence.

hot-start. A method commonly used to improve the specificity of a PCR reaction, whereby all of the reaction ingredients are prevented from interacting productively until after the first denaturation step at approximately 94°C.

hybridization. The annealing of complementary single strands of nucleic acids to form double-stranded molecules. The strands are held together by hydrogen bonds between complementary bases. *See* **annealing**.

insert. The fragment of DNA cloned into a vector.

knowledge-based. A thorough understanding of the principles underlying a technique or technology that is being transferred; for example, a solid understanding of the theory behind the technique, the role of each reagent in a solution or reaction, and the function of each piece of equipment used in a given procedure.

ligation. The annealing of two pieces of DNA by the enzyme ligase.

lysis. A process of cellular disintegration through rupture of the cell membrane.

manual amplification. Amplification that is carried out using water baths set at the required temperatures, instead of a thermocycler. The PCR reaction tubes are placed in floating racks in the baths and manually transferred between baths until the cycling process is complete.

microtiter plate. A small plastic plate uniformly indented with multiple wells (microwells).

molecular epidemiology. The use of molecular biology techniques to study the epidemiology of diseases.

mRNA. Messenger RNA, a template that carries genetic information from DNA to the ribosomes of a cell, where it is translated into protein.

mutation. Any change that alters nucleic acid sequence, permanently changing genetic structure.

nested amplification. The re-amplification of the product of a primary amplification in a second PCR, using primers that hybridize within the first product, to increase the specificity and sensitivity. With proper modification, both amplifications can be carried out in the same tube.

nuclease. An enzyme that breaks down both DNA and RNA.

nucleic acid. Large chain-like molecules of high molecular weight formed from sugars, phosphoric acid, and one of four nitrogen bases; the building blocks of genetic information. *See* **DNA** and **RNA**.

nucleotide. The basic building blocks of nucleic acids. Each nucleotide is composed of a sugar (ribose), a base (adenine, guanine, cytosine, or thymine [uracil in RNA]), and three phosphate groups. *See* **dNTP**.

oligonucleotide. A short, synthetic piece of DNA.

overhang. The single-stranded region of DNA created by cleavage of double-stranded DNA by a restriction enzyme that generates sticky ends.

participatory. A learning environment where all participants actively engage in performing every experiment with their own hands. All participants are considered equal and learn from each other in an atmosphere of reciprocal exchange.

patent. An official document conferring a right to produce, use, or commercialize an invention.

pathogen. A microorganism capable of causing disease in a susceptible host.

PCR. Polymerase Chain Reaction. A patented procedure that exponentially amplifies a piece of DNA of specific size and sequence.

PCR inhibitor. Compounds that inhibit the activity of polymerases, thereby preventing amplification.

plasma. The clear fluid (upper layer) obtained by centrifuging noncoagulated whole blood (collected in the presence of anticoagulants). Below the plasma, a layer of white blood cells (the buffy coat) is formed, while the lowest layer consists of a large pellet of red blood cells. *Compare with* **serum.**

plasmid. Circular DNA episomes that are able to replicate indefinitely outside the host chromosome.

polymerase. An enzyme that replicates template nucleic acid in the direction 5′ to 3′. This enzyme requires a primer with a free 3′ hydroxyl (OH) group for DNA synthesis.

polymorphism. In a genetic context, the variation in nucleic acid sequence. The differences can be recognized by the use of restriction endonucleases and specially designed PCR primers.

primer. A short piece of DNA in the form of a synthetic oligonucleotide that anneals to a complementary sequence of DNA and is extended by a polymerase. The sequence of a primer is what confers specificity to PCR amplification.

primer-dimer. Primers with sufficient homology to anneal to one another in a complex, resulting in the amplification of the complex rather than the fragment of interest.

probe. A nucleic acid segment that is labeled so that it can be followed during the course of hybridization. Probes can be used to identify DNA molecules because if the labeled fragment and target nucleic acid sequence are complementary, a double-stranded molecule will form.

processivity. Refers to the number of nucleotides that a polymerase can incorporate into the replicated strand before the enzyme falls off the template. High processivity is associated with high catalytic potency.

ramp time. The time it takes for the thermocycler or heating block to reach the desired temperature between amplification steps.

RAPD. Random amplified polymorphic DNA. An amplification technique using a single primer of arbitrary sequence to generate a unique pattern of bands from the DNA template. No prior information is needed about the target sequence.

reference method. A standard technique that is recognized by the scientific community as meeting the optimal criteria for identification of an organism and to which all other identification and characterization methods are compared. Also referred to as "gold standard."

repetitive element. Recurring sequence elements within a strand of DNA.

restriction enzyme. An enzyme (restriction endonuclease) that recognizes specific palindromic target nucleotide sequences and cleaves double-stranded DNA at or near its recognition site.

reverse transcription. The synthesis of a DNA strand from an RNA template; a process catalyzed by the enzyme reverse transcriptase. *See* **cDNA.**

RFLP. Restriction fragment length polymorphism. A method for distinguishing between strains of an organism or homologous chromosomes by detecting the presence or absence of particular restriction enzyme sites in the genome, manifested as DNA fragments of different lengths after digestion, electrophoresis, transfer to a membrane, and hybridization with a labeled probe.

RNA. A covalently linked chain of ribonucleic acids. In RNA, the 2′ position of the ribose sugar is linked to a hydroxyl group (OH) as opposed to hydrogen (H) in DNA.

RNase. An enzyme that degrades RNA into nucleotides.

secondary structures. Three-dimensional structures formed by base pairing of nucleotides within a single strand of nucleic acid, generating structures such as hairpins, cloverleafs, and hammerheads. The formation of hairpins within primers must be avoided. Secondary structures can interfere with amplification by blocking the extension of the replicated strand by the polymerase. Also, the second level of protein structure (α helix, β sheet); the primary structure in proteins is the amino acid sequence.

sensitivity. Capacity of a diagnostic test to identify as positive those patients who have the disease of interest. A good test gives positive results in diseased subjects. Using a 2 X 2 table to evaluate the sensitivity of a particular test, the sensitivity is calculated as follows: test positives/all positives = test positives/test positives + false-negatives. Sensitivity is also understood as the limit of detection of a diagnostic or analytical technique. A very sensitive technique like PCR can detect low levels of its target.

sequence. The order of nucleotides in a gene or the order of amino acids in a protein. Genetic information is contained in the sequence. Once the sequence of a stretch of nucleic acids is known, complementary primers and probes can be designed.

sequencing. Determining the exact nucleotide sequence of DNA or RNA or the exact amino acid sequence of proteins.

serology. The study of components of serum.

serotype. Subdivision of a species on the basis of its antigenic characteristics. Used to describe distinct variants of dengue virus, *V. cholerae*, *Shigella*, and other bacteria. *See* **serovar**.

serovar. Subdivision of a species on the basis of its antigenic characteristics. Used to describe subdivisions within species of *Chlamydia*, *Leptospira*, and several other microorganisms. *See* **serotype**.

serum. The clear fluid (upper layer) obtained by centrifuging coagulated whole blood. The lower layer (clot) consists of blood cells and fibrin. In this instance, no discrete layer of white cells is formed, as in plasma. *Compare with* **plasma**.

silica particles. Tiny glass particles with a positively charged property that allows them to selectively bind to nucleic acids. Effectively used for the purification of DNA.

sodium hypochlorite. The active ingredient of bleach.

Southern blot. Transfer of electrophoretically separated DNA fragments from the gel to a membrane filter. The DNA fragments are detected by hybridization with complementary nucleic acid probes, which are labeled with nonradioactive molecules or radioactive isotopes. *See* **blot**.

species. A subdivision of the genus classification. A lineage of organisms with distinguishing characteristics that can interbreed.

specific activity. The amount of a specific substrate converted by a given enzyme at 25°C, per minute per milligram of protein.

specificity. The capacity of a diagnostic test to identify as negative those who do not have the disease of interest. A good test gives negative results in healthy subjects. Using a 2 X 2 table to evaluate the specificity of a particular test, the specificity is calculated as follows: test negatives/all negatives = test negatives/test negatives + false-positives.

SSCP. Single-strand conformation polymorphism. Also known as single-strand conformational analysis (SSCA).

sticky end. The single-stranded end of a DNA fragment generated by particular restriction enzymes and resulting in a staggered cut in the DNA. Sticky ends will readily join to complementary fragments similarly produced. Also referred to as cohesive end. *Compare with* **blunt end**.

stock. The original isolate of a particular organism (e.g., bacteria, virus). Also, a concentrated preparation of a particular reagent.

strain. A lineage of organisms that differ at specific genomic loci but belong to the same species.

sustainable transfer. Transfer of knowledge and techniques in such a manner as to effect their long-term implementation. *See* **accessible** and **appropriate**.

synthesis. The generation of a complex product through a combination of simpler elements. For example, the formation of oligonucleotides or DNA from nucleotides or the formation of protein from amino acids.

Taq **polymerase.** A thermostable enzyme, originally isolated from the bacteria *Thermus aquaticus*, that is used in PCR to replicate DNA.

template. A single strand of DNA or RNA that specifies the sequence of nucleotides that is replicated by a polymerase.

thermal profile. The temperatures in the metal block of a thermocycler during cycling. The theoretical profile as programmed into the thermocycler may vary from actual amplification conditions.

thermal transfer. The passage of thermal energy (heat) from the metal block to the reaction mixture in the tubes inside the metal block of a thermocycler.

thermocycler. A programmable piece of equipment that facilitates amplification through automated temperature cycling. It contains a metal block in which the tubes with the PCR reaction mixture are placed. The temperature of the block changes in accordance with the amplification instructions.

thermolabile. Sensitive to heat. Some enzymes are denatured at high temperatures and become inactivated.

thermophilic. Adapted to surviving at high temperatures, as with some bacteria.

thermostable. Resistant to high temperatures. Some enzymes are not denatured in response to heat and retain activity.

3′ terminus. The end of a nucleic acid strand where the ribose sugar is located. The term 3′ refers to the third carbon in ribose from the nucleotide base. *See* **5′ terminus**.

transcription. An enzymatic process in which one strand of DNA is used as a template for the synthesis of complementary RNA.

transformation. The introduction of foreign DNA into competent cells (e.g., bacteria). *See* **competent cells**.

UV transillumination. Detection of nucleic acids labeled with a compound such as ethidium bromide that fluoresces under ultraviolet radiation.

variable region. Sequence of DNA that is polymorphic. *See* **conserved region**.

vector. A small, well-characterized molecule used as a vehicle to enable the replication of a cloned fragment, because it can replicate autonomously in an appropriate host. Also, an insect capable of transmitting a pathogenic microorganism.

Afterword

The publication of this book could not have come at a more propitious time. The importance of new and re-emerging diseases has been increasingly recognized. Cholera in Latin America, East Africa, and Russia; "Chicken" flu in Hong Kong; the resurgence of malaria in South Asia and Africa; the continuing global spread of dengue fever; Rift Valley Fever in Kenya—the list goes on and will continue to grow. The reasons for this emergence/re-emergence are many: changes in society (economic, civil, urbanization); changes in human behavior (sexual, travel, recreation); environmental changes (deforestation, climate changes); deterioration of the public health infrastructure (vector control, decreases in immunization); and microbial adaptation.

If a society is to minimize the impact of new and re-emerging diseases it must recognize early the presence of those diseases. The same can be said of the global response to new and re-emerging diseases. Both for national and global preparedness, WHO and others have called for the development of a surveillance system that includes, in addition to a trained cadre of epidemiologists, the development of public health laboratories with adequate equipment, supplies, and well-trained staff. Herein lies a major weakness of the global and local surveillance network. There are over 100 WHO Collaborating Centres in Diseases worldwide, of which 49 are in the United States and Canada. There are, however, only three centers for all of Asia and none in Africa. Both the number of centers and laboratory facilities/skills are lacking in the developing world—especially in countries where the ecology-human interactions are intense. Establishment of these laboratories can be an expensive undertaking, and the wealthier countries have been reluctant to pay for equipment and training. Development of low-cost technology then is critical.

It is no longer acceptable for outside scientists to "parachute" into an area and leave with coolers of samples to be tested elsewhere. Both the collection of specimens (often the weakest link in the chain) and testing for pathogens must be joint and collaborative efforts.

Herein then lies the true importance of this book. Its goal is no less than to facilitate an effective and sustained technology transfer, in this case, of PCR. The need to train local scientists and health workers in an economically and scientifically accessible technology is critical to any surveillance system. There are innumerable books on the PCR technique, but none address the topic so simply and practically. This book is technically solid and informed yet clear and straightforward in its explanations. PCR is certainly not the ultimate diagnostic technology—nor is it appropriate in all situations, but its limitations must be understood if it is to be used effectively. As important as the PCR message is, this book's approach toward technology transfer is applicable to any new technology. It can be generalized. There will, of course, be other diagnostic techniques that are developed. Their applicability and affordability must always be considered. Dipsticks to diagnose malaria and other pathogens are already being developed. We must learn to take science to where the problem is, for unless we do—that is, the global scientific community—we will have a global surveillance system in name only. We must focus on assisting those who want to develop the tools to help their own societies. Eva Harris has taken a major step in this direction with this important book.

Richard A. Cash, M.D., M.P.H.

Harvard Institute for International Development/
Harvard School of Public Health
Cambridge, MA
January 1998

Index